BIOTERRORISM

Edited by **Stephen A. Morse**

Bioterrorism
Edited by Stephen A. Morse

Published by InTech
Janeza Trdine 9, 51000 Rijeka, Croatia

Publishing Process Manager Sasa Leporic

Technical Editor Teodora Smiljanic

Cover Designer InTech Design Team

Additional hard copies can be obtained from orders@intechopen.com

Bioterrorism, Edited by Stephen A. Morse
p. cm.
ISBN 978-953-51-0205-2

For EU product safety concerns:
IN TECH d.o.o., Prolaz Marije Krucifikse Kozulić 3, 51000 Rijeka, Croatia,
info@intechopen.com or visit our website at intechopen.com.

Meet the editor

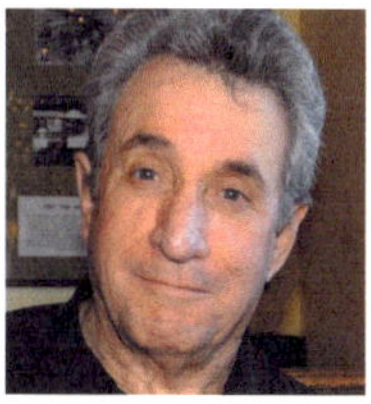

Dr Stephen A. Morse received his M.S.P.H. in environmental chemistry and biology in 1966, and a PhD in microbiology in 1969 from the University of North Carolina at Chapel Hill. He has developed his academic career at: Harvard School of Public Health and Harvard Medical School, 1971-74; Oregon Health Sciences University, 1974-84; Centers for Disease Control and Prevention (CDC): Director, Sexually Transmitted Diseases Research Program, 1984-95; Associate Director for Science, Division of Bioterrorism Preparedness and Response, 1999-2008; Associate Director for Environmental Microbiology, 2008 - present. He has published over 290 articles, books and chapters and has received numerous awards, including: the McLaughlin Award from the University of Texas Medical School at Galveston; the Harriet Hylton Barr Outstanding Alumnus Award from the School of Public Health of the University of North Carolina at Chapel Hill; and the Joseph E. McDade Citation for Lifetime Scientific Achievement, CDC. Currently, he works as Adjunct Professor at Emory University School of Medicine. He is a past member of the Board of Governors of the American Academy of Microbiology and the FBI Scientific Working Group for the forensic analysis of chemical, biological, radiological and nuclear terrorism.

Contents

Preface

Pathogenic microorganisms and their toxins have always posed a significant threat to humans, animals, and plants that become exposed and infected naturally. But now there is a newly recognized threat – the deliberate use of pathogenic microorganisms and toxins as weapons in acts of bioterrorism or in the commission of biocrimes. Long before the germ theory of disease was understood, man knew that pathogenic microorganisms and toxins were useful as weapons. However, as the twentieth century came to a close, the perceived difficulties in production, weaponization, and deployment of these biological weapons as well as a belief that moral restraints would preclude the use of these weapons gave many a false sense of security. Recently, a number of events have served to focus attention on the threat of terrorism and the potential for the use of biological weapons against the military, civilian populations, or agriculture for the purpose of causing illness, death, or economic loss. This threat is a significant concern in the United States as well as internationally.

Bioterrorist attacks occur as one of two scenarios: overt and covert. In either scenario, biologic agents could be introduced into populations by several routes, including aerosol; contamination of food, water, or medical products; fomites; or the release of infected arthropod vectors. The deliberate nature of such dissemination will often be obvious, as in the case of multiple mailed letters containing anthrax spores (ie overt). Because we currently lack the ability to conduct extensive real-time monitoring for the release of a biologic agent, a covert release of a microorganism of toxin in a population would be likely to go unnoticed for some time, with individuals exposed leaving the attack area before the act of terrorism became evident. Because of the incubation period, the first signs that a microorganism or toxin has been released may not become apparent until hours or weeks later, when individuals become ill and seek medical care.

Bioterrorism presents many challenges, particularly when compared to chemical, radiological, or nuclear terrorism. These challenges reflect the dual-use nature of many technologies that can be used for either beneficial purposes or bioterrorism; intentional threats that can coexist with similar and naturally occurring threats; the complexity of the interaction of the threat with the environment, the human immune system, the society/social structure; and rapid advances in biotechnology. Preparing for and responding to bioterrorism in the twenty-first century has brought together diverse disciplines with different backgrounds and cultures, for example intelligence agencies, public health and medical professionals, law enforcement officers, scientists, and the commercial sector. It remains a learning process.

Many biological agents can cause illness in humans, but not all are capable of affecting public health and medical infrastructures on a large scale. As part of an effort to focus public health preparedness efforts, the United States Centers for Disease Control and Prevention (CDC) developed a prioritized list of biological agents taking into consideration criteria such as high morbidity and mortality; potential for person-to-person transmission, directly or by vector; low infectious dose and high infectivity by aerosol, with a commensurate ability to cause large outbreaks; ability to contaminate food or water supplies; lack of a specific diagnostic test and/or effective treatment; lack of a safe and effective vaccine; potential to cause anxiety in the general public and in healthcare workers; and potential for weaponization. The final category assignments (A, B, or C) of agents for public health preparedness were based on an overall evaluation of the ratings the agents received in the aforementioned criteria. Agents placed in Category A (eg Yersinia pestis, botulinum neurotoxins) were considered to have a moderate to high potential for large-scale dissemination, the greatest potential for adverse public health impact with mass casualties, and a requirement for broad-based public health preparedness efforts. Agents placed in Category B (eg rickettsia, ricin, staphylococcal enterotoxins) also have some potential for large-scale dissemination with resultant illness, but generally cause less illness and death and, therefore, would be expected to have lower public health and medical impact. Biological agents that were not believed to present a high bioterrorism risk to public health but which could emerge as future threats, as scientific understanding of these agents improved were placed in Category C.

This book was written to provide a resource to scientists, epidemiologists, clinicians, and others in the field of bioterrorism defense. Not all possible topics are described. Instead, representative topics, authored by international experts provide a unique and state-of-the-art perspective on this field. The book consists of this preface and nine other chapters that address the broad areas of (1) detection capabilities (ie spatio-temporal disease surveillance; diagnostic bioterrorism response strategies; methods for detecting the presence of botulinum neurotoxins in food and other biological samples; and detection of bacillus spores by surface-enhanced Raman spectroscopy) and (2) characteristics of specific pathogenic microorganisms and toxins (ie Rickettsia and Rickettsial diseases; recent advances in the development of vaccines against Yersinia pestis; botulinum neurotoxins; ricin; and staphylococcal enterotoxins).

Dr. Stephen A. Morse
Associate Director of Science, Division of Bioterrorism Preparedness and Response,
and Director of the Environmental Microbiology Program, CDC,
USA

1

Current Methods for Detecting the Presence of Botulinum Neurotoxins in Food and Other Biological Samples

Luisa W. Cheng[1], Kirkwood M. Land[2] and Larry H. Stanker[1]
Foodborne Contaminants Research Unit, Western Regional Research Center,
[1]Agricultural Research Service, U.S. Department of Agriculture, Albany, CA,
[2]Department of Biological Sciences, University of the Pacific, Stockton, CA,
USA

1. Introduction

Botulinum neurotoxins (BoNTs) are some of the most lethal human bacterial toxins and the causative agent of botulism (Arnon et al., 2001; Simpson, 2004). The usual routes of intoxication for BoNTs are oral ingestion of clostridial spores or pre-formed toxin, manifested as infant, foodborne and adult onset botulism. An increasingly common route of intoxication is associated with intravenous drug use resulting in wound botulism. BoNTs are also classified as Select Agents and have been used as agents of bioterrorism (Arnon et al., 2001; Bigalke and Rummel, 2005). Potential methods for toxin exposure include intentional contamination of the food and drink supply, or by aerosol spread, leading to inhalational botulism.

Usually, an identification of botulism is made through clinical manifestations and diagnosis, with subsequent confirmation by laboratory identification of clostridial spores or toxin in foods, environmental or clinical samples (CDC, 1998; Lindström and Korkeala, 2006; Solomon and Lilly, 2001). The speed of recovery from botulism increases with the timely administration of antitoxin or medical interventions (Arnon et al., 2001; Simpson, 2004). Thus, sensitive and rapid toxin detection and diagnostic methods are critical for improved recovery time, as well as, facilitate the epidemiologic study of outbreaks.

Due to the potential for bioterrorism use, much effort and resources have been dedicated to the development of detection methods, treatment, and prevention of botulism. A multitude of assay formats have been developed over many years, with in some cases, reported sensitivities at the attomolar level (Grate et al., 2010). Many assays were designed for use in the validation of toxin production, for commercial purposes, or for high-throughput screening methods to identify therapeutics that inhibit toxin function. These highly sensitive methods usually detect highly purified BoNT samples and are used in research type applications. Many such assays are not usable for the detection of BoNT contamination in food or other complex samples. This chapter focuses on the diagnostic methods for toxin detection and the challenges encountered while adapting analytical methods for the detection of BoNTs in foods and other biological and environmental samples.

The biology and mechanisms of action of BoNTs are described in a previous chapter in this book, and readers should refer to the botulinum neurotoxins chapter by Webb, Roxas-Duncan and Smith, for more background reading. This chapter will briefly describe the properties of BoNTs as they relate to detection methods and will compare and contrast currentlyused methods for food and biological sample analyses and methods in development. For detailed analyses and descriptions of detection assays please also refer to excellent reviews by (Grate et al., 2010; Lindström and Korkeala, 2006; Scarlatos et al., 2005; Sharma and Whiting, 2005). We apologize to others not named here due to space constraints.

2. Overview of botulinum neurotoxin structure and function as they relate to the development of diagnostic tools

A single gram of BoNT released and subsequently inhaled can lead to the deaths of more than one million people (Arnon et al., 2001; Hill et al., 2007). BoNTs are produced by the ubiquitously distributed, gram-positive, strictly anaerobic, spore-forming bacteria *Clostridium botulinum, C. barati, C. butyricum* and *C. argentinense*. To date, seven different botulinum serotypes, indicated by letters A through G, have been identified. Serotypes A, B, E, and F have been associated with human disease (Table I).

Type of botulism	Average number of cases per year	Percent of total	BoNT Serotypes
Infant	85	66	A, B, E, F
Wound	24	19	A, B
Foodborne	19	15	A, B, E, F
Adult	0.4	0.3	A, B, F
Unknown	1.4	1	A, B, F

Table 1. Survey of U.S. human botulism cases from 2001-2009 as reported by the U.S. Centers for Disease Control and Prevention (CSTE).

BoNT serotypes can differ from each other by 34-64% at the amino acid level (Garcia-Rodriguez et al., 2011; Hill et al., 2007; Jacobson et al., 2011; Smith et al., 2007; Smith et al., 2005). Genetic variation within each serotype is sometimes significant. And 32 toxin subtypes with amino acid level differences of 2.6-32% have been identified thus far, with more likely to be identified in the future. Serotype and subtype diversity may impact antibody and molecular-based assay designs.

BoNT is synthesized as an ~150 kDa protein, also called the holotoxin, that is subsequently processed by a clostridial trypsin-like protease into two polypeptides linked by a single disulfide bond; and are thus similar to other known bacterial A-B dimeric toxins (Oguma, Fujinaga, and Inoue, 1995; Singh, 2000). The ~100 kDa fragment, known as the heavy chain (HC), facilitates toxin binding to specific host cell receptors and later, translocation of the toxin from vesicles into the cell cytosol. The ~50 kDa fragment, known as the light chain (LC), contains the enzymatic domain. The LC fragment is often used for the development of activity-based assays. HC and LC specific antibodies have been developed for toxin neutralization and toxin detection immunoassays.

BoNT holotoxin is secreted from bacteria in association with other non-toxic proteins, called neurotoxin associated proteins or NAPs, forming large protein complexes of 500-900 kDa. These large protein complexes are referred to as progenitor toxins or simply as BoNT complex (Inoue et al., 1996). Complexed BoNTs are significantly more toxic in oral intoxications (Cheng et al., 2008; Ohishi, Sugii, and Sakaguchi, 1977) than holotoxins. NAPs are thought to protect the holotoxin from gastric digestion as well as help holotoxins cross the intestinal barrier (Fujinaga et al., 2009; Niwa et al., 2007; Simpson et al., 2004). Toxin complexes that survive the gastric challenge translocate across the epithelial cell barrier (transcytosis) gaining access into the bloodstream, where the holotoxin is released. BoNT complexes are the forms that will most likely be found in natural intoxication and bioterrorism cases. Thus, the detection of toxin when associated with NAPs or the use of NAPs as detection targets in foodborne intoxications is a consideration in the design of new assays.

The target for BoNT holotoxin is the peripheral cholinergic nerve ending, resulting in flaccid paralysis (Simpson, 2004). Specific receptors for the toxin HC of BoNTs have been identified; BoNT/A binds to glycoprotein SV2; serotype F binds SV2 and gangliosides; and serotype G binds synaptotagmin I and II. Toxin binding to nerve cells is followed by receptor-mediated endocytosis and subsequent translocation of the LC (directed by the translocation domain of the HC) into the cytoplasm. The LC of different serotypes targets different SNARE proteins. BoNT serotypes A, C and E target SNAP-25, and serotypes B, D, F, and G target VAMP2, while serotype C targets syntaxin (Hakami et al., 2010). Different SNARE targets of BoNTs have been used to develop *in vitro* assays for toxin activity. Peptides with fluorescent labels and quencher molecules have been designed and used in various forms of enzymatic activity assays.

3. Challenges to the development of detection assays for botulinum neurotoxins

The development of robust and sensitive detection assays for BoNTs requires consideration of at least six factors explored in detail below.

3.1 Sensitivity

Assay sensitivity is not a simple criterion to define and is determined in part by the specific application. For example, the human lethal dose (LD) for oral intoxication is estimated at 1 μg/kg or about 70 μg for a 70 kg adult (Arnon et al., 2001; Scarlatos et al., 2005). Assays designed for evaluating food must detect at least this amount in a typical portion. Since portions vary widely between individual foods, assay sensitivity requirements may vary with specific matrixes. Foods that typically have large portion sizes would require assays with lower detection limits. Furthermore the dose to cause illness but not death might be lower. Our experience with BoNT exposure in rodents is that a level 10-fold lower than the minimal lethal dose falls into this latter category. Thus, a dose level 10-fold lower than the LD in humans, 7 μg, translates into an assay sensitivity of 70 ng/mL if a serving is typically 100 mL. A 10-fold threshold lowers the sensitivity to 7 ng/mL. In contrast, detection levels for tests used in sera or other clinical matrices should be as sensitive as possible to account for low toxin levels. For example, in oral mouse toxicity studies, only a small portion of the ingested BoNT actually survives the harsh conditions in the gut to reach the bloodstream (Cheng and Henderson, 2011; Cheng et al., 2008). The lethal toxin intravenous dose varies between 20-200 ng in an adult human with approximately 5 liters of blood (Arnon et al., 2001). Taking into account natural degradation, and clearance of toxin in sera, the assay sensitivity for diagnostic evaluation must be in the low to sub-pg/ml range.

3.2 Specificity

There are currently seven known serotypes of BoNTs, and 32 known subtypes. New subtypes are expected to be identified in the future. Amino acid sequence differences can vary as much as 70% among serotypes (Hill et al., 2007; Smith et al., 2005). This level of genetic diversity and variation can prove challenging for both molecular and antibody-based diagnostic methods. False negative results could be obtained if a gene or protein structure of the toxin differ from what established oligonucleotides/PCR primers or antibodies can recognize. At the very least, assay performance needs to be established on as many toxin sero- and subtypes as practical. Reagents generated for detection assays should ideally recognize all known subtypes of each serotype.

3.3 Matrix effects

In almost all scenarios, BoNT samples to be tested would be found in a wide variety of matrices of food, clinical (serum, sputum, feces, etc) or environmental samples (dust, soil, water, etc). Yet, most assay methods are designed, tested and optimized in buffer conditions and thus the sensitivity or application in complex matrices may be diminished. Complex matrices may contain many challenging conditions such as high fat, high protein or salt content, low or high pH; the presence of other active proteases could also interfere with detection sensitivity, increase background signal, and give false positive or negative signals. Methods to alleviate matrix interference range from simple sample dilution, pH rebalancing, addition of protease inhibitors, to specific affinity binding steps prior to detection. Extensive analysis of different matrices will be necessary to evaluate assay sensitivity and determine the best methods to circumvent matrix effects on assay performance.

3.4 Activity

The potent toxicity associated with BoNTs is attributed to their enzymatic properties. The differentiation of active versus inactive forms of the toxin is needed for proper risk assessment and should be an important consideration in assay design. An active BoNT has many roles, it must be able to bind host cell receptors, translocate across membranes and finally reach the host cell cytosol and cleave its target protein. Few assays can measure all aspects of toxin function. Immunoassays (IA) can generally detect both active and inactive toxin and may give false positive results even when no active toxin is present. However, positive results from IA requiring the presence of both HC and LC are predictive of active toxin (Stanker et al, 2008). Assays measuring endopeptidase activities of BoNTs are available but are not as sensitive and amenable to use in complex matrices. Genomic methods, while sensitive, detect the presence of toxin genes but not that of toxin. Depending on the diagnostic needs, a combination of methods may have to be used to get a full activity profile of the toxin.

3.5 Ease of use

For the widest application of an assay, it must be user-friendly and allow for a timely diagnosis. Furthermore, assays need to be validated in multiple laboratories, use equipment or tools that are readily available, and require minimal training to execute. Ideally, the assay should also be field deployable.

3.6 Cost

The cost of an assay in terms of reagent or equipment availability can be an important factor on how widely an assay is used and deployed.

4. Current diagnostic methods of toxin detection

The current "gold standard" for detection of BoNTs is the mouse bioassay. Despite many attempts and much research to replace the use of animals, it is still the best assay to model all aspects of BoNT intoxication: binding, translocation and enzymatic activity (Grate et al., 2010). In attempts to replace the mouse bioassay and improve assay time and sensitivity, both *in vitro* and *in vivo* systems have been developed for the detection of BoNTs. The development of a robust detection assay for BoNT requires that the assay meet as many of the six challenges mentioned above as possible. This section of the chapter will mainly focus on assays that can be used in food and biological samples for the detection of BoNTs.

4.1 Mouse bioassays

The mouse bioassay is still one of the most sensitive and robust methods to detect BoNTs (Schantz and Kautter, 1978; Solomon and Lilly, 2001). The mouse bioassay measures BoNT in minimal lethal dose (MLD) units, which is the lowest dose at which all tested mice die. Mice are usually injected intraperitoneally with 0.5 ml of BoNT sample in a dilution series, and then monitored over several days for signs of intoxication and death (CDC, 1998; CFSAN, 2001). Signs of intoxication include: ruffled fur, wasp-waist (Figure 1), labored-breathing, paralysis and death. Signs of intoxication can appear from a few hours post-injection to a few days depending on the dose and type of BoNT. When enough sample is available, the identity of the unknown BoNT can simultaneously be tested by the addition of neutralizing antibodies against each of the serotypes (A-G). The serotype is identified by the antibody that protects their respective mice from death. The mouse bioassay sensitivity is in the range of 20-30 pg for BoNT/A and 10-20 pg/ml for BoNT/B (Ferreira et al., 2004; Wictome et al., 1999).

While the mouse bioassay has high sensitivity, can detect different serotypes and subtypes, measures different aspects of active toxin, and is amenable to use in different matrices, it has many drawbacks. These include: long assay times, requires specialized animal facilities, trained staff, and the use of animals (with death used as an endpoint). There is also substantial variation of results observed among different research laboratories.

Alternative refined animal assays that do not use death as an endpoint such as the mouse phrenic nerve hemi-diaphragm assay have been evaluated (Rasetti-Escargueil et al., 2009). Although they may be sensitive and faster than the use of whole animals, these assays require use of sophisticated equipment and training, and are not amenable for use with large samplings of complex matrices (Grate et al., 2010). A recently developed *in vivo* assay using the toe-spread reflex model was tested for the detection of BoNT in buffer, serum and milk samples (Wilder-Kofie et al., 2011). This new assay can provide results more quickly than standard mouse bioassays. The robustness of this assay and how easily staff can be trained to perform this assay have yet to be determined.

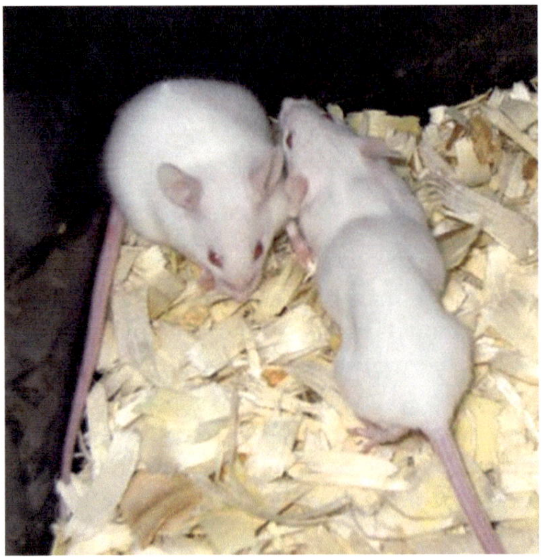

Fig. 1. Mouse bioassay. Mice were intraperitoneally treated with BoNT/A (right mouse) or phosphate buffered saline (left mouse). The intoxicated mouse shows a typical wasp-waist phenotype.

4.2 Nucleic acid based methods of detecting *C. botulinum* in food matrices and other biological samples

4.2.1 Polymerase chain reaction

The use of the polymerase chain reaction (PCR) to identify the presence of *C. botulinum* DNA was originally used to detect the presence of bacterial spores. The method could detect the presence of as few as 10^2 spores per reaction mixture for serotypes A, E and F and only 10 spores per reaction mixture for BoNT/B. To enhance sensitivity, Lindström and colleagues developed an enrichment method that could detect as few as 10^{-2} spores/gram of sample for serotypes A, B and F and 10^{-1} spores/gram of sample for BoNT/E (Lindström et al., 2001). However, one critical drawback of this method is that enrichment often requires 5 days. Furthermore, the applicability of the assay for detection of food contamination was diminished by the observation that beef could interfere with the sensitivity of the assay. Also, if contamination were to occur with the actual toxin, and not cells, this traditional PCR method would not be useful.

4.2.2 Multiplex polymerase chain reaction

It is highly desirable to analyze unknowns for multiple targets, such as different pathogens and/or associated gene products of those pathogens. This approach, known as Multiplex technology, is conceptually simple for PCR based assays. Different sets of PCR primers, each one highly specific for a gene of interest can be easily generated, allowing for the amplification of multiple targets in one reaction tube. One such multiplex method was able to discriminate among BoNT serotypes A, B, E, and F, corroborating mouse bioassay results (De Medici et al., 2009). Furthermore, Peck and colleagues developed a culture enrichment methods that when coupled with multiplex PCR, can identify strains of *C. botulinum* that are non-proteolytic (BoNT serotypes B, E, and F) (Peck et al., 2010). Importantly, this method was robust and reasonably rapid for use with food samples contaminated with *C. botulinum*.

Recently, Fach and colleagues have adapted the use of the GeneDisc Cycler (GeneSystems PCR Technology) to amplify *C. botulinum* genes encoding BoNT serotypes A, B, E, and F on different microchambers (Fach et al., 2011). This technology allows the simultaneous amplification of multiple targets along with a number of different internal controls. A number of different toxin-producing clostridia and non-toxin producing bacteria that were isolated from different food, clinical, and environmental samples and results were compared with those obtained from the mouse bioassay. Notably, all of the botulinum genes were detected correctly and no cross-reactivity was observed with either non-toxin producing bacteria or with *C. botulinum* serotypes C, D, and G. Four European laboratories evaluated this technology, examining 77 toxin producing clostridia as well as 10 food and clinical samples. In all cases, this GeneDisc Cycler was specific and reliable for identifying *C. botulinum* serotypes A, B, E, and F; and was also useful for screening naturally contaminated food and fecal samples.

4.2.3 Real-time polymerase chain reaction

Real-time or quantitative PCR is useful in studies of gene expression; specifically differential expression of genes under different environmental conditions or for comparative studies among different organisms. For detection of clostridia, real-time PCR methods that examine expression of the NTNH (non-toxic, non-hemagglutinin) genes have been developed, as well as methods to study toxin gene expression in *C. botulinum* serotypes A, B, E, and F (Fach et al., 2009). In that study, twenty-nine different strains of toxin-producing *C. botulinum* were screened, and compared with expression profiles from non-toxin producing clostridia as controls. This assay has a sensitivity of 100-fg/1000 fg total DNA in the PCR tube (equivalent to approximately 25-250 genomes). Converting this DNA concentration to its equivalent in cells/ml, suggested a detection limit of approximately 10^3 to 10^4 cells/mL. Following a 48-hour enrichment under anaerobic conditions, these investigators reported the detection of *C. botulinum* serotype A in a naturally contaminated sample of *foie gras* suspected in a botulism outbreak. Recently, pentaplex methods have been developed to simultaneous identify and discriminate among larger numbers of different serotypes using a wider array of different genes (Kirchner et al., 2010). This technology should prove to be efficient and cost-effective.

4.2.4 DNA microarrays

Microarray technology for toxin identification of contaminated food has not been widely used. This may be due to the challenge in isolating high-quality RNA samples from clostridia in food matrices. A recent oligonucleotide microarray with 62 different sequences based on known strain variable regions in the genome of *C. botulinum* strain ATCC 3502 was constructed and used to differentiate different *C. botulinum* type A strains (Raphael et al.,

2010). Regions corresponding to BoNT genes of various serotypes, and other markers components, and other markers were observed. Further development of microarray based assay approaches may provide a means to rapidly identify toxin-producing strains.

4.3 Antibodies as detection tools for BoNT contamination in food

High-affinity monoclonal antibodies (mAbs) that specifically bind individual or multiple BoNT serotypes (and subtypes) have been generated using either mouse hybridoma technology or yeast affinity maturation methods (Grate et al., 2010). These antibodies have been used extensively in traditional ELISA, bead-based, immuno-PCR, microarray assays or in sample preparation before use in a detection assay. Several such assays used in food and biological matrices are highlighted below.

4.3.1 ELISA and ELISA-based methods of detection

ELISA is a widely used detection assay format that uses anti-BoNT capture and detector antibodies usually in a sandwich type format. The read-out for the assay can be colorimetric, luminescence or other formats. Most older generation BoNT immunoassays are about 10 times less sensitive than the mouse bioassay (Ferreira et al., 2004; Scarlatos et al., 2005; Sharma and Whiting, 2005). Although not as sensitive, ELISA based methods are relatively fast, inexpensive and simple. They are also less subject to matrix effects. Sharma and colleagues designed an amplified enzyme-linked immunosorbent assay (ELISA) for detecting toxins in food matrices (Sharma et al., 2006). Specifically, toxins for serotypes A, B, E, and F could be detected in liquids, solid, and semisolid food. Assay performance in a range of foods include broccoli, orange juice, bottled water, cola soft drinks, vanilla extract, oregano, potato salad, apple juice, meats, and dairy items were evaluated. Assay sensitivity varied for each botulinum complex serotype, and were reported as 60 pg/ml for BoNT/A, 176 pg/ml for BoNT/B, 163 pg/ml for BoNT/E, and 117 pg/ml for BoNT/F. The tests readily detected 2 ng/ml of serotypes A, B, E, and F in a variety of the foods tested.

Recently, traditional format sandwich ELISA assays using highly sensitive mAbs against BoNT/A and BoNT/B have detected as low as 5 pg/mL and 25 pg/mL BoNT/A, in buffer and in a milk matrix, respectively (Stanker et al., 2008); and 100 fg and 39 pg/ml of BoNT/B in the buffer and milk matrix, respectively (Scotcher, Cheng, and Stanker, 2010). These mAbs were also used in electrochemiluminescence ELISA type assays using a Meso Scale Discovery (MSD) instrument. Detection sensitivities for BoNT/A using the MSD instrument were similar to traditional ELISAs in the buffer system but offered marked improvement in detection limits and reduction in backgrounds in liquid food matrices (Cheng and Stanker, unpublished results). The higher sensitivity and less time required for these new ELISA assays make them great alternatives or complements for the mouse bioassay.

4.3.2 Multiplex antibody-based detection systems

The multiplex technology has been applied to the development of methods to analyze multiple epitopes on a single antigen or multiple targets in a single sample. This approach uses multiple mAbs as well as polyclonal antibodies to reduce false-positive and false-negative results. The Luminex xMAP technology utilizes microsphere beads conjugated with antibodies. The antibody-bead complexes detect multiple epitopes in single sample; for instance, this technology was used to detect abrin, ricin, botulinum toxins, and staphylococcal enterotoxins in spiked food samples (Garber, Venkateswaran, and O'Brien, 2010). The study used paramagnetic beads instead of non-magnetic polystyrene beads to help in the analysis of food matrices, such as chipotle mustard, which contain large amounts of particulate matter.

4.3.3 Affinity immunochromatography column-based methods

Accurate and sensitive detection of contaminated food and other biological samples in the field is critical. To this end, Brunt and colleagues (Brunt, Webb, and Peck, 2010) have developed a number of rapid affinity immunochromatography column (AICC) assays for the detection of BoNT serotypes A, B, E, and F in food matrices. These authors reported a detection limit for BoNT/A of 0.5 ng, two fold more sensitive than earlier reported lateral flow methods. For serotypes B, E, and F, the minimum detection limit ranged from 5 ng to 50 ng. Although not as sensitive as ELISA or mouse bioassays, immunochromatographic methods generally are rapid assays, requiring only 15 to 30 minutes to complete, do not require enrichment steps, making them highly amenable to use in the field.

4.3.4 Lateral flow technology

The application of lateral flow methods for detecting toxins has led to the development of a number of kits for sensitive and rapid testing. The principle here is that capture antibodies are printed on nitrocellulose membranes. Detection antibodies are labeled with materials that can be visualized (eg., colloidal gold, or colored latex beads) The sample is added to a reagent pad containing labelled detection antibodies that bind toxin, wick across the membrane where toxin is retained, thus concentrating the labelled detection antibody. A positive reaction leads to a colorimetric change that is usually detected as a line. These assays are generally qualitative, and determine the presence or absence of toxin. Sharma and coworkers tested different commercial lateral flow devices (such as the Bot-Tox-BTA kit) for their capacities to detect toxin in food samples (Sharma et al., 2005). They were able to detect as little as 10 ng/ml of BoNT serotypes A and B and 20 ng/ml of BoNT/E in a variety of liquids such as milk products, soft drinks, and fruit juices. Results by Stanker (unpublished) show sensitivity of 0.5 and 1 ng/ml for BoNT/A in buffer and milk, respectively, in lateral flow devices using sensitive mAbs described in the ELISA section above (Stanker et al., 2008). Although simple lateral flow tests have poorer sensitivities compared to other methods, they produced rapid results, require no additional reagents or equipment, are easily interpreted, and have many applications. They can be useful for the quick screening of samples where the presence of BoNT may be more abundant.

4.3.5 Immuno-polymerase chain reaction (I-PCR)

An innovative approach for toxin detection combines antibodies with the amplification power of PCR in an assay called immuno-PCR (I-PCR). Here, instead of a secondary antibody conjugated to the detection enzyme, template DNA is conjugated to the antibody; and upon binding of antigen by the antibody, an indirect test for the presence of the BoNT is carried out using PCR. Chao et al. described a sensitive I-PCR method (femtogram amounts, 10^{-15} grams) for detection of BoNT/A. These investigators also compared standard ELISA as well as sandwich ELISA methods with the sensitivity of the I-PCR method. Both ELISA methods were sensitive for toxin detection down to 50 fg, and the I-PCR method was between 10^3 to 10^5 times more sensitive (Chao et al., 2004; Wu et al., 2001). For more background on the basic principles of I-PCR, the reader is referred to Niemeyer and colleagues (Niemeyer, Adler, and Wacker, 2005). The use of I-PCR for highly sensitive detection of BoNT in food matrices or other biological backgrounds has yet to be developed.

4.4 Activity based assays for detecting food contamination

Rapidly distinguishing between the presence and absence of active versus inactive toxin is critical for intervention. Since BoNTs are zinc metalloproteases, enzyme-substrate assays have been developed using knowledge of the human targets for these enzymes. Activity assays range from mixing toxin with recombinant versions of host targets (such as SNAP-25) and then using immunoblotting to detect cleavage of those substrates, to measuring fluorescence emitted from cleavage of fluorogenic peptide substrates. One such peptide, called SNAPtide, used in an assay with a reverse phase HPLC with a fluorescence detector, can detect as low as 5 pg/mL of BoNT/A in skim milk (Christian, Suryadi, and Shine, 2010). Other peptide substrates: VAMPtide and SYNTAXtide, useful for their cognate BoNTs have been developed. The levels of substrate cleavage correlate well with toxin activity.

Other investigators have looked for other indications of substrate cleavage by BoNTs. For instance, Nuss and colleagues generated antibodies that specifically recognize the full-length version of human SNAP25 and not the cleaved form (Nuss et al, 2010). Use of this antibody to confirm the absence of toxin activity (by detecting only the intact, full length substrate) might be useful to confirm the absence of bioactive forms of the toxin.

Other activity-based approaches have used physical methods such as surface plasmon resonance to detect cleavage of substrates. For instance, Ferraci and colleagues have demonstrated that cleavage of the BoNT/B substrate VAMP2, a membrane SNARE protein associated with synaptic vesicles, can be measured using real-time surface plasmon resonance; vesicle capture is detected by specific antibodies coupled to microchips (Ferracci et al., 2010). This assay is functional in low ionic strength buffers and stable over a wide range of pH values (5.5-9.0). Cleavage of VAMP2 was detected within 10 minutes with 2 pM of native BoNT/B holotoxin. Contamination of liquid food products such as carrot juice, apple juice, and milk with low picomolar amounts of BoNT/B toxin is revealed within 3 hours. BoNT/B activity was detected in sera samples from botulism patients but not in healthy patients or in patients with other neurological diseases.

4.4.1 Cell-based assays and their possible use in detecting food contamination

Cell-based assays measure BoNT receptor biding, translocation and enzymatic activity and can be viable alternatives to the mouse bioassay. A number of different neuronal and non-neuronal derived cell lines have been generated for use in BoNT assays. These include: rat spinal cord cells (Pellett et al., 2007); chick embryo neuronal cells (Stahl et al., 2007); neuroblastoma cells N2A (Eubanks et al., 2007); and BE(2)-M17 cells (Hale et al., 2011). The read-out for most of the cell-based assays for detection of BoNT/A is the cleavage of SNAP-25. Antibodies for SNAP-25 allow immunoblot detection of cleavage products, specifically detecting a decrease in size of endogenous SNAP-25 protein.

Investigators continue to examine different parameters in order to develop a more robust cell-based assay. The U.S. Food and Drug Administration recently approved a cell-based assay developed by Allergan for use as possible replacement of the mouse bioassay. Details of the assay have yet to be published. Cell -based assays may yet prove valuable for toxin detection in food.

4.5 Combining assay methods to increase detection sensitivity

Detection methods can exploit the power of sensitive antibodies for enrichment or sample preparation, as well as the signal amplification ability of enzymatic assays. Two recent approaches are highlighted below.

4.5.1 ALISSA (assay with a large immunosorbent surface area)

The ALISSA utilizes a two-step approach; first, an antibody-mediated step concentrates toxin onto a large bead surface. Captured toxin molecules are then subjected to a SNAPtide protease assay (Bagramyan et al., 2008). When compared to other established methods for toxin detection in food matrices, the ALISSA assay can detect toxin concentrations as low as 50 fg/mL, more sensitive than the mouse bioassay or either immunoassay or SNAPtide assay alone. The use of this method to evaluate a number of different food matrices suggests that it may be useful in food contamination studies.

4.5.2 ENDOPEP-MS: antibodies, activity assays, and mass spectrometry

The ENDOPEP-MS method uses antibodies to concentrate and extract BoNT serotypes A, B, E, and F from test samples. The concentrated toxins are then subjected to an endopeptidase activity-based assay to generate target cleavage products. Finally, mass spectrometry is used to identify cleavage target products (Kalb et al., 2005; Kalb et al., 2006). This approach has been successful in identifying BoNT serotypes A, B, E, and F in a variety of food and clinical sample matrices with sub-mouse bioassay sensitivities. To advance this technique even further, a single, high-affinity mAb (4E17.1) that can simultaneous identify BoNT serotypes A, B, E and F has been developed (Kalb et al., 2010). The use of this mAb reduced assay time while maintaining assay sensitivity. The use of mass spectrometry can give fast and definitive results. With the future development of low cost equipment, this method may be more readily available to investigators.

5. Conclusion

Detection of BoNT presents a unique set of challenges. The high toxicity of BoNT requires detection methods capable of toxin measurement in the low to sub pg/mL range. PCR methods can readily detect the presence of low levels of *C. botulinum* DNA but do not detect the presence or absence of the toxin. In many cases, such as blood samples, only toxin may be present. Current methods for toxin detection rely on 1) the gold standard mouse bioassay, or 2) *in vitro* tests such as molecular tests, immunoassays and/or activity-based assays. Recent improvements in the generation of high-affinity mAbs have resulted in immunoassays with sensitivities equal to or lower than the mouse bioassay. However these tests generally do not distinguish active from inactive toxin. Activity-based assays can detect active toxin but generally have poorer detection limits than immunoassays. New assays must also be carefully validated in individual food matrices or for as many toxin subtypes as possible, in order to establish assay performance standards. With refinement of the methods described above, the prospect of an assay that is sensitive, cost effective, and fast could be possible for use in food or other biological samples. Furthermore, these new strategies for assay development can easily be extended to other toxins and pathogens.

6. Acknowledgment

Due to space constraints, the authors apologize for not being able to devote enough attention to many worthy assay methods. We thank our colleagues for insightful comments and discussions. Thomas D. Henderson II for help with background research. KML was funded by the Department of Biological Sciences and the Office of Grants and Sponsored Programs, the University of the Pacific. LWC and LHS were funded by the United States Department of Agriculture, Agriculture Research Service, CRIS project 5325-42000-048-00D, the National Institute of Allergy And Infectious Diseases Service Grant U54 AI065359, and DHS agreement 40768. The USDA is an equal opportunity provider and employer.

7. References

Arnon, S. S., Schechter, R., Inglesby, T. V., Henderson, D. A., Bartlett, J. G., Ascher, M. S., Eitzen, E., Fine, A. D., Hauer, J., Layton, M., Lillibridge, S., Osterholm, M. T., O'Toole, T., Parker, G., Perl, T. M., Russell, P. K., Swerdlow, D. L., and Tonat, K. (2001). Botulinum toxin as a biological weapon: medical and public health management. *Jama* 285(8), 1059-70.

Bagramyan, K., Barash, J. R., Arnon, S. S., and Kalkum, M. (2008). Attomolar detection of botulinum toxin type A in complex biological matrices. *PLoS ONE* 3(4), e2041.

Bigalke, H., and Rummel, A. (2005). Medical aspects of toxin weapons. *Toxicology* 214(3), 210-20.

Brunt, J., Webb, M. D., and Peck, M. W. (2010). Rapid affinity immunochromatography column-based tests for sensitive detection of Clostridium botulinum neurotoxins and *Escherichia coli* O157. *Appl Environ Microbiol* 76(13), 4143-50.

CDC (1998). Center for Disease Control and Prevention. Botulism in the United States (1899-1996). Handbook for epidemiologists, clinicians and laboratory workers. *U.S. Department of Health and Human Services, CDC. Atlanta, Ga.*

CFSAN (2001). Center for Food Safety and Applied Nutrition. Bacteriological analytical manual (BAM). U.S. Food and Drug Administration, Washington, D.C.

CSTE Council of State and Territorial Epidemiologists. 2001-2009. Botulism Surveillance Summary. http://www.cdc.gov/nationalsurveillance/botulism_surveillance.html

Chao, H. Y., Wang, Y. C., Tang, S. S., and Liu, H. W. (2004). A highly sensitive immuno-polymerase chain reaction assay for *Clostridium botulinum* neurotoxin type A. *Toxicon* 43(1), 27-34.

Cheng, L. W., and Henderson, T. D., 2nd (2011). Comparison of oral toxicological properties of botulinum neurotoxin serotypes A and B. *Toxicon* 58(1), 62-7.

Cheng, L. W., Onisko, B., Johnson, E. A., Reader, J. R., Griffey, S. M., Larson, A. E., Tepp, W. H., Stanker, L. H., Brandon, D. L., and Carter, J. M. (2008). Effects of purification on the bioavailability of botulinum neurotoxin type A. *Toxicology* 249(2-3), 123-9.

Christian, T., Suryadi, K., and Shine, N. (2010). Ultra Sensitive HPLC Detection Assay for Botulinum Neurotoxin Type A. *Presented at the 47th Annual Interagency Botulinum Research Coordinating Committee Meeting, November 2010 in Atlanta, GA.*

De Medici, D., Anniballi, F., Wyatt, G. M., Lindström, M., Messelhausser, U., Aldus, C. F., Delibato, E., Korkeala, H., Peck, M. W., and Fenicia, L. (2009). Multiplex PCR for detection of botulinum neurotoxin-producing clostridia in clinical, food, and environmental samples. *Appl Environ Microbiol* 75(20), 6457-61.

Eubanks, L. M., Hixon, M. S., Jin, W., Hong, S., Clancy, C. M., Tepp, W. H., Baldwin, M. R., Malizio, C. J., Goodnough, M. C., Barbieri, J. T., Johnson, E. A., Boger, D. L., Dickerson, T. J., and Janda, K. D. (2007). An in vitro and in vivo disconnect uncovered through high-throughput identification of botulinum neurotoxin A antagonists. *Proc Natl Acad Sci U S A* 104(8), 2602-7.

Fach, P., Fenicia, L., Knutsson, R., Wielinga, P. R., Anniballi, F., Delibato, E., Auricchio, B., Woudstra, C., Agren, J., Segerman, B., de Medici, D., and van Rotterdam, B. J. (2011). An innovative molecular detection tool for tracking and tracing *Clostridium botulinum* types A, B, E, F and other botulinum neurotoxin producing Clostridia based on the GeneDisc cycler. *Int J Food Microbiol* 145 Suppl 1, S145-51.

Fach, P., Micheau, P., Mazuet, C., Perelle, S., and Popoff, M. (2009). Development of real-time PCR tests for detecting botulinum neurotoxins A, B, E, F producing *Clostridium botulinum, Clostridium baratii and Clostridium butyricum. J Appl Microbiol* 107(2), 465-73.

Ferracci, G., Marconi, S., Mazuet, C., Jover, E., Blanchard, M. P., Seagar, M., Popoff, M., and Leveque, C. (2010). A label-free biosensor assay for botulinum neurotoxin B in food and human serum. *Anal Biochem* 410(2), 281-8.

Ferreira, J. L., Eliasberg, S. J., Edmonds, P., and Harrison, M. A. (2004). Comparison of the mouse bioassay and enzyme-linked immunosorbent assay procedures for the detection of type A botulinal toxin in food. *J Food Prot* 67(1), 203-6.

Fujinaga, Y., Matsumura, T., Jin, Y., Takegahara, Y., and Sugawara, Y. (2009). A novel function of botulinum toxin-associated proteins: HA proteins disrupt intestinal epithelial barrier to increase toxin absorption. *Toxicon* 54(5), 583-6.

Garber, E. A., Venkateswaran, K. V., and O'Brien, T. W. (2010). Simultaneous multiplex detection and confirmation of the proteinaceous toxins abrin, ricin, botulinum toxins, and Staphylococcus enterotoxins A, B, and C in food. *J Agric Food Chem* 58(11), 6600-7.

Garcia-Rodriguez, C., Geren, I. N., Lou, J., Conrad, F., Forsyth, C., Wen, W., Chakraborti, S., Zao, H., Manzanarez, G., Smith, T. J., Brown, J., Tepp, W. H., Liu, N., Wijesuriya, S., Tomic, M. T., Johnson, E. A., Smith, L. A., and Marks, J. D. (2011). Neutralizing human monoclonal antibodies binding multiple serotypes of botulinum neurotoxin. *Protein Eng Des Sel* 24(3), 321-31.

Grate, J. W., Ozanich, R. M., Jr., Warner, M. G., Marks, J. D., and Bruckner-Lea, C. J. (2010). Advances in assays and analytical approaches for botulinum-toxin detection. *Trends in Analytical Chemistry* 29(10), 1137-1156.

Hakami, R. M., Ruthel, G., Stahl, A. M., and Bavari, S. (2010). Gaining ground: assays for therapeutics against botulinum neurotoxin. *Trends Microbiol* 18(4), 164-72.

Hale, M., Oyler, G., Swaminathan, S., and Ahmed, S. A. (2011). Basic tetrapeptides as potent intracellular inhibitors of type A botulinum neurotoxin protease activity. *J Biol Chem* 286(3), 1802-11.

Hill, K. K., Smith, T. J., Helma, C. H., Ticknor, L. O., Foley, B. T., Svensson, R. T., Brown, J. L., Johnson, E. A., Smith, L. A., Okinaka, R. T., Jackson, P. J., and Marks, J. D. (2007). Genetic diversity among Botulinum Neurotoxin-producing clostridial strains. *J Bacteriol* 189(3), 818-32.

Inoue, K., Fujinaga, Y., Watanabe, T., Ohyama, T., Takeshi, K., Moriishi, K., Nakajima, H., Inoue, K., and Oguma, K. (1996). Molecular composition of *Clostridium botulinum* type A progenitor toxins. *Infect Immun* 64(5), 1589-94.

Jacobson, M. J., Lin, G., Tepp, W., Dupuy, J., Stenmark, P., Stevens, R. C., and Johnson, E. A. (2011). Purification, modeling, and analysis of botulinum neurotoxin subtype A5 (BoNT/A5) from *Clostridium botulinum* strain A661222. *Appl Environ Microbiol* 77(12), 4217-22.

Kalb, S. R., Garcia-Rodriguez, C., Lou, J., Baudys, J., Smith, T. J., Marks, J. D., Smith, L. A., Pirkle, J. L., and Barr, J. R. (2010). Extraction of BoNT/A, /B, /E, and /F with a single, high affinity monoclonal antibody for detection of botulinum neurotoxin by Endopep-MS. *PLoS One* 5(8), e12237.

Kalb, S. R., Goodnough, M. C., Malizio, C. J., Pirkle, J. L., and Barr, J. R. (2005). Detection of botulinum neurotoxin A in a spiked milk sample with subtype identification through toxin proteomics. *Anal Chem* 77(19), 6140-6.

Kalb, S. R., Moura, H., Boyer, A. E., McWilliams, L. G., Pirkle, J. L., and Barr, J. R. (2006). The use of Endopep-MS for the detection of botulinum toxins A, B, E, and F in serum and stool samples. *Anal Biochem* 351(1), 84-92.

Kirchner, S., Kramer, K. M., Schulze, M., Pauly, D., Jacob, D., Gessler, F., Nitsche, A., Dorner, B. G., and Dorner, M. B. (2010). Pentaplexed quantitative real-time PCR assay for the simultaneous detection and quantification of botulinum neurotoxin-producing clostridia in food and clinical samples. *Appl Environ Microbiol* 76(13), 4387-95.

Lindström, M., Keto, R., Markkula, A., Nevas, M., Hielm, S., and Korkeala, H. (2001). Multiplex PCR assay for detection and identification of *Clostridium botulinum* types A, B, E, and F in food and fecal material. *Appl Environ Microbiol* 67(12), 5694-9.

Lindström, M., and Korkeala, H. (2006). Laboratory diagnostics of botulism. *Clin Microbiol Rev* 19(2), 298-314.

Niemeyer, C. M., Adler, M., and Wacker, R. (2005). Immuno-PCR: high sensitivity detection of proteins by nucleic acid amplification. *Trends Biotechnol* 23(4), 208-16.

Niwa, K., Koyama, K., Inoue, S., Suzuki, T., Hasegawa, K., Watanabe, T., Ikeda, T., and Ohyama, T. (2007). Role of nontoxic components of serotype D botulinum toxin complex in permeation through a Caco-2 cell monolayer, a model for intestinal epithelium. *FEMS Immunol Med Microbiol* 49(3), 346-52.

Nuss, J. E., Wanner, L. M., Tressler, L. E., and Bavari, S. (2010). The osmolyte trimethylamine N-oxide (TMAO) increases the proteolytic activity of botulinum neurotoxin light chains A, B, and E: implications for enhancing analytical assay sensitivity. *J Biomol Screen* 15(8), 928-36.

Oguma, K., Fujinaga, Y., and Inoue, K. (1995). Structure and function of Clostridium botulinum toxins. *Microbiol Immunol* 39(3), 161-8.

Ohishi, I., Sugii, S., and Sakaguchi, G. (1977). Oral toxicities of Clostridium botulinum toxins in response to molecular size. *Infect Immun* 16(1), 107-9.

Peck, M. W., Plowman, J., Aldus, C. F., Wyatt, G. M., Izurieta, W. P., Stringer, S. C., and Barker, G. C. (2010). Development and application of a new method for specific and sensitive enumeration of spores of nonproteolytic *Clostridium botulinum* types B, E, and F in foods and food materials. *Appl Environ Microbiol* 76(19), 6607-14.

Pellett, S., Tepp, W. H., Clancy, C. M., Borodic, G. E., and Johnson, E. A. (2007). A neuronal cell-based botulinum neurotoxin assay for highly sensitive and specific detection of neutralizing serum antibodies. *FEBS Lett* 581(25), 4803-8.

Raphael, B. H., Joseph, L. A., McCroskey, L. M., Luquez, C., and Maslanka, S. E. (2010). Detection and differentiation of *Clostridium botulinum* type A strains using a focused DNA microarray. *Mol Cell Probes* 24(3), 146-53.

Rasetti-Escargueil, C., Jones, R. G., Liu, Y., and Sesardic, D. (2009). Measurement of botulinum types A, B and E neurotoxicity using the phrenic nerve-hemidiaphragm: improved precision with in-bred mice. *Toxicon* 53(5), 503-11.

Scarlatos, A., Welt, B. A., Cooper, B. Y., Archer, D., DeMarse, T., and Chau, K. V. (2005). Methods for detecting botulinum toxin with applicability to screening foods against biological terrorist attacks. *Journal of Food Science* 70(8), 121-130.

Schantz, E. J., and Kautter, D. A. (1978). Standardized assay for *Clostridium botulinum* toxins. *Journal of the AOAC* 61(1), 96-99.

Scotcher, M. C., Cheng, L. W., and Stanker, L. H. (2010). Detection of botulinum neurotoxin serotype B at sub mouse LD(50) levels by a sandwich immunoassay and its application to toxin detection in milk. *PLoS One* 5(6), e11047.

Sharma, S. K., Eblen, B. S., Bull, R. L., Burr, D. H., and Whiting, R. C. (2005). Evaluation of lateral-flow *Clostridium botulinum* neurotoxin detection kits for food analysis. *Appl Environ Microbiol* 71(7), 3935-41.

Sharma, S. K., Ferreira, J. L., Eblen, B. S., and Whiting, R. C. (2006). Detection of type A, B, E, and F *Clostridium botulinum* neurotoxins in foods by using an amplified enzyme-linked immunosorbent assay with digoxigenin-labeled antibodies. *Appl Environ Microbiol* 72(2), 1231-8.

Sharma, S. K., and Whiting, R. C. (2005). Methods for detection of *Clostridium botulinum* toxin in foods. *J Food Prot* 68(6), 1256-63.

Simpson, L. L. (2004). Identification of the major steps in botulinum toxin action. *Annu Rev Pharmacol Toxicol* 44, 167-93.

Simpson, L. L., Maksymowych, A. B., Park, J. B., and Bora, R. S. (2004). The role of the interchain disulfide bond in governing the pharmacological actions of botulinum toxin. *J Pharmacol Exp Ther* 308(3), 857-64.

Singh, B. R. (2000). Intimate details of the most poisonous poison. *Nat Struct Biol* 7(8), 617-9.

Smith, T. J., Hill, K. K., Foley, B. T., Detter, J. C., Munk, A. C., Bruce, D. C., Doggett, N. A., Smith, L. A., Marks, J. D., Xie, G., and Brettin, T. S. (2007). Analysis of the neurotoxin complex genes in *Clostridium botulinum* A1-A4 and B1 strains: BoNT/A3, /Ba4 and /B1 clusters are located within plasmids. *PLoS One* 2(12), e1271.

Smith, T. J., Lou, J., Geren, I. N., Forsyth, C. M., Tsai, R., Laporte, S. L., Tepp, W. H., Bradshaw, M., Johnson, E. A., Smith, L. A., and Marks, J. D. (2005). Sequence variation within botulinum neurotoxin serotypes impacts antibody binding and neutralization. *Infect Immun* 73(9), 5450-7.

Solomon, H. M., and Lilly, T. J. (2001). Chapter 17. *Clostridium botulinum. Bacteriological Analytical Manual, 8th Edition, Revision A, 1998.*

Stahl, A. M., Ruthel, G., Torres-Melendez, E., Kenny, T. A., Panchal, R. G., and Bavari, S. (2007). Primary cultures of embryonic chicken neurons for sensitive cell-based assay of botulinum neurotoxin: implications for therapeutic discovery. *J Biomol Screen* 12(3), 370-7.

Stanker, L. H., Merrill, P., Scotcher, M. C., and Cheng, L. W. (2008). Development and partial characterization of high-affinity monoclonal antibodies for botulinum toxin type A and their use in analysis of milk by sandwich ELISA. *J Immunol Methods* 336(1), 1-8.

Wictome, M., Newton, K., Jameson, K., Hallis, B., Dunnigan, P., Mackay, E., Clarke, S., Taylor, R., Gaze, J., Foster, K., and Shone, C. (1999). Development of an in vitro bioassay for *Clostridium botulinum* type B neurotoxin in foods that is more sensitive than the mouse bioassay. *Appl Environ Microbiol* 65(9), 3787-92.

Wilder-Kofie, T. D., Luquez, C., Adler, M., Dykes, J. K., Coleman, J. D., and Maslanka, S. E. (2011). An alternative in vivo method to refine the mouse bioassay for botulinum toxin detection. *Comp Med* 61(3), 235-42.

Wu, H. C., Huang, Y. L., Lai, S. C., Huang, Y. Y., and Shaio, M. F. (2001). Detection of *Clostridium botulinum* neurotoxin type A using immuno-PCR. *Lett Appl Microbiol* 32(5), 321-5.

2

Detection of Bacillus Spores by Surface-Enhanced Raman Spectroscopy

Stuart Farquharson[1], Chetan Shende[1], Alan Gift[2] and Frank Inscore[1]
[1]*Real-Time Analyzers,*
[2]*University of Nebraska, Omaha,*
USA

1. Introduction

On September 18 and October 9, 2001, two sets of letters containing *Bacillus anthracis* spores passed through the United States Postal Service's Trenton, NJ, Processing and Distribution Center (Jernigan et al., 2001). The first set was destined for Florida and New York, while the second set was destined for Washington, DC. The infection of 22 people by these spores resulted in 5 deaths: a media employee in Florida, two postal workers in DC, a hospital worker in New York, and a retired woman in Connecticut (Inglesby et al., 2002). This bioterrorism event closely followed the September 11, 2001 attack on the Pentagon building and the World Trade Center towers, which added to the nation's concern about terrorism within US borders. There was additional anxiety associated with this second attack, in that the extent of spore distribution along the east coast was unknown, and it took a long time to determine who was infected. This was even true for the letter that was mailed to Senator Tom Daschle at the Hart Senate Office (HSO) Building in DC. While the powder that fell from the letter was immediately suspected as *B. anthracis,* due to the previous week's news from Florida and New York, and collection of nasal swabs from HSO personnel was initiate within 9 hours (Hsu et al., 2002), it still took several additional days to determine who was exposed and infected (Jernigan et al., 2001,).

This delay was due to the fact that the spores must be germinated and grown in culture media to sufficient cell numbers so that they can be measured by standard methods. Presumptive *B. anthracis* was based on shape (1 to 1.5 by 3 to 5 μm rods), lack of motility, lack of a hemolysis on a sheep blood agar plate, susceptibility to β-lactam antibiotics and to γ-phage lysis, and staining for gram-positive bacteria (Center for Disease Control and Prevention, CDC, 2001). The time consuming component of this analysis is the culture growth of cell colonies. Simply put, the fewer the initial number of spores, the less likely a sample will produce detectable colonies. Only samples collected from surfaces or individuals that had a high probability of being contaminated produced colonies that were evident in 24 hours. Furthermore, tests were initially limited to individuals within the vicinity of where the letter was opened, which proved insufficient, as three postal workers at the Brentwood, DC, Processing and Distribution Center became infected, two fatally (Jernigan et al., 2001; Sanderson et al., 2002). Upon notification of their hospitalization, the CDC initiated collection of several hundred environmental (mostly surface) samples from associated facilities and several thousand nasal swab samples from visitors to these facilities, including first responders, and their employees. According to the team at the National Institutes of Health, who processed nearly 4000 samples, current methods of culture growth and analysis were "extremely time-consuming and labor-intensive" (Kiratisin et al., 2002).

From these bioterrorist attacks, it became clear that considerably faster methods of analysis are required. This would expedite assessment of the extent of attack, including the path of such letters from destination back to origination. More importantly, it would minimize fatalities, since it was learned that if exposure is detected within the first few days, the majority of victims can be treated successfully using Ciprofloxacin, doxycycline and/or penicillin G procaine (Bell et al., 2002).

At the time of the attack two rapid methods were used, immunoassay kits and polymerase chain reaction (PCR) analyzers. Immunoassay methods use competitive binding of the bioagent (as an antigen) and its labeled conjugate for a limited number of antibodies. These methods can be relatively fast (<20 minutes) with modest sensitivity. The latter was not an issue for the Senator Daschle letter, which contained billions of spores (Kennedy, 2001). However, as yet no well-defined anthrax antigen has been identified (Bell et al., 2001; Kellogg, 2010), and as a result, the false-positive rates remain unacceptably high. Consequently, immunoassay development has shifted to detecting the *B. anthracis* proteins involved in infection. This includes the protective antigen and lethal factor (Bell et al., 2002; Mabry et al., 2006; Tang et al., 2009). But these immunoassays require several days after the onset of infection for these proteins to reach detectable concentrations, even with the use of time-resolved fluorescence detection, which may not provide sufficient time to substantially improve the odds of successful treatment (Tang et al., 2006).

During the 2001 bioterrorism event NIH employed Applied Biosystems (Foster City, CA) to use PCR to sequence the 16S rRNA *B. anthracis* gene (Kiratisin et al., 2002). However, the specificity of this gene for *B. anthracis* was in doubt as Bacilli are highly homologous to the extent that *B. anthracis*, *B. cereus* and *B. thuringiensis* may belong to one species (Helgason et al., 2000, Sacchi et al., 2002). Since the attacks, more definitive *B. anthracis* gene sequences have been identified. Specifically, the genes within the toxin encoding pXO1 plasmid and the capsule-encoding pXO2 plasmid are being targeted for analysis. The development of "real-time" PCR systems that combine the use of primers to separate these organism-specific nucleic acid sequences and polymerases to amplify the sequences (Bell et al., 2001 & 2002; Thayer, 2003), resulted in the installation of such systems at some 300 regional US Postal offices through 2006 at a cost of $600 million (Shane, 2004; Leingang, 2004).

While, PCR and immunoassays continue to be developed, other methods are also being developed that rapidly assess the extent of contamination in the event of an attack, such as fluorescence, luminescence, mass spectrometry, and Raman spectroscopy (Nudelman et al., 2000; Pellegrino et al., 2002; Hathout et al., 2003; Farquharson et al., 2004, respectively). These methods focus on portability and sensitivity, rather than on specificity.

Most of these methods have been focusing on the detection of calcium dipicolinate (CaDPA) or its derivatives as a *B. anthracis* signature since it has been reported that CaDPA represents 10 to 15% by weight of these spores (Fig. 1; Janssen et al., 1958; Murrell at al., 1969; Hindle & Hall, 1999; Ragkousi at al., 2003; Liu et al., 2004; Phillips & Strauch, 2002). This is a valid approach, first because only 13 genera of spore-forming bacteria contain CaDPA (Berkeley

& Ali, 1994), but only *Bacillium* and *Clostridium* are common (and of interest; Phillips & Strauch, 2002), and second, the most widespread, potentially interfering spores, such as pollen and mold spores, do not. Relatively fast methods have been developed to chemically extract the acid of CaDPA, dipicolinic acid (DPA; Pellegrino et al., 2002), and then to detect it directly by mass spectrometry (Beverly et al., 1996; Hathout et al., 2003), fluorescence (Nudelman et al., 2000), or indirectly by luminescence (Pellegrino et al., 2002; Rosen et al., 1997). Although mass spectrometry provides a relatively high degree of discrimination and sensitivity, it still requires significant time due to sample preparation. Hot dodecylamine (DDA) has been used to extract DPA and form a highly luminescent complex with terbium (Pellegrino et al., 2002). Although measurements have been performed in as little as five minutes, it was found that as many as three concentration-dependent complexes can form, each with different lifetimes. This, coupled with the fact that the Tb^{3+} cation produces the same luminescence spectrum, makes determinations of low spore concentrations problematic. Furthermore, the combination of heat and the DDA surfactant severely degrade the spore, generating cell debris. This requires sample cleanup and in this particular case, $AlCl_3$ has to be added to remove phosphates that would interfere with the photoluminescent measurement.

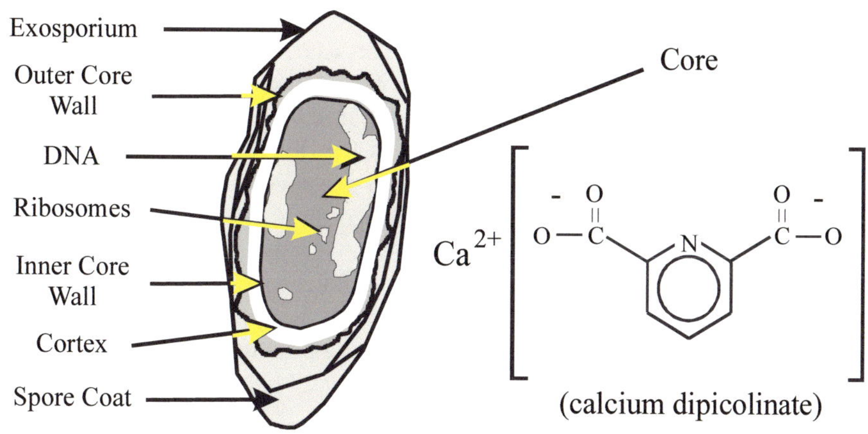

Fig. 1. Illustration of a Bacillus spore with major components indicated, and chemical structure of calcium dipicolinate. Deprotonated dipicolinic acid is shown within the brackets.

An alternative method, Raman spectroscopy (RS), is attractive in that very small samples can be measured without preparation. The sample need only be placed at the focal spot of the excitation laser and measured. Moreover, the rich molecular information provided by Raman spectroscopy usually allows unequivocal identification of chemicals and biologicals. As early as 1974 the Raman spectrum of *Bacillus megaterium* was measured and shown to be dominated by CaDPA (Woodruff et al., 1974). However, the spectrum was collected using pure spores and took hours to acquire. Since that time, considerable improvements in Raman instrumentation have led to laboratory measurements of single Bacillus spores and field measurements of spores captured from a mail sorting system (Esposito et al., 2003; Farquharson et al., 2004). Unfortunately, the single spore measurements required the use of a microscope system and time consuming efforts to locate the spores, while the field measurements required milligrams of sample.

Two approaches are widely used to improve the sensitivity of Raman spectroscopy; resonance Raman spectroscopy and surface-enhanced Raman spectroscopy (SERS). The former method involves laser excitation at or near the wavelength of a molecular electronic absorption to substantially increase the interactions between the radiation and molecular states, and was used more than a decade ago to analyze Bacillus spores (Ghiamati, 1992). The value of this technique is limited by the extremely low energy conversion of ultraviolet lasers, which require substantial power supplies and thus confine measurements to laboratory settings.

SERS involves the absorption of incident laser photons within nanoscale metal structures, generating surface plasmons, which couple with nearby molecules (the analyte) and thereby enhance the efficiency of Raman scattering by six orders of magnitude or more (Jeanmaire & Van Duyne, 1977; Weaver et al., 1985). More than a decade ago, we began investigating the potential of SERS to measure *B. anthracis* ssp. spores, beginning with the first measurement of the biomarker dipicolinic acid (Farquharson, 1999). In this chapter we summarize our efforts to develop a field portable analyzer that uses a simple digesting agent to extract DPA from *B. anthracis* spores for detection by SERS.

The approach and ultimately the success of these efforts not only depend on the instrumentation, but also on the specific terrorist scenario being addressed. This has significant implications for the choice of sampling. For example, detecting a plume of spores released from an airplane is very different than detecting spores in envelopes passing through a mail sorting machine. Here the focus is the detection of spores on surfaces to assess the extent of an attack. For this application specificity at the *Bacillus* spp. level is sufficient, i.e. it is not critical to differentiate between the various *Bacillus* spp. At present there are no guidelines defining the required sensitivity. However, an extensive number of surface samples were collected from the Brentwood, DC, mail Processing and Distribution Center and their analysis can be used as a guide to estimate sensitivity requirements (Sanderson et al., 2004). This analysis determined that the highest concentrations of spores, not surprisingly, were in the immediate vicinity of delivery barcode sorter machine number 17, which processed both letters. Analysis of dust above, within 30 meters, and 30-60 meters of this machine recorded average values of 310, 67, and 10 CFU/in^2. Since the last average value included measurements that detected "zero" spores, it lacks the certainty of the other values. Consequently, and somewhat subjectively, we have chosen the middle value, 67 CFU/in^2 (10 spores/cm^2), as a minimum requirement for measurement sensitivity. This value should not be construed as a definition of lethality.

Additional measurement requirements include the ease of sampling and speed of analysis. Based on the 2001 attacks, we consider a minimum requirement of 500 measurements per 24 hours as reasonable. Of course more than one analyzer could be used to accomplish this, but the fewer the analyzers, the lower the cost and the number of operators. If one analyzer is used, then the required measurement time would be less than 3 minutes. This would include the time to collect, deliver, measure, and analyze the sample. This suggests that sampling should involve a method or device to rapidly collect the sample (e.g. a wet swab or vacuum system) and deliver it to the measurement compartment of the analyzer. It also suggests that the analyzer should be portable to minimize or eliminate sample delivery time.

With these criteria in mind, we have developed a three-step method to detect dipicolinic acid extracted from surface spores by surface-enhanced Raman spectroscopy. The first step employs acetic acid to break apart the spores and release CaDPA into solution as DPA. The second step employs single-use, disposable, sol-gel filled capillaries to separate the DPA from other cell components and simultaneously deliver it to the SER-active metal particles. The third step employs a portable Raman analyzer to measure the SER spectrum and to identify and quantify the spores, if present. Development of this three-step method and measurements of *Bacillus* ssp. spores on surfaces are presented.

2. Experimental

Dipicolinic acid (2,6-pyridinedicarboxylic acid), acetic acid (glacial, 99.7%), dodecylamine (DDA), and all chemicals used to produce the silver-doped sol-gels were obtained at their purest commercially available grade from Sigma-Aldrich (Milwaukee, WI) and used as received. Calcium dipicolinate was prepared from disodium dipicolinate (Na_2DPA), which was prepared from DPA according to previous publications (Ghiamati, 1992). *Bacillus cereus, B. subtilis,* and *B. megaterium* were grown on nutrient agar plates at 30°C for 7 days (Ghiamati, 1992). The vegetative cells were placed into distilled water and lysed by osmotic pressure. The resultant spores were collected by scraping them into distilled water and pelleting them by centrifugation at 12,100 x g for 10 minutes. The spore pellet was re-suspended in distilled water and lyophilized, and scraped into glass vials for Raman spectral measurements. Approximately 1 gram each, determined to be 99% pure by microscopic observation, was produced for this study. The density of the spores varied from 0.06 to 0.11 g/mL, indicating a high amount of entrained air.

Calibrated samples of *B. cereus* spores were prepared by weighing 1-5 mg specks, dispersing them in 10 mL water using sonication and vortexing. Sonication was accomplished using an Ultrasonik 300 (Neytech, Burlington, NJ), while vortexing was accomplished using a Vortex-Genie 1 (Scientific Industries, Bohemia, NY). The spores per volume water were calibrated by using a Brite-line, phase-contrast hemocytometer counting grid (AO Scientific Instruments, Buffalo, NY) and imaged using an Olympus BX 51 microscope (Olympus America, Center Valley, PA) fit in-house with a Sony Cyber-shot 2.1 digital camera.

An initial stock solution of 20 mg of DPA in 20 mL HPLC grade water (Fischer Scientific, Fair Lawn, NJ) was prepared for the pH study. The pH of this solution was 2.45 as verified using a pH electrode (Corning 314 pH/Temperature Plus, Corning, NY) that had been calibrated with pH 4.00, 7.00, and 10.00 buffer solutions (Fischer Scientific). For all pH measurements a single 2-mL glass vial coated with silver-doped sol-gel was used (*Simple SERS Sample Vial*, Real-Time Analyzers, Inc. (RTA), Middletown, CT). The vial was never moved from the sample holder to ensure that the same portion of silver-doped sol-gel was examined. Two pH series were performed. First, 2 mL of the stock solution was added to the vial and measured. Then the 2 mL solution was returned to the stock solution and made basic using 0.1 M KOH. Prior to re-addition of the solution to the SER-active vial, the vial was first rinsed three times with distilled water, then twice with the new solution prior to SERS measurement. This procedure was followed to obtain spectra at pH 3.55, 4.33, 4.87, 5.59, 10.69 and 11.66. Next the solution was brought to a pH of 2.00 by adding 0.1 M HNO_3, and the spectrum was recorded. Again KOH was added drop wise to make the solution more basic. Spectra were obtained at pHs of 3.83, 5.10, 7.35 and 8.22. Next HNO_3 was added drop wise so that spectra could be obtained at pHs of 2.19, 1.71, 1.35 and 1.17. Throughout this process, no more than 20 drops of acid or base were added, and therefore the concentration was diluted by no more than 10%.

For concentration measurements, a second stock solution of DPA was prepared as above and used to prepare all lower concentration samples by serial dilution using HPLC grade water. Initial spore experiments employed 78 ^oC, 50 mM dodecylamine to digest the spores and release dipicolinic acid for measurement. Pre-weighed spore particles were placed on a glass plate for these measurements. Final spore measurements employed room temperature acetic acid to digest the spores. Pre-weighed spores were used to prepare a stock solution for calibration using a counting grid (see below), from which a known number of spores were dried on a glass plate. For both digesting chemicals, after 1 min exposure, the degraded spore sample was drawn into a SER-active capillary (*Simple SERS Sample Capillary*, RTA) for measurement.

The SER-active vials were prepared according to published procedures (Farquharson & Maksymiuk; 2003), using a silver amine precursor to provide the metal dopant and an alkoxide precursor to provide the sol-gel matrix. The silver amine precursor consisted of a 5/1 v/v ratio of 1N $AgNO_3$ to 28% NH_3OH, while the alkoxide precursor consisted of a 2/1 v/v ratio of methanol to tetramethyl orthosilicate (TMOS). The alkoxide and silver amine precursors were mixed in an 8/1 v/v ratio, then 140 µL were introduced into 2 mL glass vials, which were then spin-coated. After sol-gel formation, the incorporated silver ions were reduced with 0.03M $NaBH_4$. The SER-active capillaries were prepared in a similar manner with the following modifications. The alkoxide precursor employed a combination of methyltrimethoxysilane (MTMS) and TMOS in a v/v ratio of 6/1, which was mixed with the amine precursor in a v/v ratio of 1/1. Approximately 15 µL of the mixed precursors were then drawn into a 1-mm diameter glass capillary coating a 15-mm length. After sol-gel formation, the incorporated silver ions were again reduced with dilute sodium borohydride.

All Raman spectroscopy measurements were performed using 785 or 1064 nm laser excitation and Fourier transform Raman spectrometers (RTA, model *RamanID-785* and *-1064*; Farquharson et al., 1999). For pure Na_2DPA, CaDPA, and the spore samples 1064 nm excitation was used, for pure DPA and DPA solutions both 785 and 1064 nm laser excitation were used, while for all DPA SERS measurements, solutions or extractions, 785 nm laser excitation was used. Fiber optics were used to deliver the excitation beam to the sample probe and the scattered radiation to the interferometer (2 m lengths of 200 and 365 µm core diameter, respectively, Spectran, Avon, CT).

For 1064 nm excitation, a 24 mm diameter f/0.7 aspheric lens focused the beam to a 600 µm spot on the sample and to collect the scattered radiation back along the same axis. An f/2 achromat was used to collimate laser beam exiting the source fiber optic, while a 4 mm prism was used to direct the beam through an f/0.7 aspheric lens that focused the beam to a 600 micron spot on the sample. The scattered radiation was collected back along the same optical axis, while a second f/2 lens focused the beam into the collection fiber optic. A short pass filter was placed in the excitation beam path to block the silicon Raman scattering generated in the source fiber from reflecting off sampling optics and reaching the detector. A long pass filter was placed in the collection beam path to block the sample Rayleigh scattering from reaching the detector. For 785 nm excitation, a similar optic probe was used, except a dichroic filter was used to reflect the laser light to sample and pass the Raman scattered radiation to the collection fiber. In this case the beam was focused to a 300 µm spot on the sample. Also, appropriate short and long pass filters were used for this wavelength. All spectra presented were collected using 8 cm^{-1} resolution.

In the case of Raman spectral measurements of spores, the samples were placed on a glass slide with the probe aimed downward. In the case of SER-active vials or capillaries, the samples were mounting horizontally on an XY positioning stage (Conix Research, Springfield, OR), so that the probe aimed upwards and the focal point of the aspheric lens was just inside the vial or capillary.

For the SERS concentration and extraction measurements, nine spectra were recorded along the length of the capillary with 1 mm spacing. As a practical approach to minimizing the variability associated with the SER activity as a function of sample position, the three high and three low intensity spectra were discarded, while the three median spectra were averaged and reported. Relative standard deviations for all concentrations are reported as percent standard deviation in Table 2. SER spectra were collected in 1-min or less as indicated in figure captions.

3. Results and discussion

The present application begins with a Raman spectral analysis of Bacillus spores with regards to contributions from calcium dipicolinate. The primary CaDPA peaks occur at 659, 821, 1014, 1391, 1446, 1573, 3062, and 3080 cm^{-1} in the spore spectrum (Fig. 2), and can be assigned to a ring CC bend, an out-of-plane CH bend, the symmetric pyridine ring stretch, a symmetric OCO stretch, a symmetric ring CH bend, an asymmetric OCO stretch, and the CH symmetric and asymmetric stretches, respectively (Table 1, Farquharson et al., 2004).

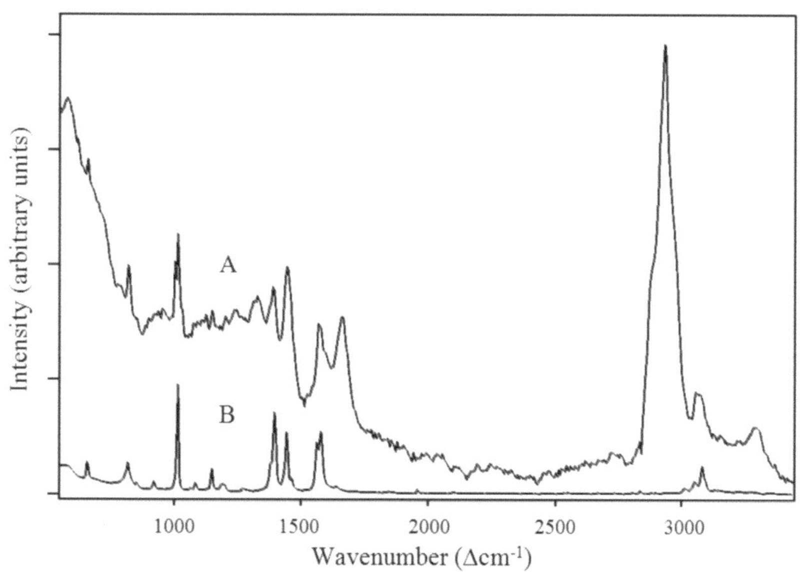

Fig. 2. RS of A) *Bacillus cereus* spores and B) calcium dipicolinate. Spectral conditions: 500 mW of 1064 nm at the sample, 5 min acquisition time, 8 cm^{-1} resolution.

The remaining peaks can be assigned to protein modes associated with the peptidoglycan cell wall, such as amino acids and peptide linkages (amide modes; Woodruff et al., 1974; Ghiamati, 1992; Grasselli et al., 1981; Bandekar, 1992; Austin et al., 1993). The former include peaks with little intensity at 821, 855, 900 cm^{-1}, which are assigned to several CC bending modes, as well as the phenylalanine modes that appear at 1003 and 1598 cm^{-1}. The latter include the amide I peak at 1666 cm^{-1}, which is primarily a C=O stretch, and amide III combination peaks at 937, 1241, and 1318 cm^{-1}, which are various CC and CN stretching combinations (peak positions are given for *B. cereus*). In several cases, protein and CaDPA vibrational modes occur at or close to the same frequency, such as the 821 and 1446 cm^{-1} peaks.

Next, the amount of CaDPA available in a spore that could be measured as DPA was considered. Although it is often stated that *Bacillus* ssp. spores contain 10-15% calcium dipicolinate by weight (Janssen et al., 1958; Liu et al., 2004), this value has been reported as low as 1% (Halverson, 1961). Since this amount will be used to calculate the number of spores measured, it is important to have as accurate a number as possible. For this reason, the Raman spectra of *Bacillus subtilis, B. megaterium*, and *B. cereus* were acquired (Fig. 3). In fact it was found that the most obvious differences between the spectra for the three *Bacillus* species are the CaDPA peaks. In particular, the 1014 cm^{-1} peak noticeably changes intensity, especially when compared to the neighboring phenylalanine peak at 1003 cm^{-1}. If it can be assumed that the composition of these *Bacilli* is very similar, then it may be assumed that the relative phenylalanine concentration is nearly constant and its Raman peak can be used as an internal intensity standard. (The amide I peak at 1666 cm^{-1} could also be used.) Using the ratio of the CaDPA and phenylalanine peak heights suggests then that the salt concentrations for *B. megaterium* and *B. cereus* are 1.85 and 2.05 times that of *B. subtilis.* In the latter case, a recent study using resonance Raman spectroscopy of the same sample

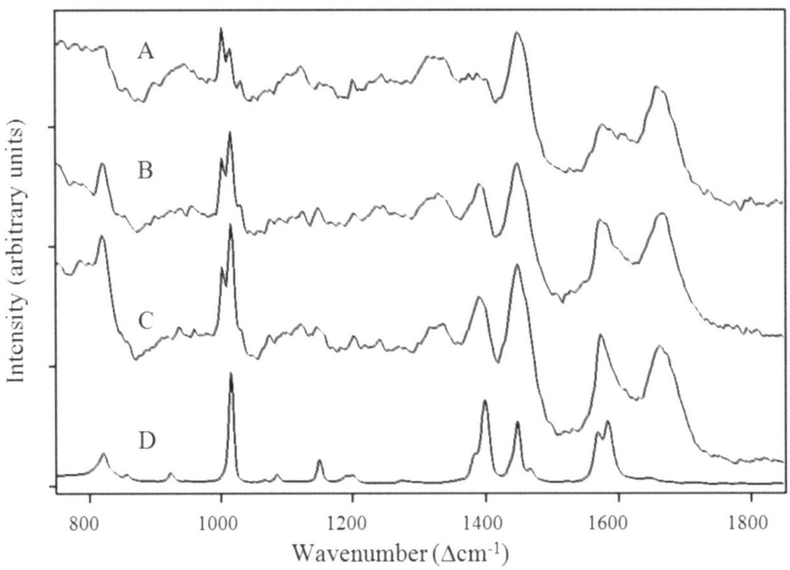

Fig. 3. RS of A) *B. subtilis*, B) *B. megaterium*, C) *B. cereus*, and D) CaDPA. Spectral conditions as in Fig. 2.

concluded that the CaDPA peak intensity corresponded to 6-7 weight percent (Nelson et al., 2004). This suggests that the CaDPA weight percent for the *B. megaterium* and *B. cereus* spore samples are 11-13 and 12.5-14.5 wt%, respectively, or in the case of DPA, 9-11 and 10-12 wt% (based on MW). It should be noted that the differences between these *Bacillus* spp. does not imply that the CaDPA concentrations are species specific. It is more likely that experimental conditions during the original growth of the bacteria, such as time, temperature, and available nutrients, influenced the extent of sporulation. Consequently, any calculations of the number of spores based on DPA content should assume a range of at least 5-13 weight percent of the spores. As a practical matter 10±5% will be used here.

For comparison purposes, the spectra of CaDPA and DPA are shown in Fig. 4, along with Na_2DPA, while the observed spectral peaks with vibrational mode assignments are listed in Table 1. The assignments for both CaDPA and DPA, based on literature (Carmona 1980; Hameka et al., 1996), were used to assign the peaks observed for Na_2DPA. Both DPA and Na_2DPA contain unique peaks with significant intensity at 760 and 1730 cm^{-1}, respectively. Since neither peak is observed in the spectrum of CaDPA, it can be concluded that this sample does not contain either chemical as an impurity.

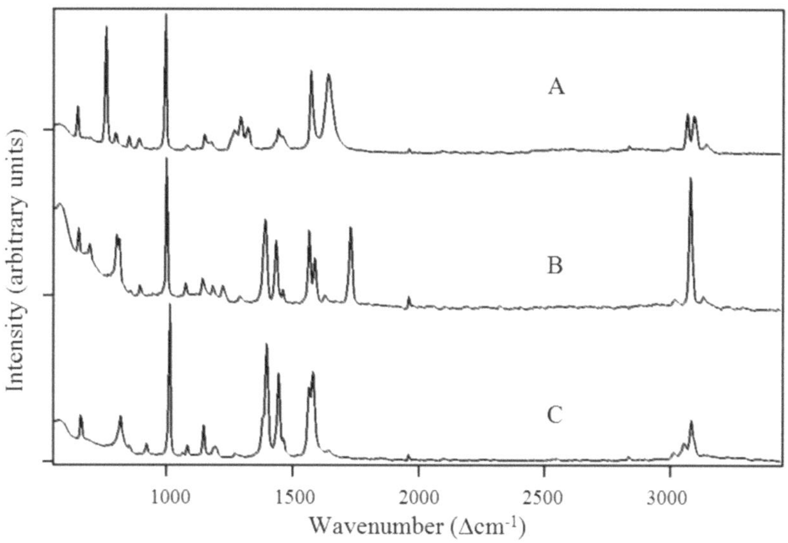

Fig. 4. RS of A) dipicolinic acid B) disodium dipicolinate, and C) calcium dipicolinate. Spectral conditions as in Fig. 2.

Next, dipicolinic acid was analyzed by SERS. The assignment of SERS peaks to vibrational modes is less straightforward than for RS peaks due to the metal-to-molecule surface interactions that shift and enhance various vibrational modes to different extents. Furthermore, it is usually found that RS spectra of analytes in solution more closely match the SER spectra than in the solid-state. However, it is usually beneficial to acquire and examine both when making assignments. Since DPA dissolves in water only sparingly, 1N KOH was used to dissolve 80 mg/mL. The RS spectrum of the solution phase is largely the same as the solid phase except for some minor changes in peak frequencies, intensities, and widths (Table 1). Notably, the 760 cm^{-1} peak in the solid phase is completely absent in the solution phase, while a new peak at 1386 cm^{-1} appears in the solution phase. The former

B. Cereus	CaDPA	Na_2DPA	DPA solid	DPA solution	SERS	Tentative Assignments
	403	413			405	
	433		425		458	CC ring bend[a]
	478	499	489			C-CO_2 str[a]
		575	573		567	
659	661	650	646	652	657	CC ring bend[a]
		696				
			760		(795)	HO-C=O in-plane def[b]
		805	801			
821	820	814		822	812	CC str[d], CaDPA CH out-of-plane def[b]
855	857	856	853		858	CC str[d]
900		897				CC str[d]
925	923					CaDPA
937						CC str + amide III[d]
1003						phe sym ring str.[c,d]
1014	1015	1003	997	1001	1006	sym ring breath[c]
					1029	
1077	1086	1079	1085	1087		trigonal ring breathing[b]
1150	1150	1147	1153	1154	1157	CH bend[a]
	1199	1185	1179	1191	1184	
		1227			1230	
1241						amide III (b)[c,d]
	1274	1256	1271			CC str[b]
		1293	1296		1285	
1318						CH_2 bend, amide III[d]
			1324			C=O str
1377sh	1383					CH bend[a]
1391	1398	1393		1386	1381	OCO sym str[c]
1446	1447	1437	1445	1438	(1426)	CH_2 bend,[d] CaDPA ring CH bend[a] or CC str[b]
	1466	1464	1461		1466	ring CC str
1573	1568	1569	1575	1572	1567	OCO asym str
1583	1583	1589			(1590)	CC ring str
1598sh						phe sym ring str.[c,d]
	1643	1634	1643			carboxylate[e]
1666						amide I[c,d]
		1704/30				C=O str (doublet)
2879sh						CH_3 sym str[f]
2934						CH_2 antisym str[f]
2968sh						CH_3 antisym str[f]
	3019	3021				
3062	3060		3070			aromatic CH sym str[f]
3080	3088	3084	3098			CH antisym str[f]
		3137	3150			CH str[f]
3302						amide NH str[c,d]

Table 1. Tentative Raman vibrational mode assignments for dipicolinates. a is from Hameka et al., 1996; b is from Carmona, 1980; c is from Woodruff et al., 1974; d is from Bendaker, 1992, e is from Ghiamati et al., 1992; f is from Grasselli et al., 1981 and Austin et al., 1993.

peak is likely associated with carboxylic acid groups (e.g. HO-C=O deformation), while the latter peak is likely associated with deprotonated carboxylic acid groups (e.g. O-C-O stretch). The latter assignment is consistent with a sample pH of 10 due to the 1N KOH. The former assignment is supported by the fact that the peak does not disappear when DPA is dissolved in the aprotic solvents dimethylsulfoxide or N,N-dimethylformamide.

The SER spectrum of 1 g/L DPA in water is more like the solution than solid phase as shown in Fig. 5. The quality of this SER spectrum is considerably better than the first reported SER spectrum of dipicolinic acid obtained on a silver electrode in an electrolytic cell (Farquharson et al., 1999). In fact, not only are most of the peaks of the solution phase RS spectrum observed in the SER spectrum, but peaks shift no more than 10 cm^{-1} and change little in relative intensity. These similarities suggest a weak molecule to silver surface interaction. The RS to SERS shifts of the major peaks are: 652 to 657 cm^{-1}, 822 to 812 cm^{-1}, 1001 to 1006 cm^{-1}, 1386 to 1381 cm^{-1}, 1438 to 1426 cm^{-1}, 1572 to 1567 cm^{-1}. The SERS peaks are assigned according to CaDPA above and literature as follows (Ghiamati et al., 1992; Woodruff et al., 1974): the 1006 cm^{-1} peak is assigned to the symmetric ring stretch, the 1381 cm^{-1} peak to the symmetric O-C-O stretch, the 1426 cm^{-1} peak to the symmetric ring C-H bend, and the 1567 cm^{-1} peak to the asymmetric O-C-O stretch. The greatest difference between the RS and SER spectra is the appearance of a new peak in the latter spectrum at 795 cm^{-1} (see below).

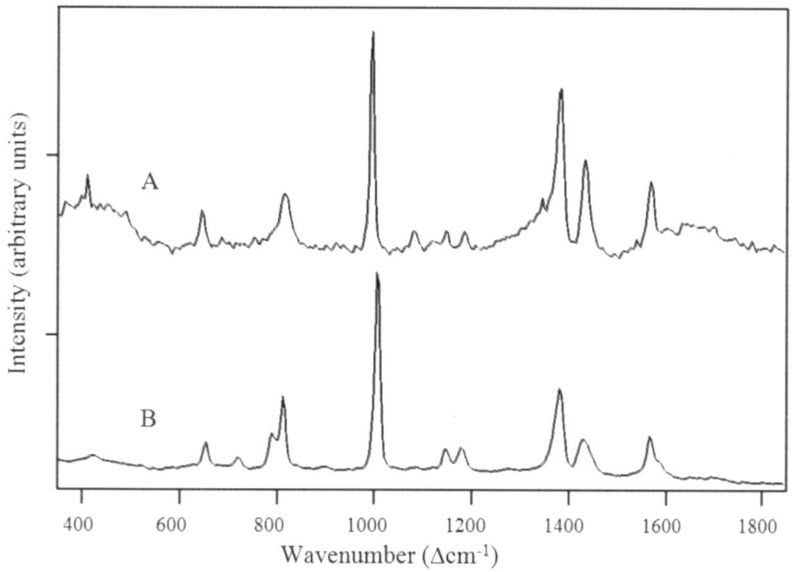

Fig. 5. A) RS of 80 mg DPA in 1 mL 1N KOH in a glass capillary. B) SERS of 1 mg DPA in 1 mL water in a silver-doped sol-gel filled glass capillary. Spectral conditions: A) 450 mW of 785 nm, 5 min acquisition time and B) 150 mW of 785 nm, 1-minute acquisition time; both 8 cm^{-1} resolution.

Next the pH dependence of both the measurement and analyte was considered. This could be significant if an acid or a base is used to digest spores and extract the CaDPA. It is widely known that the pH of the solution can have an effect on the SER signal (Laserna et al., 1988; Dou et al., 1999), particularly in the case of metal colloids where pH affects the extent of aggregation (Laserna et al., 1988), which in turn affects the plasmon field and the Raman signal enhancement. Other SER-active media are more tolerable to pH changes, such as metal coated spheres and posts, or silver-doped sol-gels, as used here. Although these sol-gels may not be affected by pH, the analyte is a diprotic acid and the neutral and ionic forms of DPA, DPA^-, or $DPA^=$, must be considered. These species may interact with the silver quite differently and consequently influence the amount that each vibrational mode is enhanced. For example, it might be expected that $DPA^=$ will interact more strongly with electropositive silver increasing the chemical component of the SERS mechanism. Furthermore, added enhancement might be expected for the vibrational modes of the deprotonated carboxylic acid groups that participate in this interaction, or for modes that are favorably aligned perpendicular to the surface due to this interaction.

The relative concentrations of DPA, DPA^-, and $DPA^=$ can be determined at any pH as long as the pK_as are known and the initial concentration. According to Lange's Handbook of Chemistry, the pK_as are 2.16 and 6.92 (Dean 1979), and the deprotonation reactions are:

$$DPA \leftrightarrow DPA^- + H^+ \qquad pK_{1a} = 2.16 \qquad \text{Reaction 1}$$

$$DPA^- \leftrightarrow DPA^= + H^+ \qquad pK_{2a} = 6.92 \qquad \text{Reaction 2}$$

The relative concentrations can then be determined by expressing [DPA] and $[DPA^=]$ in terms of $[DPA^-]$ using Reactions 1 and 2, and summing all three to equal the total starting concentration, here 1 g/L, viz:

$$[DPA] + [DPA^-] + [DPA^=] = 1\ g/L \tag{1}$$

substituting from Reactions 1 and 2:

$$([H^+][DPA^-])/K_{1a} + [DPA^-] + (K_{2a}[DPA^-])/[H^+] = 1\ g/L \tag{2}$$

rearranging:

$$[DPA^-] = 1\ g/L\ /(1+[H^+]/K_{1a} + K_{2a}/[H^+]) \tag{3}$$

As shown in Fig. 6, at pH less than pK_{1a} DPA dominates, at pH between the pK_as DPA^- dominates, and above pK_{2a} $DPA^=$ dominates.

Fig. 7 shows SER spectra of DPA for pH 4.87, 5.59, 7.35, 8.22, 10.69, and 11.66 with spectra of the 800 cm^{-1} region for pH 1.35, 1.71, 2.19 and 3.83 (inset). Overall there is only a modest decrease in intensity for most of the peaks as a function of pH. For example, the 1006 cm^{-1} peak assigned to the pyridine ring stretching mode decreases by ~7% from pH 2 to 11. The greatest changes observed, yet still modest, are in the peak intensities at 795, 812, 1567, and 1590 cm^{-1} between pH 1.3 and 5.5. These peaks change intensity as pairs. The 795 cm^{-1} peak loses intensity as the pH becomes basic, while the 812 cm^{-1} peak gains a little intensity. Similarly, the 1567 cm^{-1} peak loses intensity as the pH becomes basic, while the 1590 cm^{-1} peak gains intensity. The intensities of the former pair are plotted as a function of pH in Fig. 6. The peak heights were divided by the peak height of the 1006 cm^{-1} peak at each pH and then scaled with the lowest value set to 0 and the highest to 1 g/L. As can be seen the 795 cm^{-1} peak tracts the DPA concentration, while the 812 cm^{-1} peak tracts the DPA^- concentration. The former peak is likely associated with carboxylic acid groups, just as in the case of the 760 cm^{-1} peak in the solid phase RS spectrum of DPA.

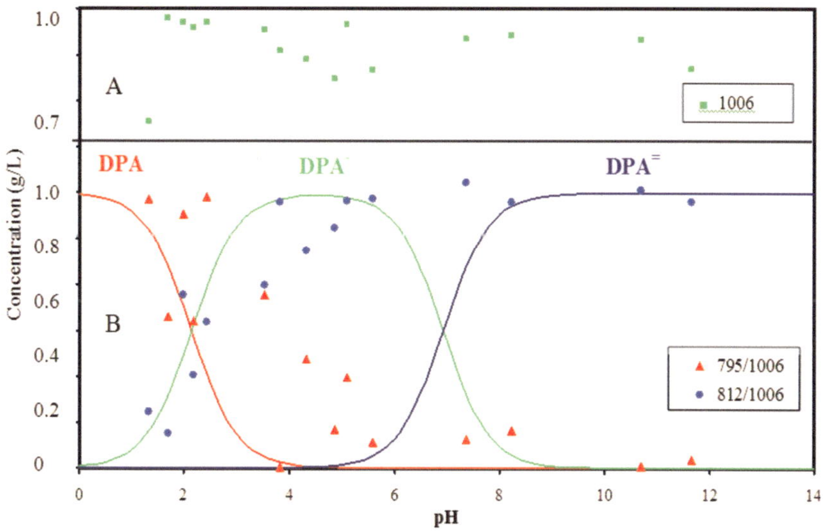

Fig. 6. DPA and its anion concentrations as a function of pH (lines). A) The 1006 cm^{-1} peak intensity is shown as measured, but scaled to a 0 to 1 g/L concentration range. B) The 795 and 812 cm^{-1} peak intensities are normalized to the 1006 cm^{-1} peak intensity and then scaled. These two peaks appear to represent DPA and $DPA^{=}$, respectively, but both with DPA^{-} character.

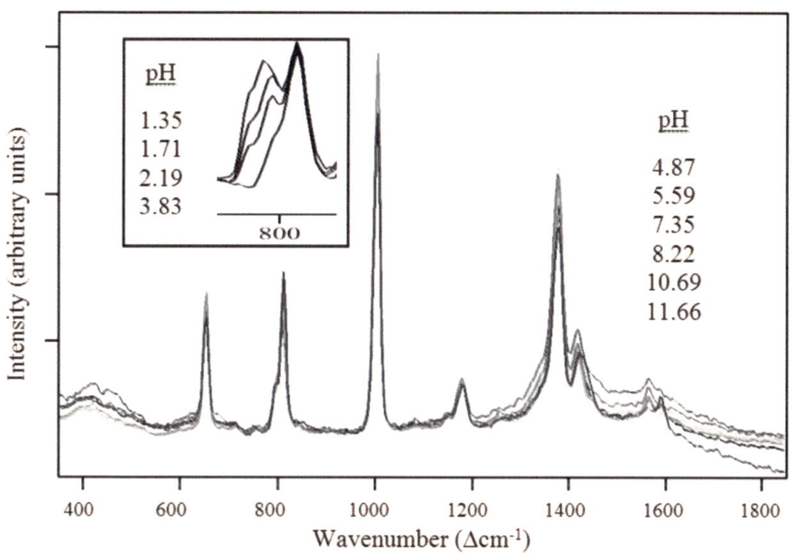

Fig. 7. SERS of 1 mg/mL dipicolinic acid as a function of pH. The spectral intensities have been normalized to the 812 cm^{-1} peak. Inset: Expanded view of low wavenumber region. Spectral conditions: 100 mW of 785 nm, 44 sec acquisition time, 8 cm^{-1} resolution.

However, a 35 cm^{-1} shift is somewhat inconsistent with a weak analyte-to-surface interaction. It is also apparent in Fig. 6 that the concentrations of DPA and DPA^{-} based on the 795 and 812 cm^{-1} peak intensities are shifted to the basic side of the predicted curves. This shift may be due to the silver surface influencing the carboxylic acid dissociation energy. Or the peaks may contain contributions from the $DPA^{=}$ species. Although clarifying this point will require further measurements, the most important conclusions from this data is that the SER intensity for most of the prominent DPA peaks change little as a function of pH, and that the silver-doped sol-gels do not appear to influence the measurement to any significance.

Next, the response of the SER intensity for DPA as a function of concentration was examined. A preliminary calibration curve was prepared by measuring 100, 50, 20, 10, 5, 2, 1, 0.5, 0.2, 0.1, 0.05, 0.02, and 0.01 mg/L samples. Fig. 8 shows SER spectra for 100, 1, and 0.01 mg/L samples measured using 100 mW of 785 nm and 1-min acquisition time. It can be seen that even at 10 μg/L the signal-to-noise ratio is quite good. The SER intensity was taken as the peak height at 1006 cm^{-1} minus the value at 950 cm^{-1} as the baseline. For each concentration, a different capillary was used. Spectra were measured at nine points along the length of each capillary and the median values are plotted in Fig. 9. It is obvious that the response is not linear, in that the peak heights change from 0.2 to 1.5, while the concentration changes over 4 orders of magnitude. This Langmuir isotherm response is typical for SERS substrates where signal intensity is a function of available silver surface area (Mullen & Carron, 1994).

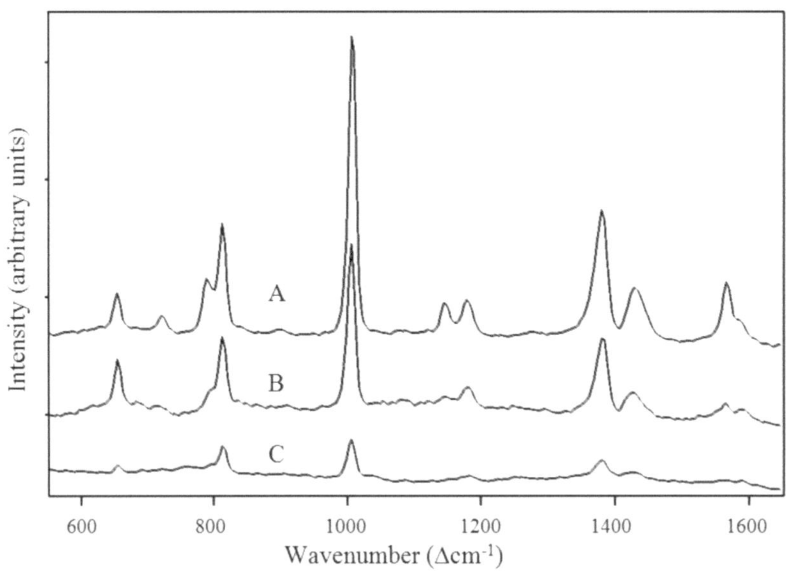

Fig. 8. SERS of DPA in water at A) 100, B) 1, and C) 0.01 mg/L (100 pg in 10 μL sample) using the SER-active capillaries, 100 mW of 785 nm and 1 min acquisition time.

All of these values were also used to estimate limits of detection (LOD), defined as the concentration that produces a signal three times as intense as the baseline noise. The signal was taken as the height of the 1006 cm^{-1} peak, while the noise was the relative standard deviation of baseline noise measured between 50 and 150 cm^{-1}. The LODs are for 1-min measurements using 100 mW of 785 nm laser excitation and 8 cm^{-1} resolution. As Table 2 indicates, the lower the measured concentration, in general, the lower the predicted LOD. Note that the lowest concentration sample, 10 μg/L (0.01 mg/L), suggests that 0.7 μg/L can

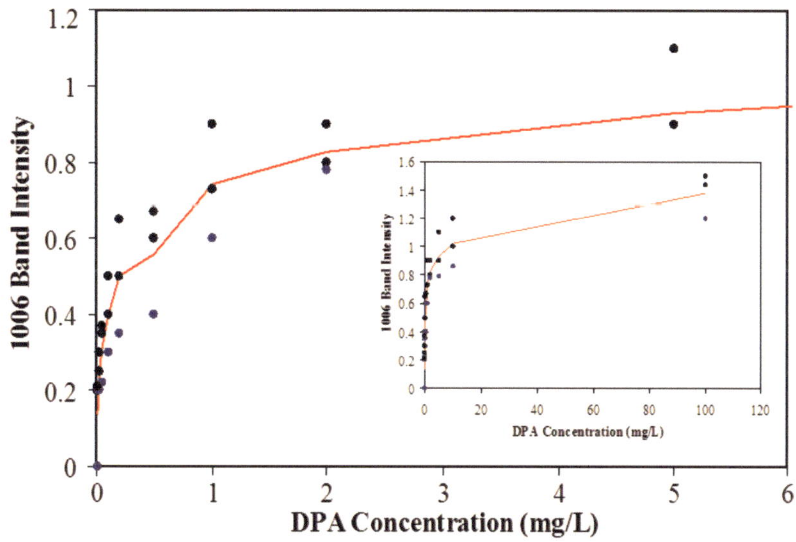

Fig. 9. Plot of SER intensity for 1006 cm^{-1} peak of DPA as a function of concentration using 100 mW of 785 nm and 1-min acquisition time. Line connects average value at each concentration. Inset includes 10 and 100 mg/L data.

be measured (S/N equaled 33 for the 1006 cm^{-1} peak). This is consistent with the fact that attempted measurements of 1 μg/L samples did yield spectra, but not in every case. It is also worth noting that only 10 μL samples were used to generate the spectra, or in the case of the 10 μg/L sample, the actual sample was 100 pg DPA in 10 μL water.

Conc mg/L	spores in 0.1 mL	Signal (ave)	Std Dev	RSD (%)	Noise	S/N	LOD factor	LOD mg/L	LOD spores/0.1 mL
0.01	**1229**	**0.14**	0.12	86.68	0.0033	41.4	13.8	7.24E-04	**89**
0.02	**2457**	**0.25**	0.05	20.00	0.0042	59.5	19.8	1.01E-03	**124**
0.05	**6143**	**0.31**	0.08	25.99	0.0043	72.9	24.3	2.06E-03	**253**
0.1	**12,285**	**0.40**	0.10	25.00	0.0047	85.1	28.4	3.53E-03	**433**
0.2	**24,570**	**0.50**	0.15	30.00	0.005	100.0	33.3	6.00E-03	**737**
0.5	**61,425**	**0.56**	0.14	25.17	0.006	92.8	30.9	1.62E-02	**1986**
1	**122,850**	**0.74**	0.15	20.24	0.0067	110.9	37.0	2.70E-02	**3322**
2	**245,700**	**0.83**	0.06	7.78	0.008	103.3	34.4	5.81E-02	**7133**
5	**614,251**	**0.93**	0.16	16.90	0.0067	138.8	46.3	1.08E-01	**13276**
10	**1,228,501**	**1.02**	0.17	16.75	0.0096	106.3	35.4	2.82E-01	**34687**
100	**12,285,012**	**1.38**	0.16	11.50	0.0122	113.1	37.7	2.65E+00	**325820**
~1*	**100,000**	**0.70**	0.14	20.11	0.0055	126.7	42.2	2.37E-02	**2368**
~0.22**	**22,000**	**0.45**	0.10	23.20	0.0159	28.3	9.4	2.33E-02	**2332**

* Approximate concentrations for dodecylamine surface measurements, see below.
** Approximate concentrations for acetic acid surface measurements, see below.

Table 2. Estimated limits of detection in terms of mg DPA per L water and corresponding spores per 0.1mL DDA.

Finally, an enhancement factor (EF) for DPA can be estimated by comparing the measurement conditions and signal intensities for the 10 μg/L SERS and 80 g/L RS. The spectra are plotted on the same scale in Fig. 10. The 1006 cm^{-1} peak heights are nearly identical at 0.20 and 0.173 (arbitrary units), while the laser power at the sample and collection time were somewhat different at 150 and 450 mw, and 1 and 5 minutes for the SERS and RS, respectively. In both cases, 1-mm capillaries were used to hold the samples, and the same sample optics were used. Taking the concentration into account yields an estimated enhancement factor of $2.4x10^7$. It is difficult to determine the precise number of molecules in the field of view for the sol-gel, and this number may represent better than average enhancement, i.e. better than 10^6, or it may reflect the ability of the sol-gel to concentrate the sample. In either case, the measurement of 10 μg/L suggests that 10 ng of spores in a 100 μL solution of a digesting chemical can be measured; assuming all of the CaDPA is made available as DPA (10%). Recent estimates suggest that this mass corresponds to 1000 spores (Inglesby et al., 2002).

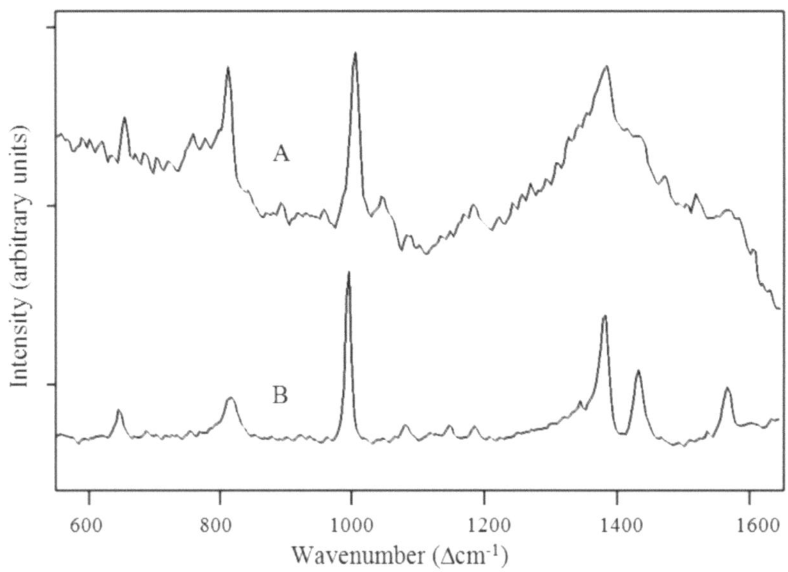

Fig. 10. A) SERS and B) RS of DPA plotted on the same scale, but offset. Conditions: A:B 10^{-5}:80 g/L, 150:450 mW of 785 nm, and 1:5 min acquisition time. EF = $2.4x10^7$.

Next, methods were developed to rapidly extract CaDPA as DPA from Bacillus spores. Initially, DPA was obtained from *B. cereus* spores following the procedure of Pellegrino et al. Specifically, a 2 mg sample was placed in 2 mL of 5 mM dodecylamine in ethanol that was heated and maintained at 78 °C for 40 minutes. Approximately 10 μL of this solution was drawn into a SER-active capillary and measured. Since SER spectra of DPA were readily observed, shorter heating periods, higher DDA concentrations and smaller spore masses, were examined. In due course experiments were performed in which 100 μL of 78 °C 50 mM DDA in ethanol was added to ~10 μg samples of spore specks (~ 1 million spores) placed on a surface. After 1 minute exposure, approximately 10 μL of the solution were drawn into a SER-active capillary and measured. Fig. 11 shows a representative spectrum for one of these capillaries using a 1-min acquisition time. The primary DPA peaks at 657 cm^{-1}, 810 cm^{-1}, 1006 cm^{-1}, 1382 cm^{-1}, and 1428 cm^{-1} are easily observed, even in the case of a 2-sec scan.

Furthermore, an attempted measurement of 50 mM DDA (without sample) did not produce a spectrum that might interfere with the measurement (Fig. 11C). The amount of DPA extracted was estimated to be between 0.5 and 5 mg/L by comparing the 0.7 signal intensity of the 1006 cm^{-1} peak to that measured for DPA in water (see Table 2). In fact this intensity is closest to that obtained for the 1 mg/L samples. This value can be used to estimate the number of spores in the 100 μL DDA sample. Assuming, as stated above, that a spore contains approximately 10% DPA by weight, and that 100 spores have a mass of ~1 ng, then this corresponds to 100,000 spores per 100 μL DDA or ~10% of the spores in the prepared particles. This low percentage could be due to incomplete degradation of the spores by DDA, interference from the spore cell debris, inefficient collection of the sample from the surface, or inefficient transfer of the DPA to the silver particles.

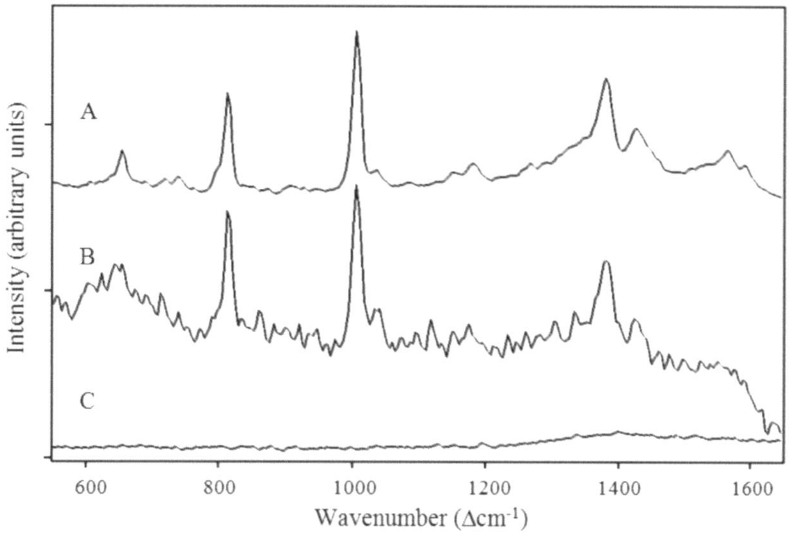

Fig. 11. SERS of DPA extracted from ~10 μg *B. cereus* particle using 100 μL of 50 mM hot DDA acquired in A) 1 minute and B) 2 seconds. C) Attempted SERS of 50 mM hot DDA in ethanol using silver-doped sol-gel coated glass capillary acquired in 1 minute. Spectral conditions: 150 mW of 785 nm, 8 cm^{-1} resolution.

Although, these initial measurements clearly demonstrated the potential of rapid spore analysis using SERS, the approach had two significant limitations. First, the sensitivity is insufficient, and second the use of a hot reagent severely limits its practical use in the field. To overcome these limitations we investigated numerous acids, bases and solvents (e.g. nitric acid, potassium hydroxide, phenol, etc.), separately and as mixtures that could digest spores rapidly at room temperature, and make available all or nearly all of the DPA for SERS detection.

Eventually, it was found that glacial acetic acid had the appropriate properties. However, reactivity of acetic acid with the sol-gel and competition with DPA for the silver surface was a concern, so a series of DPA concentration samples were prepared and measured. Fig. 12 shows a SER spectrum of 100 pg DPA in 10 μL acetic acid (10 ppb) and a SER spectrum of pure acetic acid drawn into SER-active capillaries.

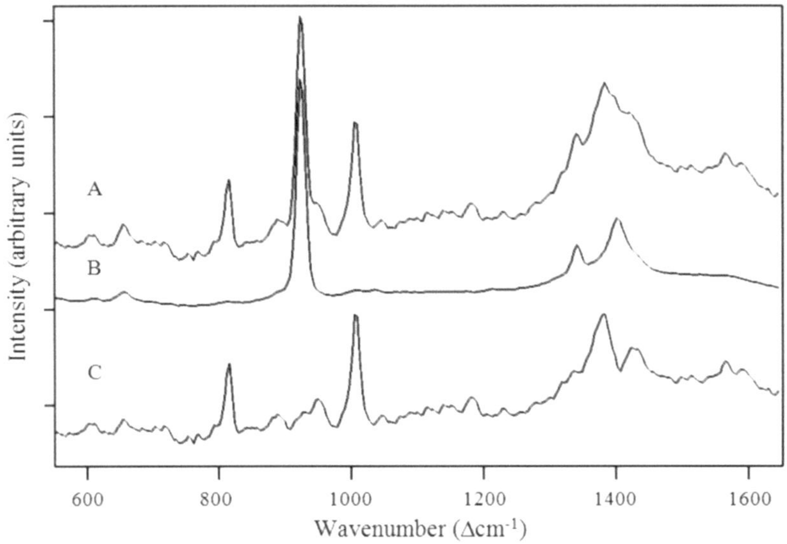

Fig. 12. A) SERS of DPA in acetic acid at 10 pg/μL, B) SERS of acetic acid, and C) difference spectrum of A-B). Spectral conditions: 85 mW of 785 nm, 1 min acquisition time, 8 cm^{-1} resolution.

Acetic acid produced several peaks, notably at 925, 1340, and 1405 cm^{-1}. Subtraction of the acetic acid spectrum reveals a standard SER spectrum of DPA (Fig. 12C). The SER spectral intensity of DPA in acetic acid as a function of concentration is very similar to that previously measured in water. In fact the 1006 cm^{-1} peak intensity, once corrected for the difference in laser power is nearly identical for the same concentration in water (compare 0.13 in acetic acid versus 0.14 in water, Table 2). Fig. 13 shows SER spectra of four orders of magnitude of DPA

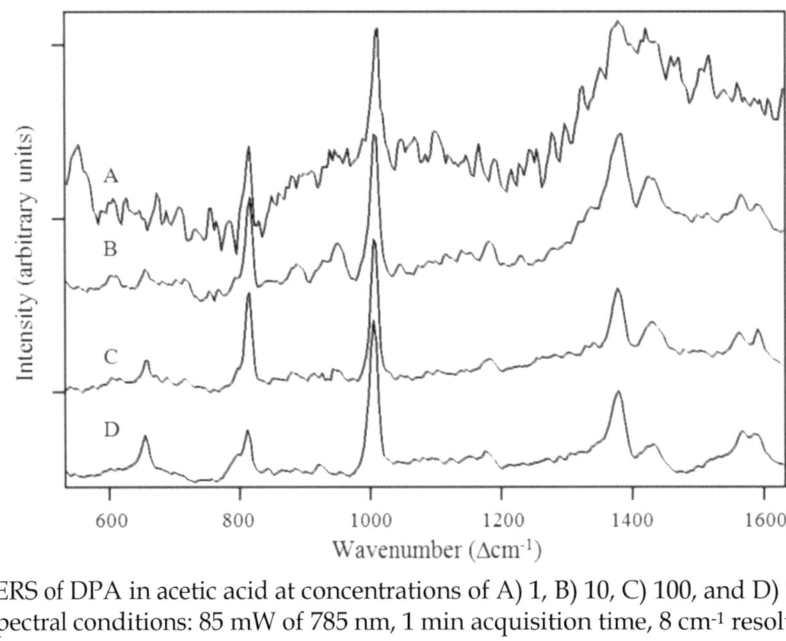

Fig. 13. SERS of DPA in acetic acid at concentrations of A) 1, B) 10, C) 100, and D) 1000 pg/μL. Spectral conditions: 85 mW of 785 nm, 1 min acquisition time, 8 cm^{-1} resolution.

concentration in acetic acid, in which the dominant 1006 cm^{-1} peak intensity is held constant and the base line noise is observed to increase with decreasing concentration.

Next, experiments were performed using acetic acid to digest spore samples on a surface, collect the DPA and detect it in SER-active capillaries. As a specific example, a 2 mg sample of spores was weighed and dispersed in 10 mL of water by vortexing. The spores per volume water were calibrated by placing 10 µL on a standard hemocytometer counting grid. Each grid holds 4 nL (0.2x0.2x0.1 mm). Microscope images of 10 grids were recorded and 870 spores were counted, which represents ~22,000 spores per µL (Fig. 14A). The original spore solution was diluted by a factor of 10 to produce a 2200 spore per µL. From this solution, a 1 µL sample was placed on a glass slide and allowed to dry producing a 2200 spores per ~0.2 cm^2 spot (Fig. 14B). Although this represents 11,000 spores/cm^2, 3-orders of magnitude greater than the target sensitivity, no attempt was made to spread the spores across the surface (i.e. identical results would likely have been obtained if the sample was allowed to dry on a 10 cm^2 area). Next, 10 µL of acetic acid was added to the spore spot (Fig. 14C). After 1 minute, 1 µL of this solution was drawn into a SER-active capillary (Fig. 14D), and a 1-minute spectrum measured (Fig. 15A). The measurement represents 220 spores/µL. The entire measurement was accomplished in less than 2.5 minutes, and at a measured pH of 2.1 the primary DPA peaks at 657 cm^{-1}, 812 cm^{-1}, 1006 cm^{-1}, 1381 cm^{-1}, and 1426 cm^{-1} are easily observed.

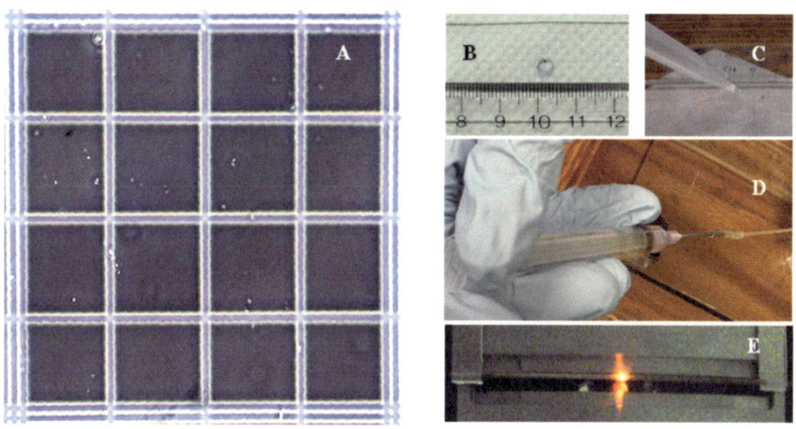

Fig. 14. A) Microscope image of initial calibration sample containing 60 spores in a 0.2 x 0.2 mm field of view (0.1 mm deep). B) 2200 spores were dried from 1 µL on the surface as (~0.2 cm^2). C) 10 µL of acetic acid was added to the spores for 1 min digestion. D) 1 µL of the solution was drawn into the chemically-selective, SER-active capillary. And E) the capillary was mounted in Raman analyzer sample compartment and the spectrum collected.

The quantitative accuracy of the measurement was further verified by comparing this 220 spores/µL spectrum to the 100 pg/µL (~100 spores/µL) solution of DPA in acetic acid spectrum. This was accomplished by using the acetic acid peak at 925 cm^{-1} as an internal intensity standard and normalizing both spectra to it. It was found that the primary peak at 1006 cm^{-1} of the spore sample is ~ twice the intensity of the reference DPA sample, consistent with the 220 spore estimate. This spectral comparison also shows that the spore spectrum contains a considerable baseline offset with significant noise (background). This is likely due to spore debris that has not been effectively excluded from the metal-doped sol-gels, and suggests that further "cleaning" the sample could improve sensitivity. The spectral background results in a modest S/N of 28, and an estimated LOD of 2330 *B. cereus* spores per 100 μL acetic acid or 1165 spores per cm^2 for the above experiment. But, as shown in Table 2, the LODs are consistently underestimated, and substantially better sensitivity should be expected.

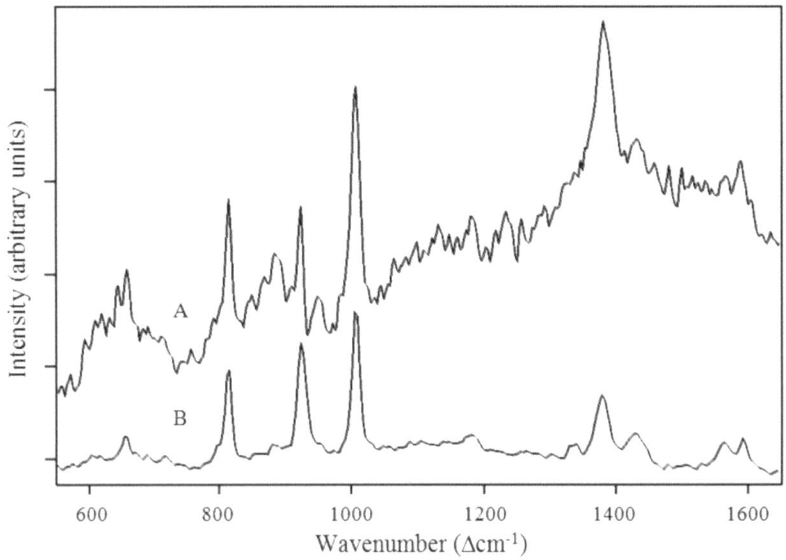

Fig. 15. SERS of A) DPA obtained from 220 *Bacillus cereus* spores using a 1-minute exposure to glacial acetic acid at room temperature and B) 100 pg/μL solution of DPA in acetic acid for comparison. Spectral conditions: 85 mW of 785 nm, 1 min acquisition time, 8 cm^{-1} resolution.

4. Conclusions

We have demonstrated that by combining rapid extraction of dipicolinic acid from *Bacillus cereus* spores with chemical identification by surface-enhanced Raman spectroscopy, Bacillus spores on a surface can be identified in 2.5 minutes. This includes the time required to dispense acetic acid onto a spore contaminated surface, draw the DPA sample by syringe into a SER-active capillary, and acquire the DPA SER spectrum. Using this method, we have measured 220 spores/μL from a 0.2 cm^2 spot containing 2200 spores (equivalent to 11,000 spores/cm^2) in 2.5 minutes, using a simple, SER-active sampling capillary, syringe and a portable Raman analyzer. Although an estimated limit of detection based on the signal-to-noise ratio suggests that 1165 spores/cm^2 could be measured, the LODs are consistently underestimated as shown in Table 2. In fact, 1 pg/μL DPA in acetic acid was consistently measured. Assuming that the *B. cereus* spores contained 10 wt % DPA and each spore has a mass of 10^{-11}g, this is equivalent to 10 spores/cm^2 for the experiment presented here. It could also be argued that the same number of spores could be spread over a 10 cm^2 region and the same amount of digesting agent would produce an equivalent SER signal. Together these arguments suggest that the present method is capable of measuring the goal of 10 spore/cm^2 and that SER-active capillaries could be used to measure surfaces and map distribution of anthrax endospores in mail distribution facilities or other environments should another verified attack occur. This would greatly aid in determining the extent of an attack, deciding who should be tested, and possibly tracing the origin of letters if used. Current research is aimed at extending the capability of this method to analysis of nasal swabs, and *B. anthracis* specific SERS-active materials.

5. Acknowledgements

The authors are grateful to Professor Jay Sperry of the University of Rhode Island for preparing spore samples and the National Science Foundation (DMI-0215819, DMI-0214280, DMI-0349687), the U.S. Army (DAAD13-02-C-0015, Joint Service Agent Water Monitor Program), and the Environmental Protection Agency (EP-D-06-084).

6. References

Austin, J.C., Jordan, T., & Spiro, T.G., (1993), UVRR studies of proteins and related compounds, In *Biomolecular Spectroscopy*, Vol 21, Clark & Hester (Eds.), John Wiley & Sons, New York, NY.

Bandekar, J., (1992), Amide modes and protein conformation, *Biochim. Biophys. Acta,* 1120, p. 123.

Bell, C.A., Uhl, J. R., & Cockerill, F. R., (2001), Direct Detection of *Bacillus anthracis* using a Real-Time PCR Method, *ASM 101st General Meeting,* Orlando, FL, May 2001.

Bell, C.A., Uhl, J.R., Hadfield, T.L., David, J.C., Meyer, R.F., Smith, T.F., & Cockerill, F.R. III, (2002), Detection of *Bacillus Anthracis* DNA by Light Cycler PCR, *J. Clin. Microbiol.,* 40, p. 2897.

Bell, D.M., Kozarsky, P.E., & Stephens, D., (2002), Clinical issues in the prophylaxis, diagnosis, and treatment of anthrax, *Emerg. Infect. Dis.,* 8, p. 222.

Berkeley, R.C.W., & Ali, N., (1994), Classification and identification of endospore-forming bacteria, *J. Appl. Bacteriol.* (Symp. Suppl.), 76, p. 1S.

Beverly, M.B., Basile, F., Voorhees, K.J., & Hadfield, T.L., (1996), A rapid approach for the detection of dipicolinic acid in bacterial spores using pyrolysis / mass spectrometry, *Rapid Commun. Mass Spectrom.,* 10, p. 455.

Carmona, P., (1980), Vibrational spectra and structure of crystalline dipicolinic acid and calcium dipicolinate trihydrate, *Spectrochim. Acta, A,* 36, p. 705.

Centers for Disease Control & Prevention, American Society for Microbiology, & Association of Public Health Laboratories. Basic diagnostic testing protocols for level A laboratories for the presumptive identification of *Bacillus anthracis,* (2001), American Society for Microbiology, Washington, D.C. Accessed Nov 2011, Available from: http://www.bt.cdc.gov/Agent/Anthrax/Anthracis20010417.pdf

Dean, J.L., (1979), *Lange's Handbook of Chemistry,* 12*th* Ed., McGraw-Hill, New York, NY.

Dou, X., Jung, Y., Cao, Z., & Ozaki, Y., (1999), Surface-Enhanced Raman Scattering of Biological Molecules on Metal Colloid II: Effects of Aggregation of Gold Colloid and Comparison of Effects of pH of Glycine Solutions between Gold and Silver Colloids, *Appl. Spectrosc.,* 53, p. 1440.

Esposito, A.P., Talley, C.E., Huser, T., Hollars, C.W., Schaldach, C.M., & Lane, S.M., (2003), Analysis of single bacterial spores by micro-Raman spectroscopy, *Appl. Spectrosc.*, 57, p. 868.

Farquharson, S., Smith, W.W., Elliott, S., & Sperry, J.F., (1999), Rapid biological agent identification by surface-enhanced Raman spectroscopy, *Proc. SPIE*, 3855, p. 110.

Farquharson, S., & Maksymiuk, P., (2003), Simultaneous chemical separation and surface-enhancement Raman spectral detection using silver-doped sol-gels, *Appl. Spectrosc.*, 57, p. 479.

Farquharson, S., Grigely, L., Khitrov, V., Smith, W.W., Sperry, J.F., & Fenerty, G., (2004), Detecting *Bacillus cereus* spores on a mail sorting system using Raman Spectroscopy, *J. Raman Spectrosc.*, 35, p. 82.

Farquharson, S., Smith, W., Carangelo, R.C., & Brouillette, C., (1999), Industrial Raman: providing easy, immediate, cost effective chemical analysis anywhere, *Proc. SPIE*, 3859, p. 14.

Ghiamati, E., Manoharan, R.S., Nelson, W.H., & Sperry, J.F., (1992), UV Resonance Raman spectra of Bacillus spores, *Appl. Spectrosc.*, 46, p. 357.

Grasselli, J.G., Snavely, M.K., & Bulkin, B.J., (1981), *Chemical Applications of Raman Spectroscopy*, John Wiley & Sons, New York, NY, Chapter 5.

Hameka, H.F., Jensen, J.O., Jensen, J.L., Merrow, C.N., & Vlahacos, C.P., (1996), Theoretical studies of the fluorescence of dipicolinic acid and its anion, *J. Molec. Struct. (Theory)*, 365, p. 131.

Hathout, Y., Setlow, B., Cabrera-Martinex, R-M., Fenselau, C., & Setlow, P., (2003), Small, acid-soluble proteins as biomarkers in mass spectrometry analysis of Bacillus spores, *Appl. Environ. Microbiol.*, 69, p. 1100.

Halverson, H.O., Ed., (1961), *Spores II*, American Society for Microbiology, Washington, D.C., p. 153.

Helgason, E., Økstad, O.A., Caugant, D.A., Johansen, H.A., Fouet, A., Mock, M., Hegna, I., & Kolstø, A.B., (2000), *Bacillus anthracis*, *Bacillus cereus*, and *Bacillus thuringiensis*-one species on the basis of genetic evidence, *Appl. Environ. Microbiol.*, 66, p. 2627.

Hindle, A.A., Hall, E.A.H., (1999), Dipicolinic acid assay revisited and appraised for spore detection, *Analyst*, 124, p. 1599.

Hsu, V.P., Lukacs, S.L., Handzel, T., et al., (2002), Opening a *Bacillus anthracis*-containing envelope, Capitol hill, Washington, D.C.: The Public Health Response, *Emerg. Infect. Dis.*, 8, p. 1039.

Inglesby, T.V., Henderson, D.A., & Bartlett, J.G., (2002), Anthrax as a biological weapon: updated recommendations for management, *JAMA*, 287, p. 2236.

Jackson, P.J., Hugh-Jones, M.E., Adair, D.M., et al., (1998), PCR analysis of tissue samples from the 1979 Sverdlovsk anthrax victims: The presence of multiple *Bacillus anthracis* strains in different victims, *Proc. Natl. Acad. Sci.*, 95, p. 1224.

Janssen, F.W., Lund, A.J., & Anderson, L.E., (1958), Colorimetric assay for dipicolinic acid in bacterial spores, Science, 127, p. 26.

Jeanmaire D.L., & Van Duyne, R.P., (1977), Surface Raman Spectroelectrochemistry, *J. Electroanal. Chem.*, 84, p. 1.

Jernigan, J.A., Stephens, D.S., Ashford, D.A, et al., (2001), Bioterrorism-Related Inhalational Anthrax: The First 10 Cases Reported in the United States, *Emerg. Infect. Dis.*, 6, p. 933.

Kellogg, M., (2010), Detection of biological agents used for terrorism: Are we ready?, *Clin. Chem.*, 56, p. 10.

Kennedy, H., (2001), Daschle letter bombshell billions of anthrax spores, *New York Daily News*, October 31, 2001.

Kiratisin, P., (2002), Large-scale screening of nasal swabs for *Bacillus anthracis*: Descriptive summary and discussion of the National Institute of Health's experience, *J. Clin. Microbio.*, 40, p. 3012.

Laserna, J.J., Berthod, A., & Winefordner, J.D., (1988), Evaluation and optimization of experimental conditions for surface-enhanced Raman detection of analytes in flow injection analysis, *Microchem. J.*, 38, p. 25.

Leingang, M., (2004), Post office installs anthrax detector, *The Enquirer (Cincinnati)*, Sept. 24, 2004.

Liu, H., Bergman, N.H., Thomason, B., et al., (2004), Formation and Composition of the *Bacillus anthracis* Endospore, *J. Bacteriol.*, 186, p. 164.

Mabry, R., Brasky, K., Geiger, R., Carrion, R. Jr., Hubbard, G. B., Leppla, S., Patterson, J. L., Georgiou, G., and Iverson, B.L.,(2006), Detection of anthrax toxin in the serum of animals infected with Bacillus anthracis by using engineered immunoassays, *Clin. Vaccine Immunol.* 13, p. 671.

Mullen, K., & Carron, K., (1994), Adsorption of chlorinated ethylenes at 1-octadecanethiol-modified silver surfaces, *Anal. Chem.*, 66, p. 478.

Murrell, W.G., Gould, G.W., & Hurst, A. Eds., (1969), *The Bacterial Spore*, Acad. Press., London, p. 215.

Nelson, W.H., Dasari, R., Feld, M., & Sperry, J.F., (2004), Intensities of calcium dipicolinate and *Bacillus subtilis* spore Raman spectra excited with 244 nm light, *Appl. Spectrosc.*, 58, p. 1408.

Nudelman, R., Bronk, B.V., & Efrima, S., (2000), Fluorescence Emission Derived from Dipicolinate Acid, its Sodium, and its Calcium Salts, *Appl. Spectrosc.*, 54, p. 445.

Pellegrino, P.M., Fell Jr., N.F., & Gillespie, J.B., (2002), Enhanced spore detection using dipicolinate extraction techniques, *Anal. Chim. Acta.*, 455, p. 167.

Phillips, Z.E., & Strauch, M.A., (2002), *Bacillus subtilis* sporulation and stationary phase gene expression, *Cell. Mol. Life Sci.*, 59, p. 392.

Ragkousi, K., Eichenberger, P., Van Ooij, C., & Setlow, P., (2003), Identification of a New Gene Essential for Germination of *Bacillus subtilis* Spores with Ca2+-Dipicolinate, *J. Bacteriol.*, 185, p. 2315.

Rosen, D.L., Sharpless, C., & McBrown, L.B., (1997), Bacterial spore detection and determination by use of terbium dipicolinate photoluminescence, *Anal. Chem.*, 69, p. 1082.

Sacchi, C.T., Whitney, A.M., Mayer, L.W., Morey, R., Steigerwalt, A., Boras, A., Weyant, R.S., & Popovic, T., (2002), Sequencing of 16S rRNA Gene: A Rapid Tool for Identification of *Bacillus anthracis*, *Emerg. Infect. Dis.*, 8, p. 1117.

Sanderson, W.T., Hein, M.J., & Taylor, L., (2002), Surface Sampling Methods for *Bacillus anthracis* Spore Contamination, *Emerg. Infect. Dis.*, 8, p. 1145.

Sanderson, W.T., Stoddard, R.R., Echt, A.S., et al., (2004), *Bacillus anthracis* contamination and inhalational anthrax in a mail processing and distribution center, *J. Appl. Microbiol.*, 96, p. 1048.

Shane, S., (2004), Post office unveils anthrax detector, *Baltimore Sun*, July 23, 2004.

Tang, S., Moayeri, M., Chen, Z., Harma, H., Zhao, J., Hu, H.,Purcell, R.H., Leppla, S.H., and Hewlett, I.K.,(2009) Detection of Anthrax Toxin by an Ultrasensitive Immunoassay Using Europium Nanoparticles, Clin.Vacc. Immun., 16, p. 408.

Thayer, A., (2003), Homeland Security: Postal Service Readies Defense - Team will install PCR-based systems to detect biohazards in mail facilities, *C&EN*, 81, p. 7.

Weaver, M.J., Farquharson, S., & Tadayyoni, M.A., (1985), Surface-enhancement factors for Raman scattering at silver electrodes: Role of adsorbate-surface interactions and electrode structure, *J. Chem. Phys.*, 82, p. 4867.

Woodruff, W.H., Spiro, T.G., & Gilvarg, C., (1974), Raman Spectroscopy In Vivo: Evidence on the Structure of Dipicolinate in Intact Spores of *Bacillus Megaterium, Biochem. Biophys. Res. Commun.*, 58, p. 197.

3

Staphylococcal Enterotoxins, Stayphylococcal Enterotoxin B and Bioterrorism

Martha L. Hale
United States Army Research Institute of Infectious Diseases, Integrative Toxicology Division, Fort Detrick, USA

1. Introduction

Staphylococcal enterotoxins (SEs) are exotoxins produced primarily by *Staphylococcus aureus,* which is a ubiquitous microorganism with world-wide distribution (Bergdoll, 1983; Dinges et al., 2000). SEs are a major cause of food poisoning and they are also potent immune activators that lead to serious immune dysfunction (Alouf and Muller-Alouf, 2003; McCormick et al., 2001). Unlike most toxins, SEs are not directly cytotoxic and cell entry is not a requirement for them to cause an effect. The Centers for Disease Control and Prevention (CDC) place one SE, staphylococcal enterotoxin B (SEB), as a select agent based on its universal availability, ease of production and dissemination, and the potential to cause moderate but widespread illnesses. Additionally, because these agents are common to the environment and the diseases they cause are similar to other diseases, Category B agents require close environmental monitoring and enhanced disease surveillance (http://www.bt.cdc.gov/bioterrorism/).

Many biothreat agents are common inhabitants of the soil and animals, and are known to cause disease in areas where they are indigenous. SEs present an additional problem in that SE-producing *S. aureus* are found throughout the world, and are known to produce a variety of illnesses, so that detection of a possible bioterrorist attack may be more problematic than those of other agents (Ahanotou, et al., 2006). The following sections describe SEB's history as a biowarfare agent and its possible use as a bioterrorism agent. To understand why it is considered a Category B agent, a description of the toxin, the main diseases caused, methods to treat the diseases, and surveillance mechanisms will also be discussed.

2. Biowarfare history

In the era of offensive biological weapons, one of the SEs, SEB, was studied, not so much for its mass destruction capabilities but, rather for its ability to incapacitate soldiers so they would be incapable of fighting or defending their posts (Croddy and Hart, 2002; Hursh et al., 1995). The United States bioweapons program studied the toxin intensively and determined that the amount of SEB required to induce incapacitation was considerably less than that of synthesized chemicals. When the toxin and chemicals were compared by expense, time, and complexity of production, SEB was far more cost-effective. A dose of 400 pg/kg body weights was estimated to incapacitate 50% of the human population exposed by an aerosol attack, while 200 ng/kg body weights would be lethal for 50% of those exposed (Ahanotu, et al., 2006; Bellamy and Freedman, 2001; Ulrich et al., 1997).

By 1966, the U.S. and its allies had produced stockpiles of various biowarfare (BW) agents, including SEB (under the code name WG) and research to establish parameters for SEB's use as an aerosolized bioweapon continued at several facilities in the U.S. and Great Britain. In the fall of 1969, President Nixon stopped the offensive BW program and by 1972, all stockpiles of agents were destroyed (Greenfield et al., 2002; Franz et al., 1997). On April 10, 1972, Great Britain, United States, and Soviet governments signed the Convention on the Prohibition of the Development, Production and Stockpiling of Bacteriological (Biological) and Toxin Weapons and on Their Destruction, which went into effect March 26, 1975.

During the latter half of the Cold War, the Defense Intelligence Agency (DIA) and the Central Intelligence Agency (CIA) suspected that the USSR was continuing to stockpile and test biological weapons and therefore, defensive research programs were established for vaccine and therapeutic development (Ulrich et al., 1997). Not only have these research programs aided in development of surveillance mechanisms, the programs have significantly contributed to a greater understanding of diseases and the development of possible therapeutic interventions.

With the end of the Cold War and dissolution of the USSR, threat of BW was greatly diminished. Other rogue nations were still stockpiling weapons and the CIA uncovered evidence that Iraq was building an arsenal of biological weapons. Although weaponized SEB was considered a high probability, it was not found when the Iraqi weapons program was dismantled (Zalinskas, 1997).

3. The toxin

SEB is one of several exotoxins isolated from *S. aureus* that are known for their emetic and superantigen traits (Bergdoll et al., 1974; McCormick et al. 2001). These exotoxins were the first superantigens to be identified, but since their discovery, additional superantigens have been isolated in other bacteria, particularly from the closely related genus, *Streptococcus*. Although staphylococcal and streptococcal superantigens are very similar, descriptions of toxin here will be limited to those toxins produced by staphylococci and the toxins will be identified as SEs or superantigens (SAG).

3.1 Description of the toxin

SEB belongs to a group of pyrogenic enterotoxins, produced primarily by *S. aureus* (McCormick et al., 2001). They are water soluble and relatively resistant to heat and proteolytic enzymes, including pepsin, trypsin, and papain (Le Loir et al., 2003). Stability does also depend upon purity of the toxin preparation, the medium's composition, and the pH. SEB is one of the most stable toxins when exposed to extreme temperature and pH, one characteristic that makes SEB an attractive bioterrorism agent (da Cunha et al., 2007; Le Loir et al., 2003; Nout et al., 1988).

Although they vary in amino acid sequence, SEs share a common three-dimensional structure that maintains their unique binding regions (Fig. 1) (Baker and Acharya, 2004; Papageorgiou et al., 1998). At least 20 serologically distinct SEs have been isolated primarily

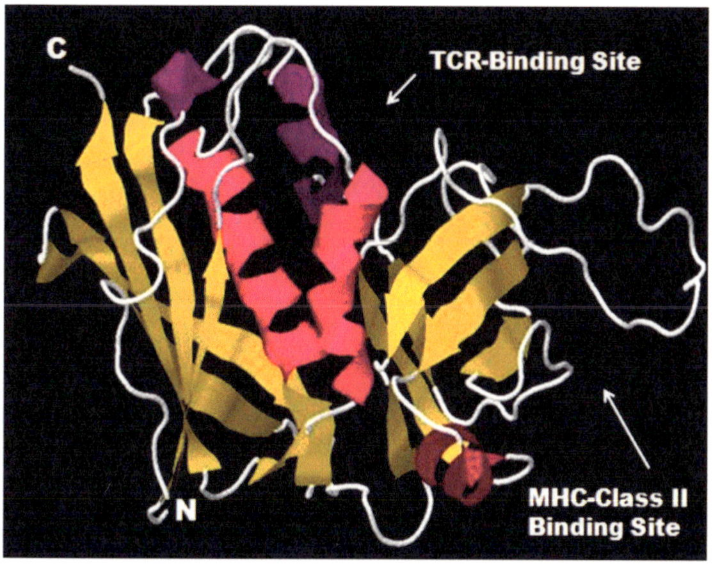

Fig. 1. Molecular structure of SEB (from PDB:3SEB using Jmol version 12.0.41) showing α-helices (magenta), β-strands (gold), and loop strucuture. The β-grasp domain is on the left, and the disulfide bond in the right. The N terminus and C terminus are labeled.

from *S. aureus* (Table 1). Using the Clustal W program, the amino acid sequences of the SEs were aligned and evolutionary distances determined. A dendrogram constructed by the near neighbor-joining method divides the toxins into three major and two minor monophyletic groups (Ono et al., 2008; Uchiyama et al., 2003). The first two groups contain the classical toxins SEA, SED, SEE (Group 1) and SEB, SEC (Group 2) in addition to newly identified SEs; Group 3 contains only newly identified toxins. There is some similarity in structure in that Groups 1, 2, and 5 have a disulfide bond while Group 3 and Group 4 (TSST-1) do not.

Many, but not all, SEs require zinc ions for functional binding to the MHC class II and for stability of its tertiary structure (Fraser et al., 1992; Ples et al., 2005); related to their amino acid sequences, the SEs bind zinc at various locations within the molecule (Brosnahan et al., 2010). Some bind zinc in the concave β sheet of the C terminal domain while others bind zinc in a cleft between the two domains. SEB and toxic shock syndrome toxin (TSST-1 do not bind zinc ions (Brosnahan and Shlievert, 2011; Ly, et al., 2001; Sundstrom, et al, 1996).

3.2 Genetic analysis of SE genes

Analysis of SE genes indicates divergence from a common ancestry. Most genes coding for the enterotoxins are found on mobile elements such as pathogenicity islands, plasmids and bacteriophages, making horizontal transfer a common occurrence (Jarraud et al., 2001; McCormick et al, 2001; Yarwood, et al., 2002). In 2001, a cluster of genes with homologies to SE genes was identified and named the enterotoxin gene cluster (egc). Since many of the genes produced SE-like proteins, Jarraud et al. (2001) suggested that the gene cluster formed an enterotoxin nursery where genomic rearrangements would lead to new SEs, a fact that has now been confirmed with the development of the new exotoxin SEG (Lindsay, 2011; Thomas et al., 2006).

Group[a]	Enerotoxin	MW (kDa)	Gene Location[b]	Emetic
1	SEA	27.1	phage	yes
	SED	26.9	plasmid (pIB485)	yes
	SEE	29.6	prophage	yes
	SEJ	31.2	plasmid (pIB485)	yes
	SEN	26.1	egc[c]	yes
	SEO	26.8	egc	yes
	SES	26.2	phage	yes
	SEP	26	phage	yes
	SHE[c]	25.1	transposon	yes
2	SEB	28.4	SaPI[d]	yes
	SEC1	27.5	SaPI	yes
	SEC2	27.6	SaPI	yes
	SEC3	27.6	SaPI	yes
	SEG	27	egc	yes
	SEIR	27	plasmid (pIB485)	yes
	SEU	27.2	egc	yes
3	SEI	24.9	egc	poor
	SEK	26	SaPI	yes
	SEL	26.8	SaPI	no
	SEM	24.8	egc	yes
	SEQ	26	SaPI	unknown
4	TSST-1	21.9	PI	no
5	SET	22.6	egc	poor

[a]Staphilococcal enterotoxins are divided into 5 monophyletic groups according to ammino acid sequence alignment (Uchiyama et al., 2003; Ono et al., 2008)
[b]Gene location of the toxin
[c]enterotoxin gene cluster
[d]Staphylococcus aureus phatogeniciti islands

Table 1. Staphylococcal enterotoxin/superantigens

As shown in Table 1, genetic elements containing SE genes vary. Most are located on mobile genetic elements (MGEs) which are DNA pieces with ends that encode genes (Lindsay, 2011). There are several types of MGEs, including plasmids, pathogenicity islands, bacteriophages, and transposons. MGEs move from one bacterium to another or between various genetic elements in the same bacterium. Mobility of the genes is thought to contribute to the number and genetic variation within this group of toxins. Interestingly, however, diversity in amino acid sequences has not affected toxin binding to its receptors, suggesting that as the proteins evolved, selective pressures maintained their binding sites by keeping a tertiary structure that supports the characteristic binding (Baker and Achara, 2004; Ulrich et al., 2007).

Expression of SE genes is highly regulated by growth phase and environmental conditions, and not all conditions are suitable for gene activation (Lindsay, 2011). With the proper medium, most toxin production occurs in late log or stationary phase (Otero et al., 1990; Rahkovic et al., 2006; Soejima et al, 2007). *S. aureus* produces regulatory proteins and small RNAs that control toxin production, probably so that in harsh conditions, the bacterium can conserve energy (Horsburg, 2008; Fournier, 2008).

One major regulator of some, but not all SE toxin production, is the accessory regulator gene (Agr) system (Lindsay, 2011). When bacteria reach a critical mass, a quorum-sensing system activates Agr, which, in turn, activates some toxin genes (SEB, for example). Other regulatory systems such as SarA can also up-regulate toxin genes indicating that regulatory pathways are complex and multiple systems probably control toxin production.

3.3 Superantigen characteristics of SEB

Marrack and Kappler (1990) coined the term "superantigen" to connote the similarities between SEs and conventional protein antigens that activate T cells by cross-linking T cells to antigen-presenting cells (APC). Both superantigens (SAG) and conventional antigens bind to the major histocompatibility class II (MHC class II) receptor located on APCs (Haffner, et al., 1996). However, conventional antigens bind to MHC class II molecules inside their antigen-binding grove and are processed into peptides expressed on the cell surface before they are presented to T cells via the T-cell receptor (TCR). In contrast, SAGs bind directly to MHC class II molecules outside the antigen-binding groove; they are not processed into peptide fragments before presentation to TCRs (Fig. 2).

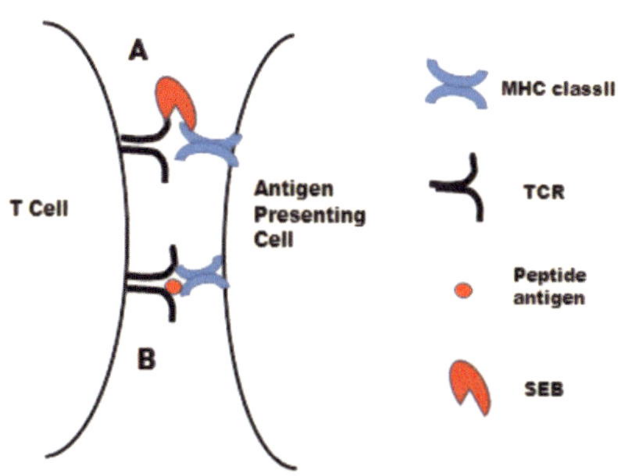

Fig. 2. Conventional antigen and SAGs bind APC and TCR. (A) SAGS bind to the outer region of the TCR Vβ and to the outer region of the MHC Class II determinant. (B) Conventional antigens are processed into peptides that are then presented to the antigen-binding region of the TCR.

While SAG must first bind to MHC class II molecules, their ability to activate large populations of T cells depends largely upon their binding to the TCR (Alber et al., 1990; Pontzer, et al., 199; Stevens, 1997; White et al., 1989). There are five different elements (Vα, Jα, Vβ, Dβ, and Jβ) that comprise the two-chain TCR receptor with each composed of a constant and variable region. The TCR uses all five elements for recognition of processed peptides on the surface of APCs (from conventional antigens). Peptide binding occurs within the peptide-binding region and requires a helper molecule such as CD4. Superantigens bind only to Vβ elements and specificity of binding results from the types of Vβ molecules present (Fig. 1). For example, SEB binds to human Vβ phenotypes 3, 12, 14, 15, 17, which differ from phenotypes bound by other SAGs (Table 2). Because many T cells contain the same Vβ phenotype, SAGs may activate up to 20% of the whole T-cell population rather than the 0.01% activation by conventional antigens.

SAGs are not restricted and can bind to both CD4 and CD8 T cells if the SAG recognizes the TCR Vβ chains, which increases the number of T cells they can affect. Superantigen-activated T cells can undergo at least five to six rounds of cell division (Nagshima et al., 2004). The massive clonal T-cell expansion results in the activation of programmed cell death in which cells responding to the specific superantigen are deleted (Choi et al., 1989; Yuh et al., 1993). Apoptosis of large numbers of T cells, clonal deletion and anergy of specific T-cell populations, and massive release of proinflammatory cytokines are all factors in the toxin's pathogenesis.

4. SE pathogenesis

There are two major diseases caused by the staphylococcal enterotoxin superantigens (SEs), and most diseases attributed to the SEs relate to chronic disease states caused by autoimmunity and repetitious stimulation by SEs. Those autoimmune diseases in which SEs are thought to play a role require more than one challenge and therefore, will probably not be a concern in a bioterrorism threat. The two diseases that are pertinent to potential bioterrorism attacks are SEB (or SEs) in the food or water supply (food poisoning) or an aerosol attack in which the toxin will be inhaled into the lungs, possibly causing toxic shock syndrome.

4.1 Food poisoning

As noted previously, *S. aureus* is a ubiquitous microorganism with a world-wide distribution, and is responsible for causing large numbers of food poisoning cases throughout the world (Bergdoll, 1989; Le Loir et al., 2003; Ortega, et al., 2010). In its normal environment, the gram-positive cocci and its toxins do not cause disease; however, when introduced into foods such as cream, mayonnaise, or similar foods, the bacteria grow rapidly secreting the exotoxins which then contaminate the food. Dack and coworkers (1930) provided the first documented report that identified a toxin from *S. aureus* as a causative agent of a food poisoning incident involving staphylococci-contaminated Christmas cake. The investigators grew the bacteria isolated from the cake and found that a sterile filtrate from the broth in which the bacteria were grown induced food poisoning when ingested by human volunteers. Thereafter, from investigations of various food poisoning outbreaks, an initial five antigenically distinct enterotoxins were identified suggesting that *S aureus* produced a family of protein toxins possessing similar properties and virulence (Casman,

1960; Bergdoll et al., 1959; Bergdoll et al., 1965; Casman et al., 1967). Since the characterization of the five serotypes, at least 20 more SEs (Table 1) have been isolated and characterized with many inducing emesis in monkeys or humans (Uchiyama et al., 2003).

Enerotoxin	TCR Vβ Specificity
SEA	1.1,5.3,6.3,6.4,6.9, 7.3,7.4,9.1,18
SEB	3,12,14,15,17,20
SEC1	3,6.4,6.9,12,13.2,14,15,17,20
SEC2	12,13.2,14,15,17,20
SEC3	3,5,12,13.1,13.2
SED	5,12
SEE	5.1,6.3,6.4,6,9,8.1,18
SEG	13.6,14,15
SHE	Vα10
SEI	1,5.1,5.2,5.3,23
SEJ	ND
SEK	5.1,5.2,6.7
SEL	5.1,5.2,6.7,16,22
SEM	18,21.3
SEN	9
SEO	5.1,7,22
SEIP	5.1,6,8,16,18,21.3
SEQ	2,5.1,5.2,6.7,21.3
SEIR	3,11,12,13.2,14
SEU	13.2,14
TSST-1	2,4

Table 2. Staphylococcal enterotoxins showing the corresponding TCR Vβ repertoires

Approximately 25% of healthy people and animals carry *S. aureus* on the skin and often food workers who carry the bacterium may contaminate food when they handle food without washing their hands or wearing gloves. The microorganism is also found in unpasteurized milk and cheese products and, being salt tolerant, grows in salty foods as well. Because they are highly resistant to heat and enzymatic inactivation, foods that do not require cooking or those prepared by hand provide greater risks of contamination with the bacteria and subsequent toxin production. The short incubation period, approximately 4-6 hr after ingestion, usually differentiates SE-induced food poisoning from those caused by bacteria such as *E. coli* or *Salmonella* species where presence of the bacteria is required for disease.

The onset is sudden and vomiting is the hallmark symptom. Other symptoms, such as diarrhea, abdominal pain, and nausea may also be present, but systemic manifestations such as fever are very uncommon (Alouf and Muller-Alouf, 2003; Kerouanton et al., 2007). Although extremely incapacitating, staphylococcal food poisoning is usually self-limiting and symptoms last about 1 day. Fatality in healthy adults is rare (0.03%); however, the rate is higher in susceptible populations (children, elderly, and immune-compromised adults) and may also depend upon the concentration of the toxin ingested (Do Carmo, et al., 2004).

SE-induced food poisoning was initially thought to be caused by the local interaction of the toxin with intestinal cells because the toxin stimulates nerve centers in the gut through serotonin (5-hydroxytryptamine or 5 HT) release from intestinal mast cells (Alouf and Muller-Alouf, 2003; Hu et al., 2007). Serotonin binds to 5-HT_3 receptors which are ligand-gated ion channels located on the afferent vagus nerve terminals. The binding of serotonin to the receptor opens the channel which signals the medulla emetic reflex center to generate nausea and an emetic response. However, such interactions do not explain the disease pathophysiology. Patients with SE intoxication can exhibit rather severe gastrointestinal damage including mucosal hyperemia, regional edema, petechiae, and purulent exudates (Ortega et al., 2010; Palmer, 1951). SEs cross the intestinal epithelial barrier and gain access to local and systemic lymphoid tissues, suggesting that activation of local immune tissue may be partially responsible for gastrointestinal damage (Hamad et al., 1997). Involvement of the immune system in pathogenesis could explain why immuno-compromised adults develop a more severe, life-threatening disease than normal healthy adults. However, emesis is not directly linked to T-cell proliferation because TSST-1, a potent immune activator, does not cause emesis. TSST-1 is more susceptible to enzymes in the digestive tract and could be the reason for its lack of emetic activity. SEs with emetic activity have a disulfide bond located at the top of the B domain and probably are responsible for stabilizing the molecule in a conformation needed to induce emesis (Brosnahan and Schievert, 2011).

4.2 Toxic shock syndrome

During the late 1970's, Todd and coworkers (1978) described an acute illness in seven children, between the ages of 8 to 17. Symptoms included high fever, hypotension, vomiting, watery diarrhea, a scarlatiniform rash, and renal failure. Although bacteria were not isolated from blood, cerebrospinal fluid, or urine, S. aureus was isolated from mucosal sites. Culture filtrates from cultures of these isolates were shown to contain a toxin that would cause a rash (Nikolksy sign) in newborn mice. Todd named the new disease toxic shock syndrome (TSS). In 1977 through 1980, 22 women between the ages of 13-24, were diagnosed with TSS (Chesney et al., 1981). Investigations showed that this TSS was the result of highly absorbent tampons, which became contaminated with *S. aureus*. A toxin, tsst-1, was isolated from the bacteria cultured from the contaminated tampon and shown to be similar to that discovered by Todd et al. (1978). The super absorbent tampons were found to introduce oxygen into the anaerobic environment of the vagina which facilitated the growth of *S. aureus* and release of TSST-1. When the absorbent tampons were taken off the market, the incidence of menstrual TSS decreased dramatically.

From these early investigations, TSS has been divided into two categories. The first, menstrual TSS, occurs primarily in young women, ages 16-25, during menstrual periods and is usually associated with tampon use. As first identified in the 1980s, TSST-1, remains the leading cause of menstrual TSS (Chesney et al, 1981; Brosnanhan and Schlievert, 2010). TSST-1 is also a major etiologic agent for the other TSS category, non-menstrual TSS, comprising 50% of the reported cases (Buchdahl et al, 1985). Two other SEs, SEB and SEC, have been identified as the causative agent in most of the remaining 50%. Since its discovery, TSS had been considered a rare, but often fatal disease. After removal of absorbent tampons from the market and efforts to inform the public about TSS, incidences of menstrual TSS dropped from 13.7% to 0.3% per 100,000 individuals in the U. S. Since 1986, reported incidences of TSS in the U.S. have remained stable with the annual incidence rate around 0.32%-0.52% per 100,000 people (DeVries, et al., 2011; Haijeh et al., 1996). Several reasons may account for the disease's rarity. One reason lies in the fact that most adults have been exposed to SEs over a period of many years, and therefore, possesses antibodies against many of the SEs. The lack of anti-SE antibodies could also explain why children and young adults are more susceptible to the disease. In addition to immunity against SEs, another problem in TSS diagnosis relates to the lack of a single diagnostic test and, therefore, diagnosis relies upon a complex analysis of clinical symptoms. Requirements for a case to be identified as TSS are rigorous, and while SEs are significant virulence factors in many infections, most infections do not meet the diagnostic criteria for TSS as established by CDC (Table 3).

TSS pathophysiology involves many intricate extracellular and intracellular signaling pathways and at this time, the exact pathways or pathways responsible for the syndrome are not known (Davis et al., 1980; Kumar et al., 2010; Pinchuk et al., 2010). Hallmark studies during the 1990s showed that the toxicity of SEB was due to massive T-cell proliferation and proinflammatory cytokine production (Marrack et al., 1990; White et al., 1989). Investigations using T-cell reconstituted immuno-deficient SCID mice confirmed the role of T-cell activation in SE-induced lethality (Miethke et al., 1992; Canaan, et al. 1999). Furthermore, these studies indicated that tumor necrosis factor alpha (TNF-α) plays a crucial role in SE-induced lethality because passive immunization with an anti-TNF-α/β monoclonal antibody protected the animals against an SE challenge (Fast et al., 1989; Miethke et al., 1992). Although the precise mechanisms by which proinflammatory cytokines induce TSS, these early studies and further investigations provide overwhelming evidence that tissue damage, shock, and multiple organ failure is caused by the production of pathological concentrations of proinflammatory cytokines and chemokines such as TNF-α, interleukin 1β (IL-1 β), interferon gamma (IFN-γ) and interleukin 6 (IL-6), and macrophage chemoattractant protein-1 (MCP-1) (Marrack et al., 1990; Williams, 1991).

Although T cells appear to play a dominant role in TSS, more recent investigations indicate that SE interactions with other cell types may also contribute to TSS pathophysiology (Das, 2000; Faulkner et al., 1997; Marrack et al., 1990; McCormick et al. 2001). Initially, the purpose of the APC MHC class II interaction with SEs was thought to provide a mechanism for T-cell activation and production of proinflammatory cytokines by T-cell populations. That MHC class II interactions play a more active role in TSS was shown by studies in which mortality from TSST-1 was not reduced in T-cell depleted rabbits (Dinges et al, 2003). In addition, TSST-1 induced proinflammatory cytokines in these animals, again suggesting that other cells may play a role in cytokine production. These studies are further supported by investigations in which the SE-MHC class II interaction by itself was shown to be sufficient to activate intracellular signaling pathways which induce downstream pro-inflammatory signaling and subsequent production of cytokines (Kisner (a) et al., 2011; Kisner (b) et al., 2011).

Clinical case definition
• Fever: temperature greater than or equal to 38.9°C • Rash: diffuse macular erythroderma • Desquamation: 1-2 weeks after onset of rash • Hypotension: systolic blood pressure less than or equal to 90 mm Hg for adults or less than fifth percentile by age for children aged less than 16 years
Multisystem involvement (three or more of the following organ systems:
• Gastrointestinal: vomiting or diarrhea at onset of illness • Muscular: severe myalgia or creatine phosphokinase level at least twice the upper limit of normal • Mucous membrane: vaginal, oropharyngeal, or conjunctival hyperemia • Renal: blood urea nitrogen or creatinine at least twice the upper limit of normal for laboratory or tract infection • Urinary sediment with pyuria (greater than or equal to 5 leukocytes per high-power field) in the absence of urinary tract infections • Hepatic: total bilirubin, alanine aminotransferase enzyme, or asparate aminotransferase enzyme levels at least twice the upper limit of normal values • Hematologic: platelets less than 100,000/mm3 • Central nervous system: disorientation or alterations in consciousness without focal neurologic signs when fever and hypotension are absent
Laboratory criteria for diagnosis
• Negative results on the following tests, if obtained: • Blood or cerebrospinal fluid cultures blood culture may be positive for *Staphylococcus aureus* • Negative serologies for Rocky Mountain spotted fever, leptospirosis, or measles
Case classification
• Probable: a case which meets the laboratory criteria and in which four of the five clinical findings described above are present • Confirmed: a case which meets the laboratory criteria and in which all five of the clinical findings described above are present, including desquamation, unless the patient dies before desquamation occurs

CSTE Position Statement Number: 10-ID-14

Table 3. CDC 1997 Definition for Toxic Shock Syndrome

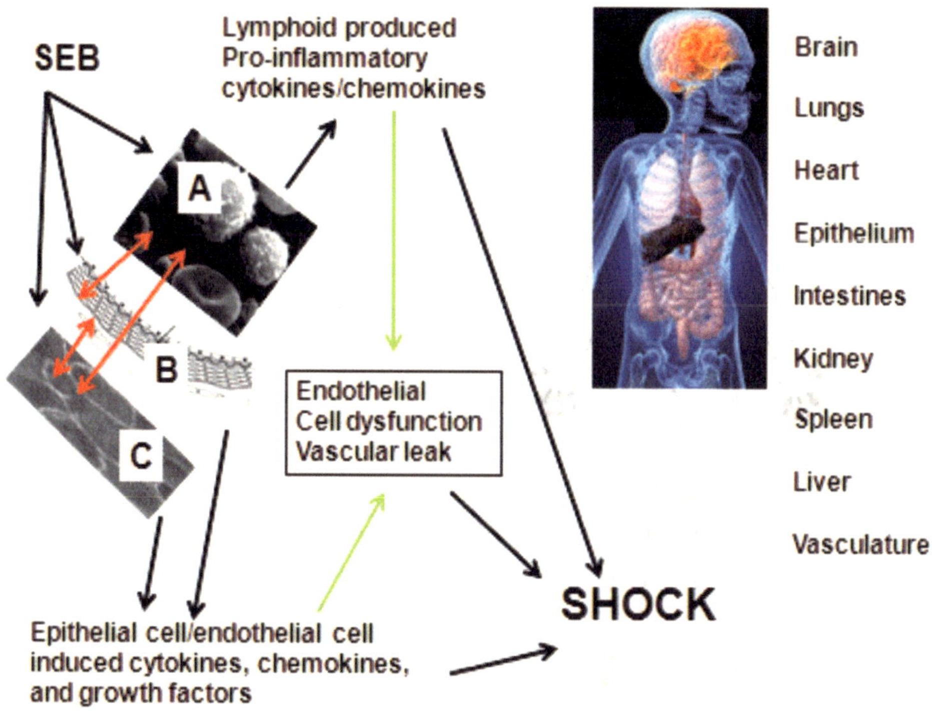

Fig. 3. Systemic SEB (SE) intoxication is a complex disease

SEB interacts with (A) lymphoid cells and induces production of proinflammatory cytokines. SEB stimulates (B) endothelial and (C) epithelial cells to release cytokines (some proinflammatory)/chemokines and growth factors. Red arrows show interactions between cell types are also affected by SEB-induced release of these factors that ultimately leads to endothelial cell dysfunction, vascular leak, and shock resulting from multi-organ failure.

SE binding to lymphoid cells has been extensively characterized and interactions of SEs with these cells are fairly well understood (Achara and Baker, 2004; Broshanan et al. 2011; Larkin et al., 2009). The complexity of the disease suggests that SEs may affect more than lymphoid cells, and recently, an epithelial binding moiety has been identified on the SE molecule (Brosnahan and Schlievert, 20011). SEs bind to epithelial cells and elicit the production of specific cytokines. SEs have also been shown to cross polarized epithelial cells *in vitro* suggesting that SEs gain systemic access to the body (Hale, unpublished data). Rajagpjalan et al. (2007) show acute activation of the systemic immune system and inflammatory response in mice that were vaginally or intranasally exposed to SEB (Rajagopalan et al. 2007; Rajagopalan et al., 2006). Since the toxin was introduced on mucosal surfaces, the only method for systemic activation would be if the toxin crossed the epithelial cell barrier and gained access to the body. Vaginal epithelial cells were also shown to bind TSST-1 and induce TNFα production while treatment of epithelial cells with TSST-1 or SEB induced production of MIP-3α and IL-8 (Brosnahan et al., 2001; Peterson, et al., 2005).

SE-induced shock causes severe damage to the endothelial vasculature and vascular leak contributes significantly to TSS pathology (Krakauer, 1994; Ortega et al. 2010). Elevated levels of vascular endothelial growth factor are observed in serum from patients with sepsis or septic shock (Karlsson et al. 2008). Because there are common features among hemorrhagic shock, septic shock, and toxic shock syndrome, factors that regulate endothelial homeostasis are probably important in its prevention. Future studies examining the interplay among lymphoid, endothelial and epithelial cells will provide more understanding of the disease and enable a logical approach for therapy.

4.3 Pulmonary complications

One of the most effective and deadly forms of a bioterrorism attack is delivery of the toxin or microorganism by aerosol exposure (Ulrich et al., 1997). Understanding SE-intoxication in humans has been difficult because there is no direct comparison between the pathogenesis of human disease and the disease caused by an intentional aerosol attack. Perhaps the most descriptive and informative reports detailed an accidental laboratory inhalational exposure of fifteen workers (Rusnak et al., 2004). Ten became symptomatic and nine were hospitalized. The onset was rapid (1 1/2 hrs to 24 hr) after exposure with the illness lasting 3-4 days. Commonly observed symptoms were fever, headache, myalgias, pulmonary symptoms, and gastrointestinal symptoms.

A Rhesus macaque animal model was used to characterize SEB intoxication by an aerosol route. In these studies, nonhuman primates (NHP) were exposed to a lethal dose (5 LD50) of aerosolized SEB in a modified Henderson head-only aerosol exposure chamber. NHPs developed gastrointestinal symptoms (anorexia, diarrhea, and emesis) within 24 hr after exposure. The gastrointestinal symptoms appeared to be self-limiting, but 24 hr later, the NHPs developed an abrupt onset of lethargy, dyspnea, and facial pallor. Usually within 4 hr, the animals died or were euthanized when moribund. Postmortem examination revealed lesions in the lungs and signs of pulmonary edema. Both large and small intestines showed petechial hemorrhaging and mucosal erosion, and lymph nodes were swollen. There was definite damage to the endothelium and endothelial cells. The authors of the study concluded that SEB is a potent stimulant in rhesus monkeys and that a similar dose in humans could produce similar symptoms. One thing to consider, however, when extrapolating from NHP to human, is that the NHP were seronegative when tested for the presence of antibodies against SEB; most humans have some degree of past exposure to the toxin and therefore would perhaps have some immunity.

Since these studies on NHP, there is evidence that links SEs exposure to asthma and respiratory problems (Kumar et al., 2010). Inflammatory reactions in the lung are induced by TNF-α and two life-threatening syndromes, vascular leak and respiratory distress develop during toxic shock (Aubert et al., 2000; Herz et al., 1999; Neuman et al., 1997). Other studies show that cytokine-mediated acute respiratory distress syndrome and inflammatory lung disease occur during SE intoxication (DeSouza et al., 2006; Fujisawa et al., 1998; Slifka and Whitton, 2002). Both conditions are critical and may be lethal without therapeutic intervention (Das, 2000; Kasai et al., 1997). Anti-inflammatory drugs reduce TNF-α and other proinflammatory cytokines which alleviates the symptoms and helps the individuals to recover from these life-threatening illnesses.

5. Animal models

A major problem in understanding the disease process of SE intoxication is the lack of appropriate animal models that mimic the human disease. There are several animal models for studying TSS, but each model has its own limitations, which need to be understood in order to use each model in furthering our understanding of the disease process.

5.1 Mouse

The mouse remains the most common model for TSS studies, although they are not sensitive to the toxin and must be sensitized with either hepatotoxins (e.g., D-galactosamine and actinomycin D) or with endotoxin to achieve an effect (Chen et al., 1991; Nagaki et al., 1991; Blank et al., 1997; Sugiyama et al., 1964). Endotoxin is a natural component of gram-negative bacteria found in the intestines and may actually contribute to shock syndromes. Although tissue damage from SE and lipopolysaccharide (LPS) may vary, acute shock caused by abnormally high levels of TNF-α and other proinflammatory cytokines results in life-threatening situations (Das, 2000; Miekthe et al, 1997; Sifka and Whitton, 2000). Thus, an animal model in which the SEB effects are magnified by sublethal concentrations of LPS provides an *in vivo* system useful for studying various facets of lethal shock. While each mouse model lacks some characteristics of the disease in humans, Krakauer et al. (2010) found that three different mouse models with different susceptibility to SEB could be used to study SEB intoxication.

T-cell deficient mice or mice engineered to have specific cytokine deficiencies show that TNF-α and T cells are both required for SE-induced lethality (Blank, et al. 1997). Transgenic mice expressing human TCR/MHC class II determinants solve some problems associated with mouse lymphoid cells binding SE and SAG-sensitive mice show a biphasic release of cytokines with early TNF-a release mediating lethal shock (Faulkner et al., 2005; Rajagopalan et al., 2002). These investigations point also to the spleen as a major source of TNF-a production during an acute (early) cytokine response. The studies support the idea that TSS is not simply due to cytokines released by T cells, but entails a series of events affecting major organs throughout the body. Recently, a humanized mouse in which T-cell immune deficient mice, SCID, were transfused with human hematopoietic fetal liver CD34+ cells that had previously been implanted with human fetal thymic and liver tissues developed long-term human innate and adaptive immune responses. When TSST-1 was injected into these mice, the mice responded immunologically in a manner similar to humans (Melkus et al., 2006) suggesting that this mouse model may overcome many of the problems associated with mouse models for SE intoxication.

5.2 Rat

Rats have been an excellent model to study TSS effects on the nervous system. Wang et al, (2004) showed activation of neuronal developmental genes after rats were given intraperitoneal injections of SEB. Activation appeared to occur through the tenth cranial nerve, the vagus, because severing this nerve prevented neuronal activation. These studies support the idea that brain-immune system communications play a role in TSS. Some sequalae of TSS relate to memory loss and confusion which would indicate involvement of the nervous system (Kusnocov and Goldfaith, 2005).

5.3 Minature swine

Because a major drawback for murine and rodent models in TSS is the lack of clinical symptoms that occur in humans, a porcine model has been developed in which 18-day-old piglets are given a lethal dose of SEB intravenously (van Gessel et al., 2004). Intoxicated piglets develop vomiting, diarrhea, febrile temperature spikes, anorexia, and hypotension similar to the clinical course of disease observed in humans and may offer an *in vivo* model with more of the symptoms observed in human TSS.

5.4 Rabbit

McCormick et al. (2003) noted that rabbits, when given SAG by a continuous perfusion, developed pyrogenic symptoms similar to humans. Investigations showed that the lethal pathology was similar to that observed in human TSS, but with newer animal models and a greater understanding of mechanisms involved in TSS, rabbits are not a major animal model for TSS.

5.5 Shrew

Most of the small animal models used to study the effects of SE-intoxication do not display an emetic response (King, 1990). Hu et al. (2003) developed an emetic model with which to study SE-induced emesis. They reported that several SE serotypes, known to induce emesis in NHP, induced emesis in the house musk shrew (*Suncus murinus*). Concentrations required to induce an emetic response were approximately 0.4 µg per animal, but the dose varied with the SE serotype. Variations in SE toxicity among the serotypes were similar to those observed in NPHs and humans, making the shrew an excellent small animal model to study emesis induced by SEs.

5.6 Nonhuman primate

NHP exhibit a similar disease progression as that observed in humans and are susceptible when given SEB orally (Boles et al., 2003; Mattix et al., 1995; Ulrich et al., 1997). Because there are limitations in the number of NHP available for studies and because of the expense involved in NHP studies, they are usually reserved for preclinical investigations. While TSS manifestations in NHPs resemble those observed in humans, there are differences between the immune systems, which may become more evident as more is learned about the disease process.

6. Therapy and prophylaxis

Most therapeutic and prophylatic measures are concerned with TSS or systemic SE intoxication because food poisoning is usually self-limiting. Although identification of unusual food poisoning incidents should be monitored as a possible biothreat action, the disease itself should not be life-threatening, and recovery occurs without serious side effects. Because therapy for food poisoning is not a serious concern, this section will address the measures to treat disease pathogenesis resulting from systemic SE intoxication.

6.1 Current therapeutic measures

At the current time, intravenous human gamma globulins (IVIG) is the primary therapeutic to treat TSS. Because there are no specific drugs available for treatment, a primary goal of any therapeutic intervention is to maintain important body functions and physiological homeostasis. Recommendations for treating TSS include first the removal of any foreign materials that might be contaminated with *S aureus* (i.e., tampons or nasal packings) and draining sites of infection to prevent further bacterial growth. Treatment with anti-microbials is also recommended if sepsis is involved. In severe cases, other therapeutic interventions that may minimize the risk of tissue damage and organ failure include fluids to prevent dehydration, dialysis if severe kidney problems occur, drugs to control blood pressure and cardiovascular function, anti-inflammatory agents, and possibly insulin, if needed. Supportive care should be aggressive and monitored carefully. Length of hospitalization may vary between 5 and 11 days (DeVries et al., 2011).

6.2 Antibody therapy for SE intoxication

As shown by studies in NHP, animals could be protected against SE intoxication using passive immunization with anti-SEB antibodies. The antibodies provided protection if given up to 4 hr after the NHPs had received 5 LD50sof aerosolized SEB (LeClaire et al., 2002). These studies showed that the antibodies were able to neutralize the toxin *in vivo* and provide protection after intoxication had occurred. Unfortunately, the antibody was a monoclonal antibody (Mab) created in a chicken, and the antibody itself may be antigenic and cause serum sickness. There are several anti-SEB Mab preparations that will not cause adverse reactions in humans. Because most Mabs are not developed using human cells, Mab development for human use will require "humanization of the Mab in order to eliminate the molecule's antigenicity (Goldsmith and Signore, 2010). Investigations using immune lymphocytes to prepare Mabs may provide therapeutics without the expense of humanization. Additionally, developing small-domain antibody fragments such as camilid antibodies may also provide therapeutic agents that, because of their size, may not be antigenic in humans (Graef et al., 2011). Further studies are needed to identify antibody reagents that will be successful therapeutics, and whether the antibody reagents will need to be combined with pharmacologic agents to enhance their efficacy.

6.3 Possible pharmacologic agents to treat SE intoxication

Over the past 20 years, there have been numerous investigations showing efficacy of various pharmacologic agents that prevent or delay lethality when animals are treated after a SE challenge, and as yet none has advanced to human clinical trials (Krakauer, 2010). Human activated protein C (hAPC) was approved for patients in severe septic shock, and had been used to treat TSS (DeVries et al. 2011). On October 25, 2011, Eli Lilly withdrew *Xigris (hAPC) because more in depth clinical trials indicated that drug did no better than a placebo in reducing mortality (*http://www.medscape.com/viewarticle/752169*)*. The complexity of TSS tends to discount development of a single drug capable of treating the disease . Because the disease affects the endothelial cell vasculature of multiple organ systems, including drugs that treat endothelial cell damage should also help to establish a therapeutic regimen for TSS.

6.4 Vaccines

To protect soldiers against SEB exposure, the U. S. Army developed a formalin-treated SEB toxoid that had some degree of success in protecting animals against a SEB challenge (Tseng et al., 1995). Due to the fact that formalin treatment did not always inactivate every toxin molecule, there was a move to develop vaccines without the need for formalin inactivation. A vaccine developed by site-specific mutagenesis provided safer and more effective vaccines. The most effective vaccine (SEBvax) was designed with mutations in the MHC class II binding region so that the vaccine no longer was capable of cross-linking T cells to APCs (Ulrich et al., 1998). The military is no longer funding development of SEBvax. The vaccine is now being used to develop a trivalent subunit vaccine that includes mutated Tst-1 and SEA proteins as well. The combination vaccine should provide protection against SEB but also against SEs more commonly associated with TSS (http://www.regionalinnovation.org/success.cfm?story=32).

7. Detection of SEs and SEB

Since September 11, 2001, The U.S. and its allies have been concerned with detection of those agents that could be dispersed by aerosol (Kman and Bachman, 2011). There are several methods used for monitoring agents of bioterrorism and surveillance occurs through an umbrella of monitoring systems. A major component of surveillance, syndromic surveillance, results from the monitoring of clinical manifestations of certain illnesses to determine if there is a higher than normal number of cases. This is usually followed by laboratory surveillance in which certain markers and laboratory data indicate the presence of a bioterrorism agent. Another type of surveillance is environmental during which the environment is continually sampled for the presence of biological agents. In situations like SEB which is not generally monitored environmentally via the BioWatch Program, syndromic and laboratory surveillance becomes extremely important for monitoring bioterrorism attacks.

SEs are stable proteins and therefore identification of the proteins using anti-SEB reagents should be possible in both the field and medical facilities. Available immunoassays are capable of identifying the protein in picogram amounts and can be used to monitor samples taken from the environment (Kahn et al. 2003; Sapsford et al., 2005). Because most humans have been exposed to SEs and have developed antibodies against them, the presence of anti-SE antibodies is of little diagnostic value, but the detection of the toxin in body fluids or from nasal swabs (after an aerosol exposure), should provide a positive confirmation (Ulrich et al., 1997).

In cases of infection with *S. aureus*, polymerase chain reaction (PCR) assays can determine the presence of the SE gene (Chiang et al., 2008; Rajkovic et al., 2006). Particularly in the case of a toxin that is known to be present in staphylococcal infections, surveillance and monitoring at the clinical level is imperative for differentiating between random outbreaks of the disease and a bioterrorist attack.

8. Category B biothreat agent

Although redefined after September 11, 2001, rogue nations have used bioterrorism for centuries as a method to harm their opponents (Bellamy and Freedman, 2001; Phillips, 2005). As described by CDC, bioterrorism agents are separated into three categories for preparedness purposes depending upon their ease of dissemination, and the ability to cause excessive morbidity and mortality (Rotz et al, 2002). Category A includes agents such as Variola major (smallpox) and *Yersinia pestis* (plague) that have been used as a weapon of mass destruction (WMD) (Henderson, 1999). As previously mentioned, Category B agents are easy to disseminate and produce moderate morbidity and low mortality. Category B agents do not meet criteria for use as a WMD, but dispersal of a Category B agent could result in regional disruptions and hysteria.

From all accounts, SEB meets the criteria for a Category B agent in that it is stable, easy to disseminate, and induces severe emesis and toxic shock. An aerosol of SEB in a crowded area could lead to an incapacitating disease in several hundred individuals. Although mortality would be low, the illness would create a serious public health impact by disrupting normal work days and cause havoc by increasing individual use of emergency rooms (Ulrich et al., 1997).

Many bioterrorism agents such as SEB are found in nature, are easy to isolate and produce in mass quantities and are usually stable in adverse environmental conditions (Ahanotu, et al., 2006). Because the agent is a common inhabitant in the environment, monitoring the agent becomes more difficult. The fact that there are accidental cases of food poisoning and occasional cases of TSS annually also complicates identifying bioterrorism incidents using SEB. In the final analysis, although SEB may not be the most favored bioterrorism agent, there is always a possibility that it will be used in an attack and, therefore, mechanisms should be in place for decontamination and treatment.

9. Summary

SEs are produced primarily by *S.aureus* which is a common inhabitant in the environment worldwide. SEs are a major cause of food poisoning and toxic shock syndrome. In the 1960s, SEB was weaponized as an incapacitating agent, and now is listed as a Category B bioterrorism agent. When inhaled, the toxin causes severe respiratory damage and endothelial dysfunction, often resulting in acute respiratory distress and severe lung damage. As yet, there is no FDA-approved vaccine or therapeutic agents to prevent or treat SEB-intoxication and with its ease of dissemination, SEB remains a serious bioterrorism agent.

10. Acknowledgements

The work was supported by funds from the Defense Threat Reduction Agency (project CBM.THRTOX.03.10.RD.020). The opinions, interpretations, conclusions, and recommendations expressed in this publication are those of the author and are not necessarily endorsed by the US Army.

11. References

Abrahmsen, L., Dohlsten, M., Segren, S., Bjork, P., Johsson, E., and Kalland, T. (1995) Characterization of two distinct MHC class II binding sites in the superantigen staphylococcal enterotoxin A. EMBO J. 14: 2978-2986.

Acharya K. R., Baker M. D., (2004) Superantigen: structure-function relationships. Int. J. Med. Microbiol. 293: 529-37.

Alber, G, Hammer, K., and Fleischer, B. (1990) Relationship between enterotoxic and T lymphocyte-stimulating activity of staphylococcal enterotoxins. *J. Immunol.* 144:4501-4506.

Alouf, J. E. and Muller-Alouf, H. (2003) Staphylococcal and streptococcal superantigens: molecular, biological, and clinical aspects. *Int. J. Med. Microbiol.* 292:429-440.

Ahanotu, E., Alvelo-Ceron, D., Ravita, T., Gaunt, E. (2006) Staphylococcal enterotoxin B as a biological weapon: recognition, management, and surveillance of staphylococcal enterotoxin. Appl. Biosafety 11: 120-176.

Aubert, V., Schneeberger D., Sauty A., Winter J., Sperisen P., Aubert J., and Spertini F. (2000) Induction of tumor necrosis factor alpha and interleukin-8 gene expression in bronchial epithelial cells by toxic shock syndrome toxin 1. Infect. Immun. 68:120-124.

Baker, M. D. and Acharya, K. R. (2004) Superantigens: structure-function relationships. *Int. J. Med. Microbiol.* 293: 529-537.

Bellamy, R. J. and Freedman, A. R. (2001) Bioterrorism. Q J Medical J. 94: 227-234.

Bergdoll, M. S., Surgalla, M. J., and Dack, G. M. (1959) Staphylococcal enterotoxin I. purification. Arch. Biochem. Biophys. 85: 62-69.

Bergdoll, M. S., Borja, C. R., and Avena, R. M. (1965) Identification of a new enterotoxin as enterotoxin C. J. Bacteriol. 90: 1481-1485.

Bergdoll, M.S., Huang, I. Y., and Schantz, E. J. (1974) Chemistry of the staphylococcal enterotoxins. J. Agric. Food Chem. 22: 9-13.

Bergdoll, M. S. (1983) Enterotoxins. In: *Staphylococci and Staphylococcal Infections* (Easman, C.S.F. and Adlam, C., eds.). Academic Press, London, UK, pp. 559-598.

Bergdoll, M. S. (1989) *Staphylococcus aureus*. In: *Foodborne Bacterial Pathogens* (Doyle, M.P., ed.). Marcel Dekker, Inc., New York, NY, USA, pp. 463-523.

Blank, C., Luz, A., Bendigs, S., Erdmann, A., Wagner, H., and Heeg, K. (1997) Superantigen and endotoxin synergize in the induction of lethal shock. Eur. J. Immunol. 27: 825-833.

Boles, J. W., Pitt, M. L., LeClaire, R. D., Gibbs, P. H., Torres, E., Dyas, B., Ulrich, R. G., Bavari, S. (2003) Generation of protective immunity by inactivated recombinant staphylococcal enterotoxin B vaccine in nonhuman primates and identification of correlates of immunity. Clin. Immunol. 108: 51-59.

Brosnahan, A. J. and Schievert, P. M. (2011) Gram-positive bacterial superantigen outside-in signaling causes toxic shock syndrome. FEBS J. 278:4649-4667.

Brosnahan, A. J., Mantz, M. J., Squier, C. A., Peterson, M. L. and Schlievert, P. M. (2009) Cytolysins augment superantigen penetration of stratified mucosa. J. Immunol. 182: 2364-2373.

Canaan, A., Marcus, H., Burakova, T., David, M., Dekel, B., Segal, H., and Reisner, Y. (1999) T cell control of staphylococcal enterotoxin B (SEB) lethal sensitivity in mice: CD4+CD459bright)/CD4+Cd45RB(dim) balance defines susceptibility to SEB cytotoxicity. Eur. J. Immunol. 29: 1375-1382.

Casman, E. P. (1960) Further serological studies of staphylococcal enterotoxin. J. Bacteriol. 79: 849-856.

Casman, E. P., Bennett, R. W., Dorsey, A. E., and Issa, J. A. (1967) Identification of a fourth staphylococcal enterotoxin, enterotoxin D. J. Bacteriol. 94: 1875-1882.

Chiang, Y. C., Liao, W. W., Fan, C. M., Pai, W. y. Chiou, C. S., and Tsen, H. Y. (2008) PCR detection of staphylococcalenterotoxins (SEs) N, O, P, Q, R, U and survey of SE types in *Staphylococcus aureus* isolates from food-poisoning cases in Taiwan. Int. J. Food Microbiol. 15: 66-73.

Chen, J. Y., Qiao, Y., Komisar, J. L., Baze, W. B., Hsu, I. C., and Tseng, J. (1994) Increased susceptibility to staphylococcal enterotoxin B in mice primed with actinomycin D. Infect. Immun. 62: 4626-4631.

Chesney, P. J., Davis, J. P., Purdy, W. K., Wand, P. J., and Chesney, R. W. (1981) Clinical manifestations of toxic shock syndrome. JAMA 246: 741-748.

Choi, Y. W., Kotzin, B., Herron,L., Callahan, J., Marrack, P., and Kappler, J. (1989) Interaction of Staphylococcus aureus toxin "superantigens" with human T cells. Proc Natl Acad Sci U S A. 86: 8941-8945.

Croddy, E. C., Hart, C., and Perez-Armendariz J., *Chemical and Biological Warfare*, (Google Books), Springer, 2002,pp. 30-31, (ISBN 0387950761

Dack, G. M., Cary, W. E., Wollpert, O., and Wiggins, H. J. (1930) An outbreak of food poisoning proved to be due to a yellow haemolytic Staphylococcus. J. Prev. Med. 4: 167-175.

da Cunha, M., Calsolari, R. A., and Junior, J. P. (2007) Detection of enterotoxin and toxic shock syndrome toxin 1genes in Staphylococcus, with emphasis on coagulase-negative staphylococci. Microbiol. Immunol. 51: 381-390.

Das, U. N. (2000) Critical advances in septicemia and septic shock. Crit. Care 4:290–296.

Davis, J. P. Chesney, P.J., Wand, P.J., and LaVenture M. (1980) Toxic-shock syndrome: epidemiologic features, recurrence, risk factors, and prevention. N. Engl. J. Med. 303, 1429-1435.

Desouza, I. A., Franco-Penteado, C. F., Camargo, E. A., Lima, C. S., Teixeira, S., Muscara, M. N., De Nucci, G., and Antunes, E. (2006) Acute pulmonary inflammation induced by exposure of the airways to staphylococcal enterotoxin type B in rats. Toxicol. Appl. Pharmacol. 15: 107-113.

DeVries, A. S., Lesher, L., Schlievert, P. M., Rogers, T., Villaume, L. G., Danilla, R., and Lynfield, R. (2011) Staphylococcal toxic syndrome 2000-2006: epidemiology, clinical features, and molecular characterization.

Dinges, M. M., Orwin, P, M., and P. M. Schlievert, P. M. (2000) Exotoxins of *Staphylococcus aureus*. Clin. Microbiol. Rev. 13: 16-34.

Do Carmo, L. S., Cummings, C., Linardi, V. R., Dias, R. S., De Souza, J. M., Sena, M. J., Dos Santos, D. A., Shupp, J. U., Poreira, R. K., Jett, M. (2004) A case study of a massive staphylococcal food poisoning incident. Foodborne Pathog. 1: 241-246.

Fast, D. J., Schlievert, P. M., and Nelson, R. D. (1989) Toxic shock syndrome-associated staphylococcal and Streptococcal pyrogenic toxins are potent inducers of tumor necrosis factor production. Infect. Immun. 57: 291–294.

Faulkner, L., Cooper, A., Fantino, C., Altmann, D.M., and Sriskandan, S. (2005) The mechanism of superantigen-mediated toxic shock: not a simple Th1 Cytokine storm. J. Immunol. *175*: 6870-6877.

Fournier, B. (2008) Global regulation of *Staphylococcal aureus* virulence genes. In: Lindsay, J. S. (ed). Staphylococcus molecular genetics. Caister Academic Press, Norfolk, UK, pp. 131-183.

Franz, D. R., Parrott, C. D., and Takafuji, E. T. (1997) The U.S. biological warfare and biological defense programs, p. 425-436. *In* Textbook of military medicine. Part I. Warfare, weaponry and the casualty, vol. 3. U.S. Government. Printing Office, Washington, D.C.

Fraser, J. D., Urban, R. G., Strominger, J. L., and Robinson, H. (1992) Zinc regulates the function of twosuperantigens. Proc. Natl. Acad. Sci. 89: 5507-5511.

Fujisawa, N., Hayashi, S., Kurdowska, A., Noble, J. M., Naitoh, K., and Miller, E. J. (1998) Staphylococcal enterotoxinA injury of human lung endothelial cells and IL-8 accumulation are mediated by TNF-α. J. Immunol. 161:5627–5632

Goldsmith, S. J. and Signore, A. (2010) An overview of the diagnostic and therapeutic use of monoclonal antibodies in medicine. Q. J. Nucl. Mol. Imaging. 54: 574-581.

Graef, R. R., Anderson, G. P., Doyle, K. A., Zabetakis, D., Sutton, F. N., Liu, J. L., Serrano-González, J., Goldman, E. R., and Cooper, L. A. (2011) Isolation of a highly thermal stable lama single domain antibody specific for *Staphylococcus aureus* enterotoxin B. BMC Biotechnol. Published online 2011 September 21. doi: 10.1186/1472-6750-11-86.

Greenfield, R. A., Brown, B. R., Hutchins, J. B., Iandolo, J. J., Jackson, R., Slater, L. N., and Bronze, M. S. (2002) Microbiological, biological, and chemical weapons of warfare and terrorism. Am. J. Med. Sci. 323: 326-340.

Haffner, A. C., Zepter, K., and Elmets, C. A. (1996) Major histocompatability complex class I serves as a ligand for presentation of the superantigen enterotoxin B to T cells. Proc. Natl. Acad. Sci. 93: 3037-3042.

Hamad, A. R. A., Marrack, P., and Kappler, J. W. (1997) Transcytosis of staphylococcal enterotoxins. J. Exp. Med. 185: 1447-1454.

Henderson, D. A. (1999) The looming threat of bioterrorism. Science 283: 1279-1282.

Herz, U., Ruckert, R., Wollenhaupt, K., Tschernig, T., Neuhaus-Steinmetz, U., Pabst, R., and Renz, H. (1999) Airwayexposure to bacterial superantigen (SEB) induces lymphocyte-dependent airway inflammation associated with increased airway responsiveness--a model for non-allergic asthma. Eur.J. Immunol. 29: 1021–1031.

Horshburg, M. J. (2008) The response of *S. aureus* to environmental stimuli. In: Lindsay, J. S. (ed). Staphylococcus molecular genetics. Caister Academic Press, Norfolk, UK, pp. 185-206.

Hursh S, McNally, R., Fanzone, J. Jr, and Mershon, M. (1995) Staphylococcal Enterotoxin B Battlefield ChallengeModeling with Medical and Non-Medical Countermeasures. Joppa, Md: Science Applications International Corp; Technical Report MB DRP-95-2.

Hu, D. L., Zhu, G., Mori, F., Omoe, M., Wakabayashi, K., Kaneko, S., Shinagawa, K., and Nakane, A. (2007)Staphylococcal enterotoxin induces emisis through increasing serotonin release in intestine and it is downregulated by cannabinoid receptor 1. Cell. Microbiol. 9: 2267-2277.

Hu, D. L., Omoe, K., Shimoda, Y., Nakane, A., and Shinagawa, K. (2003) Induction of emetic response tostaphylococcal enterotoxin in the House Musk Shrew (Suncus murinus). Infect. Immun. 71: 567-570.

Jardetzky, T. S., Brown, J. H., Gorga, J. C., Stern, L. J., Urban, R. G., Chi, Y. I., Stauffacher, C., Strominger, and J. L., Wiley, D. C. (1994) Three-dimensional structure of a human class II histocompatibility molecule complexed with superantigen. Nature 368: 711-718.

Jarraud, S., Peyrat, M. A., Lim, A., Tristan, A., Bes, M., Mougel, C., Etienne, J., Vandenesch, F., Bonneville, M., and in Staphylococcus aureus. J. Immunol. 166: 669-677.

Kasai, T., Inada K., Takakuwa T., Yamada Y., Inoue Y., Shimamura T., Taniguchi S., Sato S., Wakabayashi G., and Endo S. (1997) Anti-inflammatory cytokine levels in patients with septic shock. Res. Commun. Mol. Pathol. Pharmacol. 98:34–42.

Karlson, S, Pettila, V., Tenhunen, J., Lund, V., Hovilehto, S., and Ruokonen, E. (2008) Vascular endothelial cell growth factor in severe sepsis and septic shock. Anesth. Analg. 106: 1820-1826.

Kerouanton, A., Hennekinne, J. A., Letertre, C., Petit, L., Chesneau, O., Brisabois, A., and De Buyser, M. L. (2007)Characterization of *Staphylococcus aureus* strains associated with food poisoning outbreaks in France. Int. J. Food Microbiol. 115: 369-375.

Khan, A. S., Cao, C, J., Thompson, R. G., and Valdes, J. J. (2003) A simple and rapid fluorescence-based immunoassay for the detection of staphylococcal enterotoxin B. Mol. Cell. Probes 17: 125–126.

King, G. L. (1990) Animal models for studying vomiting. Can. J. Physiol. Pharmacol. 68: 260-268.

Kissner (a), T. L., Ruthel, G., Alam, S., Ulrich, R. G., Fernandez, S., and Saikh, K. U. (2011) Activation of MyD88 signaling upon staphylococcal enterotoxin binding to MHC class II molecules. Plos One 20: e15985.

Kissner (b), T. L., Ruthel, G., Cisney, E. D., Ulrich, R. G., Fernandez, S., and Saikh, K. U. (2011) MyD88-dependent pro-inflammatory cytokine response contributes to lethal toxicity of staphylococcal enterotoxin B in mice. Innate Immun. 17: 451-462.

Kman, N. E. and Bachmann, D. J. (2011) Biosurveillance: a review and update. Adv. Preventive Med. www.hindawi.com/journals/apm/aip/301408/ -

Krakauer, T. (2010) Therapeutic down-modulators of staphylococcal superantigen-induced inflammation and toxic shock. Toxins: 2: 1963-1983.

Krauker, T., Buckley, M., and Fisher, D. (2010) Murine models of staphylococcal enterotoxin B-induced toxic shockMil. Med. 175: 917-922.

Krakauer, T. (1994) Costimulatory receptors for the superantigen staphylococcal enterotoxin B on human vascular endothelial cells and T cells. J. Leukocyte Biol. 56: 458-463.

Kumar, S., Menoret, A., Ngoi, S., and Vella, A. T. (2010) The systemic and pulmonary immune response to staphylococcal enterotoxins. Toxins 2: 1898-1912.

Kusnecov, A. W. and Goldfarb, Y. (2005) Neural and behavorial responses to systemic immunologic stimuli: a consideration of bacterial T cell superantigens. Curr. Pharm. Des. 11: 1039-1046.

Larkin, E. A., Carman, R. J., Krakauer, T., and Stiles, B. G. (2009) *Staphylococcus aureus*: The toxic presence of a pathogen extraordinaire. Cur. Medicinal Chem. 16: 4003-4019.

LeClaire, R. D., Hunt, R. E., and Bavari, S. (2002) Protection against bacterial superantigen staphylococcal enterotoxin B by passive vaccination. Infect. Immun. 70: 2278-2285.

Le Loir, Y., Baron, F., and Gautier, M. (2003) *Staphylococcal aureus* and food poisoning. Genet. Mol. Res. 2: 630-76.

Li, Y., Li, H., Dimasi, N., McCormick, J. K. and Martin, R. (2001) Crystal structure of a superantigen bound to the high-affinity zinc-dependent site on MHC class II. Immunity 14: 93-104.

Lindsay, J. A. (2011) Genomics of *Staphylococcus*. pp. 243-267 in Genomics of Foodborne Pathogens, Weidman, M. and Zhang, W. Springer Science+Business Media, Springer, New York, New York.

McCormick, J. K., Yarwood, J. M. and Schlievert, P. M. (2001) Toxic shock syndrome and bacterial superantigens: an update. Annu. Rev. Microbiol. 55: 77-104.

McCormick, J. K. Bohach, G. A., and Schlievert, P. M. (2003) Pyrogenic, lethal and emetic properties of superantigens in rabbits and primates. Meth. Mol. Biol. 214: 245-253.

Magnotti, L. J., Upperman, J. S., Xu, D. Z. Lu, Q., and Deitch, E. (1998) Gut-derived mesenteric lymph but not portal blood increases endothelial cell permeability and promotes lung injury after hemorrhagic shock. Ann. Surg. 228: 518-527.

Marrack, P., Blackman, M., Kushnir, E., and Kappler, J. (1990) The toxicity of staphylococcal enterotoxin B in mice is mediated by T cells. J. Exp. Med. 171: 455-464.

Marrack, P. and Kappler, J. (1990) The staphylococcal enterotoxins and their relatives. Science. 248: 705-709.

Mattix, M. E., Hunt, R. E., Wilhelmsen, C. L., Johnson, A. J., and Baze, W. B. (1995) Aerosolized staphylococcal enterotoxin B-induced pulmonary lesions in rhesus monkeys (*Macaca mulatta*). Toxicol. Pathol. 23: 262-268.

Melkus, M. W., Estes, J. D., Padgett, T. A., Gatlin, J., Denton, P. W., Wege, A. K., Hasse, A. T. and Garcia, J. V. (2006) Humanized mice mount specific adaptive and innate immune responses to EBV and TSST-1. Nat. Med. 12: 1316-1322.

Miethke, T., Wahl, C., Heeg, K., Echtenacher, B., Krammer, P. H., and Wagner, H. (1992) T cell-mediated lethal shock triggered in mice by the superantigen superantigen staphylococcal enterotoxin B: critical role of tumor necrosis factor. J. Exp. Med. 175: 91–98

Nagaki, M., Muto, Y., Ohnishi, H., Yasuda, S., Sano, K., Naito, T., Maeda, T., Yamada, T., and Moriwaki, H. (1994) Hepatic injury and lethal shock in galactosamine-sensitized mice induced by the superantigen staphylococcal enterotoxin B. Gasteroenterology 106: 450-458.

Nagashima, T., Aranamai, T., Iclozan, C., and Onoe, K. (2004) Analysis of T Cell responses to a superantigen, staphylococcal enterotoxin-B. J. Clin. Exp. Hematopathol. 44: 25-32.

Neumann, B., Engelhardt, B., Wagner, H., and Holzmann, B. (1997) Induction of acute inflammatory lung injury by Staphylococcal enterotoxin B. J. Immunol. 158: 1861-1871.

Nout MJ., Notermans S., and Rombouts, FM. (1988) Effect of environmental conditions during soya-beanfermentation on the growth of *Staphylococcus aureus* and production and thermal stability of enterotoxins A and B. Int J. Food Microbiol. 31: 299-309.

Ono, H. K., Omoe, K., Imanishi, K., Iwakabe, Y., Hu, D., Kato, H., Saito, Naoyuki, Nakane, A., AUchiyama, T., andShinagawa, K. (2008) Identification and characterization of two novel staphylococcal enterotoxins, Types S and T. Infect. Immun. 76: 4999-5005.

Ortega, E., Abriouel, H., Lucas, R., and Galvez, A. (2010) Multiple roles of *Staphylococcus aureus* entertoxins: pathogenicity, superantigenic activity, and correlation to antibiotic resistance. Toxins 2: 2117-2131.

Otero, A., Garcia, M. L., Garcia, M. C., Moreno, B., and Bergdoll, M. S. (1990) Production of staphylococcal enterotoxins C1 and C2 and thermonuclease throught the growth cycle. Appl. Envion. Microbiol. 56: 555-559.

Papageorgiou, A. C., Acharya, K. R. (2000) Microbial superantigens: from structure to function. Trends Microbiol. 8: 369-75.

Papageorgiou, A. C., Tranter, H. S., and Acharya, K. R. (1998) crystal structure of microbial superantigen enterotoxin B at 1.5 A resolution: implications for superantigen recognition by MHC class II molecules and T-cell receptors. J. Mol. Biol. 277: 61-79.

Peterson, M. L., Ault, K., Kremer, M. J., Klingelhutz, A. J., Davis, C. C., Squier, C. A., and Schlievert P. M. (2005) The innate immune system is activated by stimulation of vaginal epithelial cells with *Staphylococcus aureus* and toxic shock syndrome toxin 1. Infect. Immun. 73: 2164-2174.

Phillips, M. D. (2005) Bioterrorism: a brief history. Focus on Bioterrorism. www.DCMSonline.org.

Pinchuk, I. V., Beswick, E. J., and Reyes, V. E. (2010) Stapylococcal enterotoxins. Toxins: 2: 2177-2197.

Ples, D. D., Ruthel, G., Reinke, E. K., Ulrich, R. G., and Bavari, S. (2005) Persistance of zinc-binding bacterial superantigens at the surface of antigen-presenting cells contributes to the extreme potency of these superantigens as T-cell activators. Infect. Immun. 73: 5358-5366.

Rajagopalan, G., Smart, M. K., Krco, C. J., and David, C. S. (2002) Expression and function of transgenic HLA-DQ molecules and lymphocyte development in mice lacking invariant chain. J. Immunol. 169: 1774-1783.

Rajagopalan, G., Smart, M. K., Murali, N., Patel, R., and David, C. S. (2007) Acute systemic immune activation following vaginal exposure to staphylococcal enterotoxin B—implications for menstrual shock. J. Reprod. Immunol. 73: 51-59.

Rajagopalan, G., Sen, M. M., Singh, M., Murali, N., Nath, K. A., Iijima, K., Kita, H., Leontovich, A. A., Gopinathan,U., Patel, R., and David, C. S. (2006) Internasal exposure to staphylococcal enterotoxin b elicits an acute systemic inflammatory response. Shock 25: 647-656.

Sapsfors, K. E., Taitt, C. R., Loo, N., and Frances, S. (2005) Biosensor detection of botulinum toxoid A and staphylococcal enterotoxin in food. Appl. Environ. Microbiol. 71: 5590-5592.

Schad, E. M., Papageorgiou, A., C., Svensson, L. A., and Acharya, K. R. (1997) A structrural and functional comparison of staphylococcal enterotoxin A and C2 reveals remarkable similarity and dissimilarity J. Mol. Biol. 269: 270-280.

Soejima, T., Nagau, E., Yano, Y., Yamagata, H., Dagi, H., Sinagawa, K. (2007) Risk evaluation for staphylococcal food poisoning in processed milk produced with skim milk powder. Int. J. Food Microbiol. 115: 29-34.

Slifka, M. K., and J. L. Whitton. (2000) Clinical implication of dysregulated cytokine production. J. Mol. Med. 78:74–80.

Stevens, D. L. (1997) Streptococcal toxic shock syndrome. In: Leung DYM, Huber BT, Schlievert PM, eds. Superantigens: Molecular Biology, Immunology, and Relevance to Human Disease. New York, NY: Marcel Dekker, Inc; pp. 481–501.

Suda, T., Sato, A., Sugiura, W., and Chida, K. (1995) Induction of MHC class II antigens on rat bronchial epithelial cells by interferon-gamma and its effect on antigen presentation. Lung. 173:127-137.

Sundstrom, M., Abrahmsen, I., Antonsson, P., Mehindate, K., Morad, W., Mchindate, K., and Dohlsten, M. (1996)The crystal structure of staphylococcal enterotoxin type D reveals Zn^{2+}-mediated homodimerization. EMBO J. 15: 6832-6840.

Sugiyama, H., McKissic, E. M., Bergdoll, M. S., and Heller, B. (1964) Enhancement of bacterial endotoxin lethality by staphylococcal enterotoxin. J. Infect. Dis. 114: 111–118.

Rajkovic, A., El-Mousalij, B., Uynendaele, M., Brolet, P., Zorzi, W., Heinen, E., Foubert, E., and Debevete, J.(2006) Immunoquantitative real-time PCR for detection and quantification of staphylococcal enterotoxin B in foods. Appl. Environ. Microbiol. 72: 6593-6599.

Rotz, L. D., Khan, A. S., Lillibridge, S. R., Ostroff, S. M., and Hughes, J. M. (2002) Public health assessment of potential biological terrorism agents. *Emerg. Infectious Dis.* 8: 225-30.

Rusnak, J. M., Kortepeter, M., Ulrich, R., Poli, M., and Boudreau, E. (2004) Laboratory exposures to staphylococcal nterotoxin B. Emerg. Infect Dis.10: 1544- 1549.

Thomas, D. V., Jarraud, S., Lemercier, B., Cozon, G., Echasserieau, K., Etienne, J., Gougeon, M. I., Lina, G., and Vandensch, F. (2006) Staphylococcal enterotoxin-like toxins U2 and V, two new staphylococcal superantigens arising from recombination within the enterotoxin gene cluster. Infect. Immun. 74: 4724-4734.

Todd, J., Fishaut, M., Kapral, F., and Welch, T. (1978) Toxic-shock syndrome associated with phage-group 1 staphylococci. Lancet 2: 1116-1118.

Tseng, J., Komisar, J. L., Trout, R. N., Hunt, R. E., Chen, J. Y., Johnson, A. J., Pitt, L., and Ruble, D. L. (1995) Humoral immunity to aerosolized staphylococcal enterotoxin B (SEB), a superantigen, in monkeys vaccinated with SEB toxoid-containing microspheres. Infect. Immun. 63: 2880-2885.

Uchiyama, T., Imanishi, K., Miyoshi-Akiyama, T, and Kato, H. (2006) In: The Comprehensive Sourcebook of Bacterial Protein Toxins, J. E. Alouf and M. R. Popoff, Eds: Academic Press, Paris, pp. 830-843.

Ulrich, R. G., Olson, M. A., and Bavari, S. (1998) Development of engineered vaccines effective against structurally related bacterial superantigens. *Vaccine* 16: 1857-1864.

Ulrich, R. G., Sidell, S., Taylor, T. J., Wilhelmsen, C. L., and Franz, D. R. (1997) Staphylococcal enterotoxin B and related pyrogenic toxins, p. 621-631. *In* Textbook of military medicine. Part I. Warfare, weaponry and the casualty, vol. 3. U.S. Government. Printing Office, Washington, D.C.

van Gessel Y. A., Mani, S., Bi, .S, Hammamieh, R,, Shupp, J.W., Das, R., Coleman, G.D., and Jett, M. (2004) Functional piglet model for the clinical syndrome and postmortem findings induced by staphylococcal enterotoxin B. *Exp. Biol. Med.* 229: 1061-1071.

Wang, B. R., Zhang, X. J., Duan, X. L., Guo, X., and Ju, G. (2004) Fos Expression in the rat brain after intraperitoneal injection of Staphylococcus enterotoxin B and the effect of vagotomy. Neurochem. Res. 29: 1667-1674.

Wen, R., Cole, G. A., Surman, S., Blackman, M. A., and Woodland, D. L. (1996) Major histocompatability complex class II-associated peptides control the presentation of bacterial superantigens to T cells. J. Exp. Med. 183: 1083-1092.

White, J., Herman, A., Pullen, A. M., Kubo, K., Kappler, J. W., and Marrack, P. (1989) The V beta-specific superantigen staphylococcal enterotoxin B: stimulation of mature T cells and donal deletion in neonatal mice. Cell. 56: 27-32.

Williams, J. (2001). CBRNE—Staphylococcal enterotoxin B. http://www.emedicine.com/.

Wood, A., Todd, C. I., Cockayne, A., and Arbutnott, J. P. (1991) Staphylococcal enterotoxins and the immune system. FEMS Microbiol. Immunol. 3: 121-133.

Yarwood, J. M., McCormick, J. K., Paustian, M. L., Orwin, P. M., Dapur, V., and Schlievert, P. M. (2002) Characterization and expression analysis of *Staphylococcus aureus* pathogenicity island3. Implications for the evolution of staphylococcal enterotoxin pathogenicity islands. J. Biol. Chem. 277: 13138-13147.

Yuh, K., Siminovitch, K. A., and Ochi, A. (1993) T cell anergy is programmed early after exposure to bacterial superantigen *in vivo*. Int. Immunol. 5: 1375-1382.

Zalinskas, R. A. (1997) Iraq's biological weapons. The past as furure? JAMA 278: 418-82.

Zhang, W. J., Sarawar S., and Nguyen P. (1996) Lethal synergism between influenza infection and staphylococcal enterotoxin B in mice. J. Immunol 157: 5049–5060.

4

Diagnostic Bioterrorism Response Strategies

Rickard Knutsson
National Veterinary Institute (SVA),
Sweden

1. Introduction

Various biological agents such as bacteria, parasites, viruses and toxins may be deliberately released and spread through feed, food, water and air to cause harm and panic (Rotz et al., 2004). These biological agents can infect humans and animals but also crops (Gullino, 2008). Bioterrorism is probably the most inter-sectoral and international challenges among Chemical, Biological, Radiological, and Nuclear (CBRN) threats. To improve the interactions between these sectors there are some key issues involving R&D, training, event exercises, early warning and effective communication strategies that need to be addressed to rapidly share event information related to detection and identification. In this perspective, diagnostic capabilities are critical components to enhance the preparedness against bioterrorism (Morse, 2004). Covert and overt incidents will lead to various alarm chains. In a covert incident, which is characterized by an unannounced release, the early response and detection will be driven by public health organizations. However, an overt incident is characterized by the fact that the perpetrator announces responsibility and the response will therefore be driven by law enforcement. A diagnostic response strategy must be able to address both types of incidents. This requires a multidisciplinary network composed of diagnostic capabilities both in law enforcement agencies and public health organizations such as environmental, agricultural, veterinary, and food. As a result, laboratory response networks have been developed in different countries. The US Laboratory Response Network (LRN) was established in 1999. Its formation was based on a presidential order (Decision Directive 39) in which the Centers for Disease Control and Prevention (CDC), Association of Public Health Laboratories (APHL), Federal Bureau of Investigation (FBI), and United States Army Medical Research Institute of Infectious Diseases (USAMRIID) was involved (Morse, 2003). The objective of the US LRN is to ensure an effective laboratory response to bioterrorism by improving the law enforcement and public health laboratory infrastructure. The US LRN links local, state and national public health laboratories, as well as agriculture, veterinary, military, water- and food testing laboratories. In addition, the LRN links also to international laboratories in Canada, Australia, Japan, United Kingdom and Germany. Several other countries have developed similar laboratory networks such as Canada (CRTI, 2007), Australia (Editorial, 2004) and South Korea (Hwang, 2008). A Swedish LRN was established in 2009 with the aim of facilitating collaboration between law enforcement, first responders and public health agencies. The Swedish Forum for Biopreparedness Diagnostics (FBD) was established in 2007. FBD is a national laboratory multiagency cooperation, consisting of partners from the National Food Administration (SLV), the Swedish Defense Research Agency (FOI), the National Veterinary Institute (SVA) and the Swedish Institute for Communicable Disease Control (SMI). The aim of FBD is to strengthen the diagnostic capacity in Sweden regarding dangerous pathogens. The various laboratory networks that have been established in different countries have more or less the same objectives: rapid detection, identification and characterization of pathogens, targeted surveillance programs, strengthen laboratory response capacities and capabilities, and recovery. This includes; harmonization of diagnostic methods, increasing diagnostic capacity, training and exercises, interactions with other networks, and coordination of diagnostic emergency response. For these reasons, a broad diagnostic portfolio is needed in order to respond to covert and overt bioterrorism incidents. Diagnostic collaboration and networks are essential for an efficient response to a bioterrorism attack. Diagnostic response strategies must consider the abilities of the network in handling of the following: laboratories expertise, index case, decision making, tracing and tracking, and crime scene investigations.

2. Strategic planning

To obtain international multisectoral cooperation, in terms of bioterrorism prevention, policy makers have an important function. Policy makers at the local, regional, national and international levels must work in the same direction. However, this is not always realistic and as a result strategic planning is crucial, and the use of planning scenarios (DHS, 2005) can enhance strategic planning (Davis et al., 2007). Interagency collaborative efforts are one of the most critical factors to ensure an efficient bioterrorism preparedness and response plan. Several intergovernmental organizations such as INTERPOL (INTERPOL, 2010), World Health Organization (WHO), Food and Agricultural Organization (FAO) and World Organization for Animal Health (OIE) have ongoing programs and activities to counter the threat of attacks on humans, animals and plants (Pearson, 2006). The Biological and Toxin Weapon Convention (BTWC) prohibits the deliberate release of agents to attack plants, animals and humans (UN, 1972). However, effective prevention and countermeasures for deliberate attacks need to be developed in harmony with measures to control either natural or accidental outbreaks of disease.

A lot of strategic planning is taking place at the national level. For example, reports by the US Congressional Research Service identifies strategic planning as one of four critical areas of bioterrorism preparedness and that agency implementation will be a key component to translate strategic goals into effective programs and polices (Gottron, 2011). The European Union has also developed strategic plans on how to counter bioterrorism and CBRN attacks that are outlined in the EU CBRN Action Plan (EC, 2009). The Action Plan will be implemented in the period 2010 to 2014. Some examples of other countries focusing on strategic planning for bioterrorism are Canada (CRTI, 2007), South Korea (Hwang, 2008). A lot of progress has been made in strengthening local, regional/state, national and international capacities to detect and respond to bioterrorism since letters containing spores of *Bacillus anthracis* were sent via the US mail in 2001 (Rotz et al., 2004) (Smith, 2004). The anthrax letters caused the CDC to revise its strategic plan for bioterrorism preparedness and response (Koplan, 2001), which is focused on the following six focus areas:

1. Preparedness planning and readiness assessment (including the National Pharmaceutical Stockpile);
2. Detection, surveillance and epidemiology capacity;
3. Laboratory capacity including diagnosis and characterization of biological agents;

4. Response and health alert network/communications and information technology;
5. Communicating Health Risks and Health Information Dissemination; and
6. Education and training (Kun et al., 2002).

The European political leadership has made efforts to improve a coordinated EU response to the bioterrorism incidents. (Sundelius et al., 2004) (Tegnell et al., 2003). The efforts have improved strategic, tactical, and operational aspects of preparedness planning and response (Brandeau et al., 2009). The strategic planning efforts have formed the basis for multisectoral R&D activities within the field of bioterrorism diagnostics and have improved the laboratory response networks and interagency cooperation.

3. Laboratory infrastructure and communication

Interagency and multi-sectoral laboratory cooperation requires a well developed infrastructure in terms of (i) communication and IT-systems, (ii) facilities, (iii) instruments/equipments and (iv) staff. A solid interagency cooperation of the public health laboratories, veterinary, agriculture, military, and water- and food-testing laboratories infrastructure must be based on strategic plans. These plans must facilitate building integrated response architectures and the promotion of coordination. Various tools, such as discrete event simulation modeling (Hupert et al., 2002) and information infrastructure tools (Kun et al., 2002) are useful in developing the interagency cooperation for laboratory bioterrorism preparedness.

Communication and IT-systems. The laboratory infrastructure must include services to inform and communicate accurate diagnostic data at different levels (Zarcone et al., 2010). A key element for bioterrorism preparedness is information exchange and diseases outbreaks reporting (Horton et al., 2002). Surveillance systems are crucial for early warning of biothreat agents and a coordinated information infrastructure between surveillance and laboratory activities is needed. It has been found that there is a need for coordination between syndromic and laboratory based surveillance (Sintchenko et al., 2009). The diagnostic response strategies must simultaneously fit both the epidemiological and criminal investigations and ongoing activities to improve capabilities to share electronic laboratory diagnostic data (Zarcone et al., 2010). Rational communication procedures are a key mechanism to effective bioterrorism preparedness (Pien et al., 2006). Appropriate and secure communication tools are especially important in the alarm chain allowing police and first responders to contact public and animal health official in terms of covert and overt bioterrorism incident (Holmdahl et al,. 2011). In addition, it is important to facilitate communication between clinicians, sentinel laboratories and US LRN reference laboratories. A failure to communicate information may lead to delayed detection and a greater pressure to handle the incident (Pien et al., 2006). An important infrastructure feature is data handling and electronic information sharing. The US LRN includes approximately 1200 users which require a central point of contact (Morse, 2003). To securely share standard laboratory results between laboratories, LRN Results Messenger (LRN RM) has been established (CDC, 2007). The need for sharing data was clearly identified during the anthrax letter incident in 2001. Approximately 125,000 samples and more than 1 million tests were reported during the event (CDC, 2007). The lack of efficient data sharing tools made it difficult for the laboratories to share data. Laboratory results are critical during an outbreak and they facilitate the decision making. Therefore, to support early detection and response the laboratory should share data (CDC, 2007). The LRN RM has been installed in more than

150 LRN laboratories including public health, military, federal, food, veterinary and international labs (CDC, 2007). It allows storage and sharing of tests results for biological LRN assays. In addition, the data management supports electronic reporting of proficiency testing results and the ability of laboratories to review their test results and their performance.

Facilities and laboratories. To respond to human, animal and plant biothreat agents a number of laboratory facilities are needed; e.g. clinical laboratories, animal laboratories, plant laboratories, environmental laboratories, military laboratories and forensic laboratories. Most biothreat agents, which are also select agents (CDC) (APHIS), require various biosafety levels due to their pathogenic characteristics. According to work biosafety regulations agents such as *Variola major* (smallpox) and viral hemorrhagic fevers (Ebola, Marburg, etc) requires work at Biosafety Level 4 (BSL-4). Other agents such as *Bacillus anthracis*, *Fransicella tularensis*, and *Yersinia pestis* require BSL-3 laboratories. Foot and Mouth Disease virus (FMD), which is an animal pathogen, also requires a BSL-3 laboratory. In total, there are various laboratory levels such as BSL-2, BSL-3, BSL-4 and BSL-2 and BSL-3 animal facilities. All of these facilities have various design features and each facility has to fulfill different functional and operational goals.

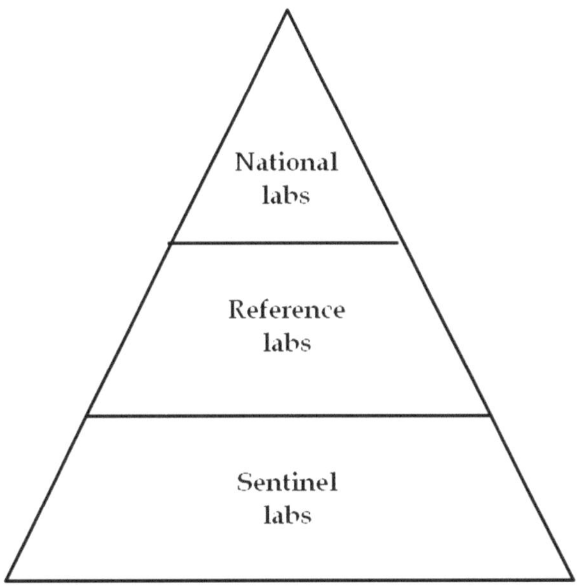

Fig. 1. The US Laboratory Response Networks in terms of operational components; National laboratories to perform definitive characterization, Reference laboratories to perform confirmatory testing and Sentinel labs to recognize and rule-out (Nauschuetz, 2005).

Instruments/equipments. The laboratories must be equipped with appropriate and evaluated instruments that also are operational in a BSL-3 or BSL-4 laboratory. The interior of these labs must also be designed for different chemical and gas decontamination methods. Many BSL-3 and BSL-4 laboratories are composed of stainless steel to allow decontamination work of highly pathogenic microorganisms, which require the highest level of cleanliness and durability. Proper biosafety cabinets, autoclaves, glove boxes and ventilation systems must continuously be monitored and tested. A lot of work in these laboratories is based on traditional methods such as labor intensive cultivation, autopsy and necropsy. However, there is a need to have alternative methods for complementary tests such as molecular based instruments in a BSL-3 level or BSL-4 environment. It is therefore important to evaluate computers, DNA extraction robots and PCR equipment from an operational point of view for these laboratories.

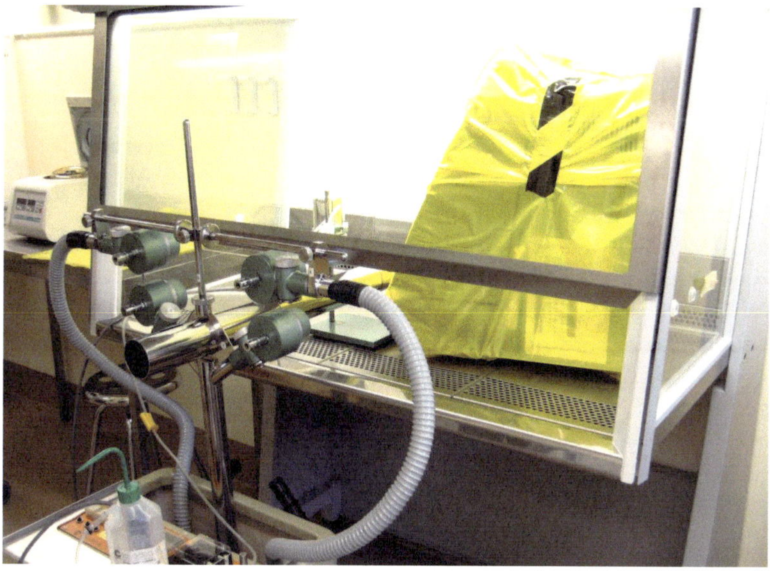

Fig. 2. The unique potassium iodide KI-discus-test, to validate a class II safety cabinet with a DNA isolation robot in a BSL-3 laboratory. The KI discus test is defined in the European Standard for microbiological safety cabinets, EN12469:2000 as a test method for validating the operator protection capabilities of the cabinet (Photo: SVA).

Staff. Having trained personnel is critical for the overall bioterrorism preparedness effort (Barden, 2002) and leadership (Marshall et al., 2010). Additional training and education is necessary to work in BSL-3 and BSL-4 labs. Minimum requirements in terms of general biosafety training include definitions of biological and bio-hazardous materials, risk groups, biosafety containment levels, controls and protective clothing including staff at sentinel laboratories (Wagar et al., 2010). Various training courses are available and one example is a Bioterrorism Preparedness Training for LRN Sentinel Laboratories offered by the National Laboratory Training Network (NLTN, 2011). It is important to have training on various diagnostic methods as well as training related to biosafety and biosecurity (Kalish et al., 2009). Joint laboratory exercises are used to evaluate the laboratory organization. Education is also crucial in the other sectors such as veterinary laboratories (Lowenstine et al., 2006).

4. Laboratory standards, certification and methods

Many regulations, practices, programs and inspections have to be met and/or fulfilled to be allowed to work on biothreat agents. This requires inspections at organizational-, facility- and personnel level. The regulations and inspections differ from country to country and from sector to sector. The US Select Agents Program clearly regulates the use and transfer of specific biological agents and the program promotes laboratory safety and security (CDC, 2010). Other countries such as the United Kingdom, France, Denmark, Japan, Australia and Canada also have programs for governing facilities and personnel working on biothreat agents (NCBI, 2009). The Biological Weapon Convention (BTWC) (UN, 1972) and the United Nations Security Council (UNSCR1540, 2004) states that each nation should take action to implement national measures to avoid misuse of biological agents. However, other groups also exist. One example is the Australian Group, which is an informal forum of countries which seeks to ensure that exports do not contribute to the development of biological weapons (AG, 2010). These various programs and conventions to avoid misuse of biological agents shall be considered for laboratories working on biothreat agents.

Laboratory standards. In 2004 the World Health Organization (WHO) published the latest edition of their biosafety manual (WHO, 2004). After publication of this manual, WHO continued to work and in 2006 they published the *Biorisk Management: Laboratory Biosecurity Guidance* (WHO, 2006). This guide integrates biosafety and biosecurity. The European Committee for Standardization/Comité Européen de Normalisation (CEN) has continued to work on the WHO Biorisk management standard, and in 2008 CEN published Laboratory Biorisk Management Standard CWA 15793:2008 (CEN, 2008). The biorisk management standard provides guidance to an organization to identify, monitor and control laboratory biosafety and biosecurity in order to ensure that organizations are well prepared to respond if biological agents are released or go missing.

Laboratory certification. For laboratories working on biothreat, BSL-3 and BSL-4 agents, it is important to have a certified laboratory to confirm that the organization and facility is working with the highest and most appropriate standards. For this reason the organization must operate within international guidelines and national regulations. Facilities working on biothreat agents require laboratory or personnel certification (Gottron, 2011). The laboratory certification process of BSL3- and BSL-4 laboratories involves compliance with a number of criteria in terms of bisafety and biosecurity. For instance, it includes a systematic review of safety processes within the laboratory such as personal protective equipment, building and system integrity and standard operating procedures (SOPs). It also includes administrative documentation and record retention systems. Therefore, to respond to a bioterrorism incident a laboratory certification process will form the basis for a well prepared and appropriate laboratory capability.

Laboratory methods and harmonized protocols. Harmonized methods and protocols are extremely important for multisectoral cooperation (Hodges et al., 2010). This means that standard protocols and reagents must be used to confirm tests. These activities can differ from country to country. To allow development of standardized and validated methods for detection and identification of biothreat agents, proficiency testing and ring trials by sending samples to different laboratories are required. For this reason a Critical Reagents Program (CRP) has been established in the US. The CRP collection includes inactivated antigens of select agent, genomic materials from biothreat agents and monoclonal and polyclonal antibodies of biothreat agents (CRP, 2011). This is a key component of laboratory preparedness as shortages of critical reagents will significantly influence the response testing (APHL, 2006). Based on validated reagents new methods can be developed, evaluated and tested (Donoso Mantke et al., 2005). The LRN laboratories use standardized protocols and reagents to detect and identify biothreat agents. The standardized protocols are developed in such a manner that they contain information for chain-of-custody requirements.

5. Development of diagnostic response strategies

Law enforcement and public health must plan together to develop diagnostic response strategies for overt and covert bioterrorism incidents. This involves joint efforts to: (i) follow-up on lessons learned from previous incidents; (ii) scenario planning, training and exercises; (iii) R&D activities; and (iv) validate and implement methods in response plans. Methods for detection and identification of microorganisms and toxins forms the basis (Skinner et al., 2009) (Musshoff et al., 2009).

Lessons learned from bioterrorism incidents and biocrimes. Several bioterrorism incidents and biocrimes have taken place, which have provided important lessons learned. For example, some more well known cases includes a salmonellosis outbreak in Oregon, a shigellosis outbreak in Dallas, the anthrax attacks of 2001 (amerithrax) and the the Aum Shinrikyo's attempt to develop biological weapons. The first case, the source of the 1984

Attackers	Motive	Year and location	Agent	Distribution and transmission mode	Reference
Rajneeshee cult	Religious motive to gain political control by influencing an election by making voters ill.	1984, The Dalles, Oregon, USA	*Salmonella typhimurium* ATCC 14028	Sallad bars/restaurants (blue cheese dressing, potato salad, lettuce)	(Torok et al., 1997)
Aum Shinrikyo	An apocalyptic cult with a motive to trigger a world war	1993, Tokyo, Japan	*Bacillus anthracis*	Aerozolization of a liquid suspension of *B. anthracis*	(Keim et al., 2001; Takahashi et al., 2004) (Olson, 1999)
Lone wolf	A laboratory employee invited other laboratory workers to eat pastries in the coffee room	1996, at a clinical laboratory in Dallas, Texas, USA	*Shigella dysenteriae* Type 2	Contamination of doughnuts and muffins	(Kolavic et al., 1997)
Lone wolf	Increase the importance of his research	2001, USA ("Amerithrax")	*Bacillus anthracis*	Letters with powder	(FBI, 2006) (Butler et al., 2002)

Table 1. Overview of some bioterrorism incidents/biocrimes (Dembek, 2007).

salmonellosis outbreak in The Dalles, Oregon, was puzzling beacuse the epidemiological investigation revealed multiple items of food were involved instead of a single suspect item (Table 1). In total, 751 salmonellosis cases were identified and 45 persons were hospitalized.

This was a deliberate outbreak perpetrated by members of the Rajneeshee cult. The cult legally obtained *Salmonella* Typhimurium ATCC 14028 and spread cultures of this organism on salad bars in area restaurants. The cause of the outbreak was found to be due to intentional contamination in October 1985, when the Federal Bureau of Investigation (FBI) investigated the cult (McDade et al., 1998). The FBI together with an Oregon public health laboratory official found an open vial of the strain in their laboratory more than a year after the outbreak took place. The culture of *Salmonella* Typhimurium ATCC 14028 found at the Rajneeshees farm was identical and indistinguishable from the outbreak strain that was isolated from clinical specimens and food items. The retrospective epidemiology was consistent and the deliberate contamination of the salad bars was confirmed (Torok et al., 1997). The case demonstrated the need for having joint cooperation between law enforcement and public health investigations. In addition, the case showed that many different food items and matrices may be responsible for a deliberate foodborne outbreak challenging the diagnostic capabilities. Various sample preparations methods for the different food items and food matrices will be needed.

In 1993 the Japanese Aum Shinrikyo cult released aerosolized spores of *B. anthracis* on two occasions. The first event took place in June when the cult sprayed *B. anthracis* from the roof of a building in downtown Tokyo. A month later the cult sprayed *B. anthracis* from a moving truck onto and around the Imperial Place and the Japan's parliament building in Tokyo (Dembek, 2007). However, none of the attacks led to any anthrax cases. In 2001, samples collected from the exterior of the exposed buildings in Tokyo were analyzed and it was found that the *B. anthracis* isolates were similar to the Sterne 34F2 strain, which is the strain used in animal vaccines for anthrax and is regarded as nonpathogenic for immunocompetent individuals. The release of this strain had little possibility of causing harm or death (Takahashi et al., 2004). From this incident one can learn that environmental sampling and proper storage is important. It also showed that microbial forensics is important as it enabled the investigators to identify the strain of *B. anthracis* released 8 years after the incident (Keim et al., 2001).

During the period between October 29th and November 1, 1996, 13 workers at a clinical laboratory in Dallas, Texas developed acute and severe diarrhea after consumption of muffins or doughnuts (Carus, 2001). The pathogen *Shigella dysenteriae* type 2 was isolated from stool samples from the infected workers. This pathogen is uncommon and no other shigellosis outbreaks occurred in the US at that time. Furthermore, no work on *Shigella* had taken place at that clinical laboratory. However, an examination of the freezer in the clinical laboratory showed some evidence of tampering with reference cultures of *S. dysenteriae* type 2. In August 1997, a laboratory technician was convicted of deliberately infecting coworkers with *Shigella dysenteriae* type 2 and sentenced to 20 years in prison (Everett, 2002). The laboratory and epidemiological investigations revealed a match of the laboratory strain to those isolated from food and clinical specimens. The tracing and epidemiological study was helped by the fact that only postproduction adulteration of the baked muffins and doughnuts could have resulted in their successful contamination.

On October 4, 2001, shortly after 9/11, an inhalation anthrax case was reported in a 63-old male in Florida (Fennelly et al., 2004). Subsequently, additional persons were identified who were infected with *B. anthracis*. Before the end of 2001, 22 cases of anthrax and 5 deaths had been reported. All of the anthrax cases were among postal workers or persons who had been in contact with contaminated mail. Exceptional collaboration was required from the different agencies involved. This event emphasized the importance of conducting public health and criminal investigations at the same time. The LRN served as a resource for identifying the agent in both environmental and clinical samples. An important lesson learned from this outbreak is that fine particles of a biological agent can become airborne, thus contaminating areas and placing persons at a risk and the need of microbial forensic (Dance, 2006).

There are many lessons to be learned from these incidents. Different types of attackers such as extremist groups and lone wolves have been involved. In addition, these incidents necessitate that forensic and epidemiological investigations occur at the same time. For example, to provide the link between isolates from clinical and various environmental and food samples with the person responsible for the deliberate spread. The need for multiple response teams has also been identified as a lesson learned.

Preparedness scenarios, training and exercises: The use of planning and preparedness scenarios between public health and law enforcement organizations will contribute to developing diagnostic response strategies. Different software tools are available for different preparedness applications. Over the last 10 years, various scenarios have been developed and used for different purposes. Modeling and bioterrorism scenarios have been used to evaluate responses to attacks with different agents causing diseases such as anthrax (Zaric et al., 2008), (Hupert et al., 2009), Foot and Mouth Disease (Schoenbaum et al., 2003), and Q-fever (Pappas et al., 2007), as well as decision making (O'Toole et al., 2001) and Bayesian approaches for estimating bioterror attacks (Ray et al., 2011). Different scenarios and exercises have been used to improve various counter measures such as a local bioterrorism exercise (Hoffman et al., 2000), an exercise on threat assessment and quantitative risk assessment (Zilinskas et al., 2004), and an exercise training bioterrorism surveillance system (Berndt, 2003). Because there are a number of published models and scenarios available these can be used to develop and improve scenarios to challenge diagnostic response strategies in terms of coordination, capabilities and capacity. Results and output from these scenarios, training and exercises can be used to initiate new R&D activities.

R&D activities. Joint R&D activities between first responders, forensic institutes and public health officials will contribute to developing appropriate methods. However this requires strategic planning and a laboratory infrastructure. Many R&D activities are performed in a specific sector, such as public health, animal health, food safety and law enforcement. Over the last few years joint diagnostic methods have been developed to counter bioterrorism. However, a lot of research has been performed without questioning the different diagnostic end-users at local, regional or national level and lessons learned from incidents and exercises have not always been considered. R&D activities have involved a broad spectra of methods such as electron microscopy (Goldsmith et al., 2009), new molecular methods (Casman, 2004), automated testing (Byrne et al., 2003) and screening (Emanuel et al., 2005), immunoassays for toxins (2008), microarray and multiplexing and nanotechnology methods (Menezes, 2011). Although technology has improved significantly since 2001 many diagnostic methods are still based on immunoassays, ELISA and PCR (Kellogg, 2010). First responders uses primarily field based immunoassays and portable PCR-assays for biothreat detection, and local and sentinel public health laboratories uses traditional culture and biochemical assays, ELISAs and molecular-based PCR methods for biothreat identification. A problem with conventional detection methods are the lack of positive controls since these methods are based on living organisms. Rapid detection methods have been well investigated (Canton, 2005) (Peruski et al., 2003). The most useful technology for identification of biothreat agents is real-time PCR. However, microarray and multiplex assays for detection of biothreat agents, such as *Bacillus anthracis, Francisella tularensis* and *Yersinia pestis* by using multiplex qPCR have recently improved (Janse et al., 2010).

Implementation in response plans. Once new diagnostic methods are developed, they need to be evaluated and validated. This is an important step and requires access to reagents for proficiency testing and ring trial evaluations. Methods need to be validated for use in real incidents. The methods must also full fill requirements for forensic applications, which adds another aspect, see Table 2.

Sample	**Monitoring and surveillance**	**Alarm (covert and/overt)**	**Laboratory Response**	**Forensics**
Animal	Animal Health and Animal surveillance	Veterinarians/ First responders	Veterinary laboratories	Forensic laboratories
Drinking water	Food and Environmental monitoring	Food inspectors/ First responders	Water and food laboratories	Forensic laboratories
Environmental	Environmental monitoring	Environmental inspectors/ First responders	Environmental laboratories	Forensic laboratories
Feed	Agricultural, Food and Animal Health	Agricultural inspectors/ First responders	Agricultural and veterinary Laboratories	Forensic laboratories
Food	Food surveillance	Food inspectors/ First responders	Food laboratories	Forensic laboratories
Human clinical	Human syndromic surveillance	Physicians/ First responders	Clinical laboratories (local, regional, national)	Forensic laboratories
Plant	Plant surveillance	Plant inspectors	Agricultural laboratories	Forensic laboratories

Table 2. A Bioterrorism response matrix outlining laboratory support and the multidisciplinary cooperation.

6. Challenges – coordination, capability and capacity

Diagnostic bioterrorism response strategies shall consider coordination/resilience, harmonization, robustness and high- resolution diagnostic tools. This includes R&D efforts of multidisciplinary detection technologies related to sampling, sample preparation, biomarker discovery, multiplexing and high resolution diagnostic typing tools (Knutsson et al., 2011). Clear mandate for coordination of response mechanisms is crucial and strong links between early warning systems provide a basis for the diagnostic bioterrorism response strategies.

Coordination - public health and forensic laboratories. Full international cooperation and efficient detection technologies are essential in order to respond efficiently to a bioterrorism event. Considering the detection needs for covert and overt bioterrorism events will require a broad range of analytical tools. There are many promising technologies on the market but still there is a need to develop emerging technologies for different end-users. This can be promoted by multidisciplinary cooperation between first responders, forensic institutes and diagnostic laboratories representing LRNs. First responders have prerequisites to use the technology for a rapid identification of the agent on site and at the crime scene. The detection technology must be user friendly and allow usage in hot, warm and cold emergency zones. Forensic institutes' major interest is to maintain chain of custody and have methods that are validated for use in court, including methods for evaluation of the results given the circumstances of the case (forensic interpretation). Public and animal health diagnostic laboratories have in general other needs. They must have a broad range of diagnostic methods available for further characterization and typing of the etiological agent. In general, joint response teams and the coordination and back-up of different laboratories are therefore crucial. The decision making procedure is very important and it has been described that in response to bioterrorism clinicians must make decisions in 4 critical domains (diagnosis, management, prevention and reporting to public health) and public health organizations must make decisions in 4 other domains (interpretation of bioterrorism surveillance data, outbreak investigation, outbreak control and communication) (Bravata et al., 2004). Early warning and coordinated rapid detection is a backbone and therefore the physicians' ability to recognize potential cases in the identification and treatment of diseases associated with bioterrorism is crucial (Bush et al, 2001), as well as for veterinarians (Davis, 2004). Bioterrorism response clinicians are essential partners to LRNs (Gerberding et al., 2002) and especially at sentinel laboratories (Pien et al., 2006). Examples of the importance of the clinicians work is clearly documented (Maillard et al., 2002) (Harris et al., 2011) and also the consequences if the diseases is not identified (Harris et al., 2011).

Capability and harmonization. To announce, for instance an anthrax outbreak (Sternberg Lewerin et al., 2010), and to make a declaration of an incident, decision makers needs validated methods. Standardized and validated PCR assays for high risk agents, such as *B. anthracis* (Wielinga et al., 2011) (Scarlata et al., 2010) and *C. botulinum neurotoxin* (Fenicia et al., 2011) are fundamental for confirming disease outbreaks. The methods should be tested in different countries and in different types of laboratories.

Capacity and robustness. Initial sampling and rapid detection is crucial (Leport et al., 2011). However, feed, food, environmental and clinical samples all contains components that may inhibit the analysis (e.g., PCR-inhibitors). Appropriate sampling (Knutsson et al., 2003) and pre PCR processing strategies are therefore needed in order to circumvent inhibition. For this purpose models to investigate PCR inhibition is an important step to study and evaluate prior to applying a method for a specific purpose (Knutsson et al., 2002) (Knutsson et al, 2002). Another important function is to have a laboratory surge capability in different areas in order to improve the robustness of the diagnostic capacity during a bioterrorism incident.

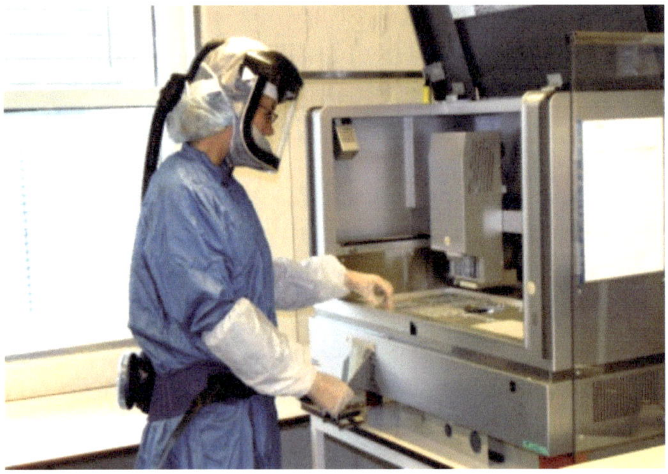

Fig. 3. Up-scaling capabilities by the use of automated DNA extractions robot in a BSL-3 laboratory (Photo: SVA).

High-resolution diagnostic tools. Multiplexing strategies for detection of several biomarkers (Lindberg et al., 2010), as well as various molecular typing methods are useful for crime scene investigation, but also for tracing and tracking the deliberate contamination. The use of massive parallel sequencing will be useful to study strain isolates from a suspicious deliberate contamination event. By applying bioinformatics it is possible to rapidly analyze large amounts of sequence data with minimal post-processing time (Segerman et al., 2011).

7. Conclusions

To obtain diagnostic bioterrorism response strategies a number of issues must be solved including strategic planning, laboratory infrastructure and standards. The laboratory work has to be strongly linked to different early warning and surveillance systems. Multiple teams as well as joint laboratory protocols are also important resources to have in place. The development of diagnostic bioterrorism response strategies should be based on lessons learned from previous attacks/incidents, planning scenarios, R&D activities and validation and implementations of methods. Laboratories must be able to detect, identify, respond and recover from covert and overt bioterrorism incidents. Key recommendations include:

- Multisectoral and international laboratory cooperation to obtain rapid detection and identification of biothreat agents
- Robust sampling and laboratory capacity for high-throughput needs
- Laboratory capabilities for diagnostic characterization needs
- Efficient IT-systems for sharing of data

8. Acknowledgements

Writing of this chapter has been supported by grants from the Swedish Civil Contingencies Agency (Anslag 2:4 Krisberedskap), Sweden (Swedish Laboratory Response Network), and the framework of the EU-project AniBioThreat (Grant Agreement:

Home/2009/ISEC/AG/191) with the financial support from the Prevention of and Fight against Crime Programme of the European Union, European Commission - Directorate General Home Affairs. This publication reflects the views of the author, and the European Commission cannot be held responsible for any use which may be made of the information contained therein. A special thanks to Communication Officer Jeffrey Skiby (DTU-Food, Denmark) for critical reading and suggestion and to Professor Birgitta Rasmusson (the Swedish National Laboratory of Forensic Science, SKL) for critical reading with a focus on forensics and Dr Gary Barker (Institute of Food Research, IFR, United Kingdom) for valuable comments on the section of diagnostic response strategies.

9. References

AG. (2010). "The Australia Group - List of Biological Agents for Export Control."

APHL (2006). Critical Shortage of LRN Reagents. Silver Spring MD, Association of Public Health Laboratories (APHL)

Barden, L. S., Delany, J.R., Glenn, S., Perry, S.R., Lipman, H., Escott, S.H., Luck, L. (2002). Training Laboratory Personnel To Identify the Agents of Bioterrorism, *Laboratory Medicine* Vol.(9): 699-703.

Berndt, D. J., Fisher, J., W, Hevner, A.R., Studnicki, J (2003). Bioterrorism Surveillance with Real-Time Data Warehousing, *Organization: IEEE Com* Vol.

Brandeau, M. L., McCoy, J. H., Hupert, N., Holty, J. E. & Bravata, D. M. (2009). Recommendations for modeling disaster responses in public health and medicine: a position paper of the society for medical decision making, *Med Decis Making* Vol.(4): 438-460.

Bravata, D. M., Sundaram, V., McDonald, K. M., Smith, W. M., Szeto, H., Schleinitz, M. D. & Owens, D. K. (2004). Evaluating detection and diagnostic decision support systems for bioterrorism response, *Emerg Infect Dis* Vol.(1): 100-108.

Bush, L. M., Abrams, B. H., Beall, A. & Johnson, C. C. (2001). Index case of fatal inhalational anthrax due to bioterrorism in the United States, *N Engl J Med* Vol.(22): 1607-1610.

Butler, J. C., Cohen, M. L., Friedman, C. R., Scripp, R. M. & Watz, C. G. (2002). Collaboration between public health and law enforcement: new paradigms and partnerships for bioterrorism planning and response, *Emerg Infect Dis* Vol.(10): 1152-1156.

Byrne, K. M., Fruchey, I. R., Bailey, A. M. & Emanuel, P. A. (2003). Automated biological agent testing systems, *Expert review of molecular diagnostics* Vol.(6): 759-768.

Canton, R. (2005). Role of the microbiology laboratory in infectious disease surveillance, alert and response, *Clin Microbiol Infect* Vol.: 3-8.

Carus, W. (2001). Working Paper: Bioterrorism and Biocrimes. The Illicit Use of Biological Agents Since 1900. F. Revision. Washington DC, Center for Counterproliferation Research, National Defense University.

Casman, E. A. (2004). The potential of next-generation microbiological diagnostics to improve bioterrorism detection speed, *Risk Anal* Vol.(3): 521-536.

CDC. (2007). "LRN Results Messenger and LIMS Integration."

CDC. (2010, http://www.bt.cdc.gov/agent/agentlist-category.asp). "CDC Bioterrorism Disease Agent List."

CEN (2008). The Laboratory Biorisk Management Standard.

CRP. (2011). "Critical Reagents Program (CRP)."

CRTI (2007). Chemical, Biological, Radiological-Nuclear and Explosives Reserach and Technology Initiative. Canada, Canadian Reserach and Technology Initiative. Annual Report 2006-2007.

Dance, A. (2008) Anthrax case ignites new forensics field. Nature Vol.454, 813.

Davis, P. K., Bankes, S.C., Egner, M.F. (2007). *Enhancing strategic planning with massive scenario generation: Theory and Experiments*, Rand Corporation.

Davis, R. G. (2004). The AbCs of bioterrorism for veterinarians, focusing on Category B and C agents, *J Am Vet Med Assoc* Vol.(7): 1096-1104.

Dembek, Z., Pavlin, J., Kortepeter, M. (2007). Epidemiology of Biowarfare and Bioterrorism. *Medical Aspects of Biological Warfare*. J. Redding, Mason, V., Wise, D., Metzgar, M., Lindsay, R., Frazier, A. Washington DC, The Office of the Surgeon General at TMM Publications.

DHS (2005). NATIONAL PLANNING SCENARIOS: Executive Summaries. F. Created for Use in National, State, &a. L. H. S. P. Activities. USA.

Donoso Mantke, O., Schmitz, H., Zeller, H., Heyman, P., Papa, A. & Niedrig, M. (2005). Quality assurance for the diagnostics of viral diseases to enhance the emergency preparedness in Europe, *Euro Surveill* Vol.(6): 102-106.

EC (2009). Communication from the commission to the european parliament and the council on strengthening chemical, biological, radiological and nuclear security in the European Unioin - an EU CBRN Action Plan. C. o. t. e. communities.

Editorial (2004). Australian Society for Infectious Diseases: Bioterrorism Response Advisory Group. Microbiology Australia. Melbourne, Australia, The Australian Society for Microbiology Inc. 25: 46.

Emanuel, P. A., Fruchey, I. R., Bailey, A. M., Dang, J. L., Niyogi, K., Roos, J. W., Cullin, D. & Emanuel, D. C. (2005). Automated screening for biological weapons in homeland defense, *Biosecurity and bioterrorism : biodefense strategy, practice, and science* Vol.(1): 39-50.

FBI (2006). Federal Bureau of Investigation. Amerithrax Fact Sheet - September 2006, http://www.fbi.gov/about-us/history/famous-cases/anthrax-amerithrax/amerithrax-fact-sheet

Fenicia, L., Fach, P., van Rotterdam, B. J., Anniballi, F., Segerman, B., Auricchio, B., Delibato, E., Hamidjaja, R. A., Wielinga, P. R., Woudstra, C., Agren, J., De Medici, D. & Knutsson, R. (2011). Towards an international standard for detection and typing botulinum neurotoxin-producing Clostridia types A, B, E and F in food, feed and environmental samples: a European ring trial study to evaluate a real-time PCR assay, *Int J Food Microbiol* Vol.: S152-157.

Fennelly, K. P., Davidow, A. L., Miller, S. L., Connell, N. & Ellner, J. J. (2004). Airborne infection with Bacillus anthracis--from mills to mail, *Emerging infectious diseases* Vol.(6): 996-1002.

Gerberding, J. L., Hughes, J. M. & Koplan, J. P. (2002). Bioterrorism preparedness and response: clinicians and public health agencies as essential partners, *JAMA* Vol.(7): 898-900.

Goldsmith, C. S. & Miller, S. E. (2009). Modern uses of electron microscopy for detection of viruses, *Clin Microbiol Rev* Vol.(4): 552-563.

Gottron, F., Shea, D.A., (2011). Federal Efforts to Address the Threat of Bioterrorism: Selected Issues and Options for Congress. C. R. Service, CRS Report for Congress.

Gullino, M., L., Fletcher, J., Gamliel, A., Stack, J.P. (2008). *Crop Biosecurity - Assuring our Global Food Supply*. Dordrecht, Springer.

Harris, M. D. & Yeskey, K. (2011). Bioterrorism and the vital role of family physicians, *Am Fam Physician* Vol.(1): 18, 20.

Hodges, L. R., Rose, L. J., O'Connell, H. & Arduino, M. J. (2010). National validation study of a swab protocol for the recovery of Bacillus anthracis spores from surfaces, *J Microbiol Methods* Vol.(2): 141-146.

Hoffman, R. E. & Norton, J. E. (2000). Lessons learned from a full-scale bioterrorism exercise, *Emerging infectious diseases* Vol.(6): 652-653.

Holmdahl, L., Granelli, K., Lorentzon, P., Danielsson, C., Knutsson, R., Myrén, S. (2011). Identifiering av larmvägar i händelse av avsiktlig smittspridning, biokriminalitet och bioterrorism, Vol.

Horton, H. H., Misrahi, J. J., Matthews, G. W. & Kocher, P. L. (2002). Critical biological agents: disease reporting as a tool for determining bioterrorism preparedness, *J Law Med Ethics* Vol.(2): 262-266.

Hupert, N., Mushlin, A. I. & Callahan, M. A. (2002). Modeling the public health response to bioterrorism: using discrete event simulation to design antibiotic distribution centers, *Med Decis Making* Vol.(5 Suppl): S17-25.

Hupert, N., Wattson, D., Cuomo, J., Hollingsworth, E., Neukermans, K. & Xiong, W. (2009). Predicting hospital surge after a large-scale anthrax attack: a model-based analysis of CDC's cities readiness initiative prophylaxis recommendations, *Med Decis Making* Vol.(4): 424-437.

Hwang, H. S. (2008). [The strategic plan for preparedness and response to bioterrorism in Korea], *J Prev Med Public Health* Vol.(4): 209-213.

INTERPOL (2010). *Bioterrorism Incident Pre-Planning & Response Guide*. Lyon, France, INTERPOL.

Janse, I., Hamidjaja, R. A., Bok, J. M. & van Rotterdam, B. J. (2010). Reliable detection of Bacillus anthracis, Francisella tularensis and Yersinia pestis by using multiplex qPCR including internal controls for nucleic acid extraction and amplification, *BMC microbiology* Vol.: 314.

Kalish, B. T., Gaydos, C. A., Hsieh, Y. H., Christensen, B. E., Carroll, K. C., Cannons, A., Cattani, J. A. & Rothman, R. E. (2009). National survey of Laboratory Response Network sentinel laboratory preparedness, *Disaster Med Public Health Prep* Vol.(2 Suppl): S17-23.

Keim, P., Smith, K. L., Keys, C., Takahashi, H., Kurata, T. & Kaufmann, A. (2001). Molecular investigation of the Aum Shinrikyo anthrax release in Kameido, Japan, *J Clin Microbiol* Vol.(12): 4566-4567.

Kellogg, M. (2010). Detection of biological agents used for terrorism: are we ready?, *Clinical chemistry* Vol.(1): 10-15.

Knutsson, R. (2011). A tracing tool portfolio to detect Bacillus anthracis, Clostridium botulinum and Noroviruses: bioterrorism is a food safety and security issue, *Int J Food Microbiol* Vol.: S121-122.

Knutsson, R., Lofstrom, C., Grage, H., Hoorfar, J. & Radstrom, P. (2002). Modeling of 5' nuclease real-time responses for optimization of a high-throughput enrichment PCR procedure for Salmonella enterica, *J Clin Microbiol* Vol.(1): 52-60.

Knutsson, R. & Rådström, P. (2003). Detection of pathogenic Yersinia enterocolitica by a swab enrichment PCR procedure, *Methods Mol Biol* Vol.: 311-324.

Knutsson, R., van Rotterdam, B., Fach, P., De Medici, D., Fricker, M., Lofstrom, C., Agren, J., Segerman, B., Andersson, G., Wielinga, P., Fenicia, L., Skiby, J., Schultz, A. C. & Ehling-Schulz, M. (2011). Accidental and deliberate microbiological contamination in the feed and food chains--how biotraceability may improve the response to bioterrorism, *Int J Food Microbiol* Vol.: S123-128.

Kolavic, S. A., Kimura, A., Simons, S. L., Slutsker, L., Barth, S. & Haley, C. E. (1997). An outbreak of Shigella dysenteriae type 2 among laboratory workers due to intentional food contamination, *JAMA* Vol.(5): 396-398.

Koplan, J. (2001). CDC's strategic plan for bioterrorism preparedness and response, *Public Health Rep* Vol.: 9-16.

Kun, L. G. & Bray, D. A. (2002). Information infrastructure tools for bioterrorism preparedness. Building dual- or multiple-use infrastructures is the task at hand for state and local health departments, *IEEE Eng Med Biol Mag* Vol.(5): 69-85.

Leport, C., Vittecoq, D., Perronne, C., Debord, T., Carli, P., Camphin, P. & Bricaire, F. (2011). [Infections at risk for epidemic or biological threat. Importance of the initial management of suspect patients], *Presse Med* Vol.(4 Pt 1): 336-340.

Lindberg, A., Skarin, H., Knutsson, R., Blomqvist, G. & Baverud, V. (2010). Real-time PCR for Clostridium botulinum type C neurotoxin (BoNTC) gene, also covering a chimeric C/D sequence--application on outbreaks of botulism in poultry, *Vet Microbiol* Vol.(1-2): 118-123.

Lowenstine, L. J. & Montali, R. J. (2006). Historical perspective and future directions in training of veterinary pathologists with an emphasis on zoo and wildlife species, *J Vet Med Educ* Vol.(3): 338-345.

Maillard, J. M., Fischer, M., McKee, K. T., Jr., Turner, L. F. & Cline, J. S. (2002). First case of bioterrorism-related inhalational anthrax, Florida, 2001: North Carolina investigation, *Emerg Infect Dis* Vol.(10): 1035-1038.

Margolis, D. A., Burns, J., Reed, S. L., Ginsberg, M. M., O'Grady, T. C. & Vinetz, J. M. (2008). Septicemic plague in a community hospital in California, *Am J Trop Med Hyg* Vol.(6): 868-871.

Marshall, S. A., Brokopp, C. D. & Size, T. (2010). Leadership principles for developing a statewide public health and clinical laboratory system, *Public Health Rep* Vol.: 110-117.

McDade, J. E. & Franz, D. (1998). Bioterrorism as a public health threat, *Emerg Infect Dis* Vol.(3): 493-494.

Menezes, G. A., Menezes, P,S., Menezes, C. (2011). Nanoscience in diagnostics: A short review, *Internet Journal of Medical Update 2011 January* Vol.(1): 16-23.

Morse, S. A., Kellogg, R.B., Perry, S., Meyer, R.F., Bray, D., Nichelson, D., Miller, J.M. (2003). Detecting Biothreat Agents: the Laboratory Response Network, *ASM News* Vol.(9): 433-437.

Morse, S. A., Kellogg, R.B., Perry, S., Meyer, R.F., Bray, D., Nichelson, D., Miller, J.M. (2004). The Laboratory Response Network. *Preparedness Against Bioterrorism and Re-Emerging Infectious Diseases*. J. Kocik, Janiak, M., Negut, M. Amsterdam, IOS Press: 26-35.

Musshoff, F. & Madea, B. (2009). Ricin poisoning and forensic toxicology, *Drug Test Anal* Vol.(4): 184-191.

Nauschuetz, W. F. (2005). Straight talk on bioterror from the Army's LRN gatekeeper, *MLO Med Lab Obs* Vol.(6): 10-11, 14, 16; quiz 18-19.

NCBI (2009). National Research Council (US) Committee on Laboratory Security and Personnel Reliability Assurance Systems for Laboratories Conducting Research on Biological Select Agents and Toxins. Responsible Research with Biological Select Agents and Toxins. Washington DC, National Academies Press

NLTN (2011). Bioterrorism Preparedness Training for Sentinel Laboratories 2011, National Laboratory Training Network: www.nltn.org/305-311.htm.

O'Toole, T. & Inglesby, T. V. (2001). Epidemic response scenario: decision making in a time of plague, *Public health reports* Vol.: 92-103.

Olson, K. B. (1999). Aum Shinrikyo: once and future threat?, *Emerg Infect Dis* Vol.(4): 513-516.

Pappas, G., Blanco, J. R. & Oteo, J. A. (2007). Q fever in Logrono: an attack scenario, *Enferm Infecc Microbiol Clin* Vol.(3): 199-203.

Pearson, G. S. (2006). Public perception and risk communication in regard to bioterrorism against animals and plants, *Rev Sci Tech* Vol.(1): 71-82.

Peruski, L. F., Jr. & Peruski, A. H. (2003). Rapid diagnostic assays in the genomic biology era: detection and identification of infectious disease and biological weapon agents, *Biotechniques* Vol.(4): 840-846.

Pien, B. C., Saah, J. R., Miller, S. E. & Woods, C. W. (2006). Use of sentinel laboratories by clinicians to evaluate potential bioterrorism and emerging infections, *Clin Infect Dis* Vol.(9): 1311-1324.

Ray, J., Marzouk, Y. M. & Najm, H. N. (2011). A Bayesian approach for estimating bioterror attacks from patient data, *Stat Med* Vol.(2): 101-126.

Rotz, L. D. & Hughes, J. M. (2004). Advances in detecting and responding to threats from bioterrorism and emerging infectious disease, *Nat Med* Vol.(12 Suppl): S130-136.

Scarlata, F., Colletti, P., Bonura, S., Trizzino, M., Giordano, S. & Titone, L. (2010). [The return of anthrax. From bioterrorism to the zoonotic cluster of Sciacca district], *Infez Med* Vol.(2): 86-90.

Schoenbaum, M. A. & Terry Disney, W. (2003). Modeling alternative mitigation strategies for a hypothetical outbreak of foot-and-mouth disease in the United States, *Prev Vet Med* Vol.(1-2): 25-52.

Segerman, B., De Medici, D., Ehling Schulz, M., Fach, P., Fenicia, L., Fricker, M., Wielinga, P., Van Rotterdam, B. & Knutsson, R. (2011). Bioinformatic tools for using whole genome sequencing as a rapid high resolution diagnostic typing tool when tracing bioterror organisms in the food and feed chain, *Int J Food Microbiol* Vol.: S167-176.

Sintchenko, V. & Gallego, B. (2009). Laboratory-guided detection of disease outbreaks: three generations of surveillance systems, *Arch Pathol Lab Med* Vol.(6): 916-925.

Skinner, C., Thomas, J., Johnson, R. & Kobelski, R. (2009). Medical toxicology and public health--update on research and activities at the Centers for Disease Control and Prevention, and the Agency for Toxic Substances and Disease Registry: introduction to the Laboratory Response Network-Chemical (LRN-C), *J Med Toxicol* Vol.(1): 46-49.

Smith, L. A. (2004). Bioterrorism: what level is the threat and are vaccines the answer?, *Expert Rev Vaccines* Vol.(5): 493-495.

Sternberg Lewerin, S., Elvander, M., Westermark, T., Nisu Hartzell, L., Karlsson-Norstrom, A., Ehrs, S., Knutsson, R., Englund, S., Andersson, A. C., Granberg, M., Backman, S., Wikstrom, P. & Sandstedt, K. (2010). Anthrax outbreak in a Swedish beef cattle herd - 1st case in 27 years: Case report, *Acta Veterinaria Scandinavica* Vol.(1): 7.

Sundelius, B. & Gronvall, J. (2004). Strategic dilemmas of biosecurity in the European Union, *Biosecur Bioterror* Vol.(1): 17-23.

Takahashi, H., Keim, P., Kaufmann, A. F., Keys, C., Smith, K. L., Taniguchi, K., Inouye, S. & Kurata, T. (2004). Bacillus anthracis incident, Kameido, Tokyo, 1993, *Emerg Infect Dis* Vol.(1): 117-120.

Tegnell, A., Bossi, P., Baka, A., Van Loock, F., Hendriks, J., Wallyn, S. & Gouvras, G. (2003). The European Commission's Task Force on Bioterrorism, *Emerg Infect Dis* Vol.(10): 1330-1332.

Torok, T. J., Tauxe, R. V., Wise, R. P., Livengood, J. R., Sokolow, R., Mauvais, S., Birkness, K. A., Skeels, M. R., Horan, J. M. & Foster, L. R. (1997). A large community outbreak of salmonellosis caused by intentional contamination of restaurant salad bars, *JAMA* Vol.(5): 389-395.

UN (1972). Convention of the Prohibition of the Development, Production and Stockpiling of Bacteriological (Biological) and Toxins Weapons and on thier Destruction. U. Nations. London, Moscow, Washington. Entered into force 26 March 1976.

UNSCR1540 (2004). United Nations Security Council Resolution 1540, United Nations.

Wagar, E. A., Mitchell, M. J., Carroll, K. C., Beavis, K. G., Petti, C. A., Schlaberg, R. & Yasin, B. (2010). A review of sentinel laboratory performance: identification and notification of bioterrorism agents, *Arch Pathol Lab Med* Vol.(10): 1490-1503.

WHO (2004). Laboratory Biosafety Manual. Geneva, World Health Organisation. 3rd.

WHO (2006). Biorisk management - Laboratory biosecurity guidance. Geneva, World Health Organisation.

Wielinga, P. R., Hamidjaja, R. A., Agren, J., Knutsson, R., Segerman, B., Fricker, M., Ehling-Schulz, M., de Groot, A., Burton, J., Brooks, T., Janse, I. & van Rotterdam, B. (2011). A multiplex real-time PCR for identifying and differentiating B. anthracis virulent types, *Int J Food Microbiol* Vol.: S137-144.

Zarcone, P., Nordenberg, D., Meigs, M., Merrick, U., Jernigan, D. & Hinrichs, S. H. (2010). Community-driven standards-based electronic laboratory data-sharing networks, *Public Health Rep* Vol.: 47-56.

Zaric, G. S., Bravata, D. M., Cleophas Holty, J. E., McDonald, K. M., Owens, D. K. & Brandeau, M. L. (2008). Modeling the logistics of response to anthrax bioterrorism, *Med Decis Making* Vol.(3): 332-350.

Zilinskas, R. A., Hope, B. & North, D. W. (2004). A discussion of findings and their possible implications from a workshop on bioterrorism threat assessment and risk management, *Risk analysis: an official publication of the Society for Risk Analysis* Vol.(4): 901-908.

5

Recent Advancement in the Development of Vaccines Against *Y. pestis* – A Potential Agent of Bioterrorism

Riyasat Ali and D.N. Rao
Department of Biochemistry, All India Institute of Medical Sciences, New Delhi, India

1. Introduction

A bioterrorism attack- is the deliberate release of biological agents such as viruses, bacteria, or toxins used to cause illness or death in people, animals, or plants (CDC). These agents are typically found in nature, but it is possible that they could be changed to increase their ability to cause disease, make them resistant to current therapeutics, or to increase their ability to be spread into the environment. Biological agents can be spread through the air, through water, or in food. Terrorists may use biological agents because they can be extremely difficult to detect and may not cause illness for several hours to several days. Some bioterrorism agents, like Variola major and *Yersinia pestis*, can be spread from person to person, while others e.g. *Bacillus anthracis* are not (Bioterrorism review, 2009). Biological agents make attractive weapons because they are relatively easy to obtain and carry from place to place, can be easily dispersed, and can cause widespread fear and panic beyond the actual physical damage they can cause. Many of the agents that could be used for bioterrorism have been divided into three categories A, B, and C, for public health preparedness based on various characteristics of the microbes or the diseases they cause.

Category A includes the most "dangerous" and highest priority for public health preparedness. Some of these pathogens can be transmitted from person-to-person, cause diseases with a high mortality rate and are likely to cause public panic and social disruption. Category A agents include *B. anthracis* (anthrax), Variola major (smallpox), *Francisella tularensis* (tularemia), *Y. pestis* (plague), *Clostridium botulinum* neurotoxin (botulism), and Viral hemorrhagic fever viruses (e.g. arenaviruses, filoviruses, bunyaviruses, and flaviviruses).

This chapter will discuss the Category A agent *Y.pestis*,the disease it causes,and recent efforts to develop vaccines.

Plague, a zoonotic disease caused by the gram-negative bacillus *Y. pestis* is primarily a disease of rodents, with transmission occurring through infected fleas. Human disease is acquired through rodent flea vectors, as well as respiratory droplets from animal to humans and humans to humans.

2. History of plague

The first reported pandemic of plague has been referred to as the "Great Plague of Justinian" (Sticker, 1908; Hirst,1953). This pandemic began around 532 AD in Egypt and spread through the Middle East and the Mediterranean basin, reaching Turkey, Constantinople, Greece, Italy, and the territories of France and Germany. The second pandemic, which is also known as the Black Death, began in 1334 in China and then spread westward along the trade routes to the Black Sea and eventually to Constantinople. The disease, which spread slowly and inevitably from village to village by infected rats and humans, or more quickly from country to country by ships, eventually killed 20 to 30 million people in Europe (Gottfried,1983). The third pandemic probably originated in the Chinese province of Yunnan around 1855 and spread to the southern coast of China, causing several smaller outbreaks. Larger epidemics occurred when the disease finally reached Canton and Hong Kong in 1894, thus marking the beginning of the third pandemic. Plague spread rapidly throughout the world through all inhabited continents, except Australia. Rats aboard the faster steamships that had replaced slow-moving sailing vessels in merchant fleets carried the disease. Between 1894 and 1903, plague entered 77 ports on 5 continents. During the early years of the third pandemic, the death toll in India and China alone was 12 million. In United State, plague was introduced in 1900. Between 1900 and 1924, most plague cases in the U.S. occurred in port cities along the Pacific and Gulf coasts (Link, 1955). More recently, a plague epidemic caused the death of several hundred residents in the Surat city of India between September and October 1994 (Perry and Fetherstone 1997).

The recent increase in the number of human plague cases together with the reappearance of epidemics in countries such as Malawi, Mozambique, and India has led to its designation by WHO as a re-emerging infectious disease (World Health Organization 2002, World Health Organization 2003). As of 30 July 2010, the Ministry of Health in Peru confirmed a total of 17 cases of pneumonic plague in Ascope province of Department La Libertad. The onset of symptoms for the last reported case of pneumonic plague was on 11 July 2010. During the investigations, 10 strains of *Y. pestis* were isolated from humans, rodents and domestic cats. In 2009, the Chinese Ministry of Health, reported a cluster of pneumonic plague cases in the remote town of Ziketan, Qinghai province. The first case was a 32 year old male herdsman, who developed fever and haemoptysis. Between 1990 and 2005, a total of 107 cases of plague were reported in the U.S.(Centers for Disease Control and Prevention, 2006). Recently there have been reports of 14 deaths potentially due to pneumonic plague in Madagascar (http://www.promed mail.org).

2.1 Plague as a biological weapon

In 1346, during the siege of Kafa (now Feodossia, Ukraine) the attacking Tartar forces catapulted the bodies of warriors who had died of plague into the besieged city as a weapon. It has been speculated that this operation may have been responsible for the advent of the Black Death in Europe (Wheelis, 2002; Lederberg, 2001). In World War II, Unit 731 of the Japanese army, developed plague-infected fleas in China resulting in outbreaks of plague (Harris, 1994). Later, to eliminate dependency on the flea vector, the U.S. and the Soviet Union biological weapons programs developed methods to aerosolize *Y.pestis*. The World Health Organization (WHO) has estimated that, if 50 kg of *Y. pestis* were released as an aerosol over a city of 5 million people, 150,000 would get pneumonic plague infection of which 36,000 would die (WHO 1970). The plague bacilli would remain viable as an aerosol for 1 hour for a distance of up to 10 km.

3. Clinical characteristics of plague

Plague can be broadly classified into three forms:

3.1 Bubonic plague

This is the classic form of the disease, which is characterised by swollen lymph nodes called buboes. Common symptoms are fever, headache, and chills occurring within 2 to 6 days of exposure to the organism either by flea bite or by contamination of open wounds with infected material. Gastrointestinal complications such as nausea, vomiting, and diarrhoea are common (Iteman et al., 1993, von Reyn et al., 1977). Buboes typically occur in the inguinal and femoral regions but may also occur in other regions of the body (Butler, 1989; Conrad et al., 1968). Bacteraemia or secondary plague septicaemia is frequently seen in patients with bubonic plague (Gage et al., 1992). In humans, the mortality of untreated bubonic plague is approximately 60%, but this is reduced to less than 5% with prompt, effective therapy.

3.2 Septicaemic plague

Primary septicaemic plague occurs mainly in patients with positive blood cultures but no palpable lymphadenopathy. Clinically, septicaemia caused by *Y.pestis* resembles that caused by other gram-negative bacteria. Common symptoms include chills, headache, malaise, and gastrointestinal disturbances. Patients with septicaemic plague are more likely to experience abdominal complications than compared those with bubonic plague. Even with treatment, the mortality of septicaemic plague may range from 30 to 50% (Crook and Tempest 1992, Hull et al., 1987, Poland and Barnes, 1979); untreated septicemic plague is virtually 100% fatal.

3.3 Pneumonic plague

Pneumonic plague is an infection of the lungs due to either inhalation of the organism (i.e., primary pneumonic plague), or dissemination to the lungs via the blood stream (i.e., secondary pneumonic plague). Pneumonic plague is the only form of the disease which is readily spread from person to person via respiratory droplets through close contact (2 to 5 ft) with an infected individual. It progresses rapidly from a flu-like illness to pneumonia with coughing and the production of bloody sputum. The incubation period for primary pneumonic plague is between 1 and 3 days. The last case of pneumonic plague in the U.S., resulting from person-to-person transmission occurred during the 1924 - 1925 epidemic in Los Angeles (Meyer, 1961). Between 1970 and 1993, 12% of U.S. plague patients developed pneumonia secondary to either the bubonic or septicemic form of the disease (Doll, 1994); In recent decades, 28% of human plague cases resulting from exposure to infected domestic cats in the U.S. presented as primary pneumonic plague. The mortality rate for untreated pneumonic plague is nearly 100%. Recent data from Madagascar epidemic indicates that mortality associated with respiratory involvement was 57%.

4. Microbiology

The genus *Yersinia*, a member of the family Enterobacteriaceae, consists of eleven species, of which three are pathogenic for humans: *Y. pestis; Y. pseudutuberculosis* and *Y. enterocolitica. Y. pestis,* is a gram-negative, non-motile, non-spore forming coccobacillus measuring 0.5 to 0.8 µm in diameter and 1 to 3 µm in length. The organism grows at 4 to 40^0 C with optimum growth at 28 to 30 ^{0} C; the optimum pH range is 7.2 to 7.6 but extreme pH (5 to 9.6) can be tolerated (Brubaker, 1972; Holt et al., 1994; Poland and Barnes, 1979; Poland et al., 1994). The lipopolysaccharide of *Y.pestis* is characterized as rough, possessing core components but lacking the extended O-group side chains. There is no true capsule; however, a carbohydrate-protein surface component, termed capsular antigen or fraction 1 (F1) is produced during growth above 33^0C (Barnes and Quan, 1992; Brubaker et al., 1972; Poland et al., 1994).Three biotypes (or biovars) of *Y. pestis* can be differentiated based on the conversion of nitrate to nitrite and fermentation of glycerol: *Antiqua, Orientalis* and *Mediaevalis*. Biotype *Antiqua* is positive for both characteristics, bitype *Orientalis* converts nitrate to nitrite but does not ferment glycerol, and biotype *Mediaevalis* ferments glycerol but does not form nitrite. Strains of the three biotypes exhibit no difference in their virulence or pathology in animals or humans (Brubaker et al., 1972; Poland et al., 1979). It is thought that *Antiqua* was responsible for the First Pandemic, *Mediaevalis* for the Second Pandemic, and *Orientalis* for the Third Pandemic. The majority of *Y. pestis* strains contain three virulence plasmids of 9.5, 70 to 75, and 100 to 110 kb (Ben-Gurion and Shafferman, 1981; Ferber and Brubaker, 1981; Filippov et al., 1990). In strain KIM and its derivatives, these plasmids are referred to as pPCP1 (pesticin, coagulase, plasminogen activator), pCD1 (calcium dependence), and pMT1 (murine toxin).

4.1 Life cycle

Plague primarily affects rodents. Transmission between rodents is associated with their fleas. While infection can occur by direct contact or ingestion, these routes do not normally play a role in the maintenance of *Y. pestis* in animal reservoirs. The rat flea (*Xenopsylla cheopis*), the classic vector for plague, ingests blood from an infected rodent (Hinnebusch and Schwan 1993). A bacterial load of 10^4 CFU/ml of rodent blood would ensure ingestion of at least 300 *Y. pestis* organisms. *Y.pestis* is cleared by some fleas but multiplies in the midgut (stomach) of others. Two days after an infected blood meal, the stomach exhibits clusters of brown specks containing *Y. pestis*. These develop into cohesive dark brown masses containing bacilli, a fibrinoid-like material, and probably hemin which extend throughout the stomach and into the proventriculus and esophagus. By 3 to 9 days after the infected blood meal, the bacterial masses may completely block the proventriculus, extend into the esophagus, and prevent newly ingested blood from reaching the stomach. As the hungry flea repeatedly attempts to feed, the blood sucked from the mammal mixes with bacilli and is regurgitated into the mammalian host (Bacot, 1914; Bacot, 1915; Bahmanyar, 1976; Bibikova 1977; Cavanaugh 1971, 1956). At higher environmental temperatures (> 28 to 30^0 C), blockage of fleas decreases and clearance of the infection increases, possibly due to the temperature regulation of hemin storage and/or Pla protease. (Burroughs, 1947; Cavanaugh, 1971; Cavanaugh, 1980; Kartman, 1969). The normal digestive process of fleas involves maintaining the blood meal as a liquid, which is subsequently degraded primarily by proteolytic enzymes (Wigglesworth, 1984). The fate of the blocked flea is death from starvation and dehydration (Bacot, 1914; Bibikova, 1977).

Y. pestis spreads from the site of the flea bite to the regional lymph nodes and multiplies, resulting in the formation of primary and sometimes secondary buboes (swollen lymph node). The bacilli can spread into the bloodstream (bacteremia), where they are preferentially removed by the spleen and liver. Growth of the organisms continues in the blood, liver, and spleen and eventually spreads to other organs (Pollitzer, 1954). Development of a bacteremia of sufficient degree and duration is essential for effective transmission in nature. Infection of the flea via the blood from a bacteremic rodent completes the cycle. If bubonic plague progresses to the pneumonic form in humans, the potential for respiratory droplet spread and a primary pneumonic plague epidemic occurs (Poland and Barnes, 1979; Poland et al., 1994). This type of epidemic is currently uncommon due to the advent of effective antibiotics and modern public health measures.

5. Diagnosis

Clinical diagnosis of disease is based on patient symptoms and exposure history. Bubonic plague is characterized by painful, swollen lymph node(s), fever, and a history of exposure to fleas, rodents, or other animals. It is very difficult to diagnose septicemic plague without a blood culture because of its resemblance to other gram-negative septicemias. Likewise, pneumonic plague has been mistaken for other pulmonary syndromes (Centers for Disease Control and Prevention. 1994). Recent data indicate that pneumonic plague should be suspected in symptomatic persons with a history of exposure to infected pets, especially cats (Craven et al., 1993; Doll et al., 1994; Gage et al., 1992).

Specimens for laboratory diagnosis include blood, bubo aspirates, and sputum, which can be stained with Gram, Giemsa, Wright, or Wayson stain (Poland et al., 1979). A positive fluorescent-antibody assay directed against purified F1, a capsular antigen expressed predominantly at 37^0 C can be used as presumptive evidence of a *Y. pestis* infection (Du and Forsberg, 1995; Poland et al., 1979). To confirm a diagnosis of plague by bacteriological means, it is necessary to isolate the organism. Other methods for diagnosing plague include: enzyme linked immunosorbent assays (ELISA) (Cavanaugh et al., 1979; Williams et al., 1984), polymerase chain reaction (PCR) assays (Norkina OV 1994), and DNA hybridization (McDonough et al., 1988). ELISAs have been used to measure levels of either F1 antigen or antibodies to F1 in serum (Williams et al.,1984). PCR-gel electrophoresis based methods have been developed for detecting *Y. pestis* in fleas and other specimens (Hinnebusch and Schwan, 1993; Norkina et al., 1994, Tsukano et al., 1996). Real-time PCR assays in various formats have also been developed for detecting and identifying *Y. pestis* (Higgins et al., 1998; Iqbal et al., 2000; Lindler and Tall, 2001; Loiez et al., 2003; Tomaso et al., 2003; Chase et al., 2005; Woron et al., 2006). Real-time PCR based methods are more specific, and require less time and labor than conventional PCR assays. Real-time PCR methods include SYBR Green (Saikaly et al., 2007), molecular beacons (Varma-Basil et al., 2004), TaqMan probes (Loiez et al., 2003; Chase et al., 2005) and minor groove binding (MGB) probes (Skottman et al., 2007), and target specific sequences on the chromosome and (or) plasmids. However, PCR based diagnosis is expensive compared to immunoassays, which may be useful for mass screening during epidemics.

6. Treatment

Patients suspected of having bubonic plague should be placed in isolation until two days after starting antibiotic treatment to prevent the potential spread of the disease. Antibiotics such as streptomycin, gentamicin, oxytetracyclne, tetracycline and chloramphenicol have been used to treat primary infection (Meyer, 1950). Due to the toxicity associated with streptomycin, patients are not usually maintained on this antibiotic for the full 10-day course but shifted to one of the other antibiotics, usually tetracycline. The tetracyclines are also commonly used for prophylaxis, while chloramphenicol is recommended for the treatment of plague meningitis (Becker et al.,1987). Newer antibiotics have been used to successfully treat experimental plague infections in mice (Bonacorsi et al., 1994). Recently, the quinolone levofloxacin was found to be effective against *Y.pestis, B.anthracis,* and *F. tularensis* (Peterson et al., 2010).

7. Immunology of *Y. pestis*

Yersinia spp like many other gram-negative bacterial pathogens, employ a specialized secretory apparatus called the type III secretion system (TTSS) to interact with host cells (Cornelis et al., 1998; Cornelis, 2000). The TTSS is a multicomponent secretion apparatus that injects specialized proteins (effectors) into the cytosol of the host cell where they interact with a variety of host proteins to manipulate cellular functions to ultimately benefit the pathogen (Galan and Collmer, 1999). The *Yersinia* effector proteins called Yops– (**Y**ersinia **O**uter membrane **P**roteins) and other proteins involved in the TTSS are encoded on a 70-kb plasmid (Cornelis et al., 1998). The functions of the Yops are currently under intense study and fall into two general categories: proteins facilitating the translocation of Yops into the host cells, and those actually secreted into the cytosol. Notably, YopD, YopB, and LcrV (low calcium response protein V) appear to function in the translocation of other Yops into the cytosol whereas YopE, YopH, YopJ (Yop P in *Y. enterocolitica*), YopM, YopO, and YopT function within the host cell. Yops are virulence factors that can interfere with phagocytosis, inhibit the antimicrobial oxidative burst, inhibit the production of inflammatory cytokines (e.g. TNF-α,), and promote apoptosis in macrophages and neutrophils (Cornelis et al.,1998, 2000). Like TTSS effectors of other bacterial pathogens, Yops function by mimicking activities of host cellular proteins and either activate or inhibit cellular processes to promote the pathogen's survival and replication (Staskawicz et al., 2001).

LcrV, is an important virulence factor (Sing et al., 2002; Fields et al., 1999; Lee et al., 2000). It forms the tip of TTSS and helps to translocate effector proteins to host cells. LcrV can also be secreted into the environment (Fields et al., 1999) where it has been shown to down regulate host protective immune responses in an IL-10 mediated manner (Sing et al., 2002). Thus, pretreatment of wildtype peritoneal macrophages with recombinant LcrV (rLcrV) inhibited zymosan induced TNF-α production. The anti-inflammatory effect of macrophages was found to be IL-10 dependent because it could be reversed by neutralizing antibodies specific to IL-10.There was no effect of neutralizing antibodies against IL-4 or TGF-β, two other cytokines known to inhibit inflammatory responses of macrophages (Sing et al., 2002). The cell receptors responsible for LcrV-induced IL-10 production were identified as CD14 and TLR2 (Sing et al., 2002). IL-10 secretion in response to rLcrV was abrogated in CD14- and TLR2- deficient macrophages. Furthermore, the TLR2 stimulating region of LcrV mapped to a short N-terminal 19 amino acid sequence (Sing et al., 2002). CD14 / TLR2 mediated production of IL-10 by LcrV was further established by the observation that TLR2-deficient mice were more resistant to *Y. enterocolitica* infection than their wild-type parents (Sing et al., 2002).

Y. pestis replicates extracellularly; whether its virulence relies upon intracellular replication remains a question of debate. *Y. pestis* replicates within macrophages/ dendritic cells as well as *in vitro* (Cavanaugh et al., 1959; Janssen et al., 1969; Straley et al.; 1984; Pujal et al., 2005). Nevertheless, detailed kinetic studies of mice infected intranasally (Lathem et al., 2005) and rats infected intradermally (Sebbane et al., 2005), failed to observe significant numbers of intracellular organisms *in vivo*. However, *Y.pestis* bacilli were detected in spleen cells and in CD11b-expressing macrophages when mice were infected subcutaneously (Lukaszewski et al., 2005). In addition, studies of pneumonic plague in nonhuman primates have documented the presence of intact *Y. pestis* within alveolar macrophages (Finegold et al., 1969; Davis et al., 1996). Electron microscopy confirmed the presence of alveolar macrophages containing intact bacilli in the lungs of aerosol-infected macaques (Finegold et al., 1969).

Although, the growth of *Y. pestis* within phagocytes, plays an important pathogenic role, extracellular bacilli predominate during the late stages of infection although intracellular organisms have also been detected at that time (Finegold et al., 1969; Davis et al., 1996; Lukaszewski et al., 2005). These findings suggested that cells of the monocyte/macrophage lineage offer *Y. pestis* a protected intracellular niche that provides sufficient time for the pathogen to grow within mammals by upregulating expression of capsular F1 protein, LcrV and Yops (Cavanaugh et al., 1959).

One to 4 hours after infection of macrophages, *Y. pestis* rapidly expresses virulence markers such as Yops, F1 antigen, and V antigen. By 1 to 2 days postinfection, the virulence-associated proteins begin to paralyse host immune mechanisms by inducing apoptosis, suppressing the production of proinflammatory cytokines (e.g. TNF-α), inhibiting Fc receptor-mediated phagocytosis, and preventing neutrophil chemotaxis (Perry and Fetherston, 1997). Inside macrophages, *Y. pestis* F1 protein (fraction 1 antigen) forms a capsule around the bacterium. This capsule enhances resistance to engulfment by both macrophages and neutrophils, probably by preventing interactions of receptors that could facilitate uptake of the pathogen (Du et al., 2002). It was also observed that *Y. pestis* produces a less-acylated (tetra-acylated) lipid A at 37 °C, which results in poor induction of host toll-like receptor (TLR) 4-mediated innate immune responses and ultimately poor activation of human macrophages (Kawahara et al., 2002; Kolodziejek et al., 2010). When *Y. pestis* KIM1001, which expresses a poorly TLR4-stimulating LPS, was modified to strongly induce TLR4, it became avirulent (Montminy et al., 2006).

A fimbrial structure in *Y. pestis*, PsaA (pH 6 antigen) is induced at 37°C in acidic media, an environment similar to that of the macrophage phagolysosome (Lindler and Tal, 1993; Price et al., 1995). PsaA selectively binds to apolipoprotein B (*apoB*)-containing lipoproteins (LDL) in human plasma (Makoveichuk et al., 2003), which may prevent recognition by the host immune system (Huang XZ 2004, Makoveichuk et al., 2003).

Infection by *Y.pestis* leads to a global depletion of NK cells and decreased secretion of IFN-γ, resulting in reduced macrophage function. These immunomodulatory effects depend on the effector YopM (Kerschen et al.,2004). Phagocytes (macrophages and neutrophils) are the main target cells of the Yops. YopH, YopE, YopT, and YopO inhibit the phagocytosis of Yersiniae, either by interfering with the host cell actin regulation of Rho GTPases (YopE, YopT, and YopO) or specifically and rapidly inactivating host proteins associated with signalling from the receptor to actin (YopH) (Aepfelbacher and Heesemann, 2001; Aepfelbacher et al., 2005; Andersson et al., 1996; Iriarte et al., 1998; Rosqvist et al., 1990). YopH can suppress the production of reactive oxygen intermediates by macrophages and PMNs (Green et al., 1995). Moreover, Yops also inhibit the proinflammatory responses elicited by infected cells. YopP inhibits TNF-α and IL-8 release by macrophages, and epithelial, and endothelial cells, respectively (Boland and Cornelis 1998). TNF-α is a potent proinflammatory cytokine, released by activated macrophages and plays a crucial role in limiting the severity of the bacterial infection. In addition to YopP, YopM interacts with protein kinase C-like 2 and ribosomal protein S6 kinase, which are also involved in proinflammatory signalling (McDonald et al., 2003). The suppression of the production of proinflammatory factors not only reduces the activation of NK cells and phagocytes, but also destroys the inflammatory environment needed for adaptive immunity.

7.1 Current vaccine strategy

There is a need for a safe and effective plague vaccine to counter the threat of bioterrorism. Researchers have been trying for more than 100 years to develop such a vaccine (Titball and Williamson, 2004). The first vaccine consisting of a heat-killed broth of densely grown, fully virulent *Y. pestis* was developed in 1897 (Haffkine, 1897; Taylor, 1933). This formulation was found to be effective against bubonic plague but had undesirable side effects, such as high grade fever, in the majority of human recipients and severe adverse reactions limited its acceptance (Taylor, 1933). This vaccine was not effective against the pneumonic form of disease (Taylor, 1933; Lien-Teh, 1926). Later, Meyer and colleagues (1974, 1970) developed a more refined whole-cell plague vaccine comprised of formalin-killed *Y. pestis* organisms suspended in a saline solution. Ultimately, a vaccine of this type was licensed and sold as Plague Vaccine, USP, and was used to protect U.S. military personnel against bubonic plague during the Vietnam War (Meyer, 1970; Cavanaugh et al., 1974). However, these vaccines also caused significant adverse effects, including fever, headache, malaise, lymphadenopathy, erythema and induration at the site of injection (Meyer KF et al., 1974). In addition, they generally failed to protect mice and nonhuman primates against pulmonary *Y. pestis* challenge (Titball and Williamson, 2004; Meyer et al.,1974; Meyer et al.,1970; Kolle and Otto 1904).

In 1904, Kolle and Otto showed that relatively small quantities of live-attenuated *Y. pestis* were sufficient to protect rodents. Later, Strong (1906, 1908) reported that live-attenuated vaccines protected humans from bubonic plague. In subsequent years, this formulation was used to immunize millions of people in Indonesia, Madagascar and Vietnam (Girard, 1963). The results suggested that these vaccines were fully protective in humans against both the bubonic and pneumonic form of plague (Titball and Williamson, 2004; Meyer et al., 1970; Girard, 1963). Unfortunately, the live attenuated vaccines were found to be unstable, sometimes killing experimental animals (i.e., nonohuman primates) due to the retention of significant virulence (Welkos et al., 2002; Meyer et al., 1970; Meyer et al., 1974; Russell et al., 1995). In addition, they also produced frequent side effects in humans such as, debilitating fever, malaise and lymphadenopathy (Meyer et al., 1974). These safety concerns have limited the use of live-attenuated plague vaccines in the U.S. and Europe.

Current vaccines are based on variants of a pigmentation-negative *Y. pestis* strain EV76. Strain EV76 produces a robust T-cell response that contributes to protection against pneumonic plague in a murine model (Sha et al., 2008). Despite safety concerns and a high degree of immune variability among vaccine recipients, the NIIEG line of strain EV 76 is still in use today (Zilinskas, 2006). However, uncertainty about the reversal of virulence makes the EV76 live attenuated option much less appealing than the development of new vaccines.

To overcome the problems associated with the EV76 strain, researchers are trying to find non-pathogenic substitutes by replacing it with a plasmid-expressed gene that could engender protection. In that context, an *Escherichia coli*-derived plasmid encoding the lipopolysaccharide LpxL, which was over-expressed in the EV76 strain, was chosen because of its immunogenicity and ability to activate TLR-4 (Szaba et al., 2008).

The *E.coli lpxL* gene was introduced into the *Y. pestis* chromosome, which encodes a hexa-acylated lipid A. LpxL is a potent TLR-4 agonist, capable of inducing a strong innate immune response. Immunization with this strain resulted in 100 % protection from subsequent subcutaneous and intranasal challenges (Sun et al., 2011). Genes for additonal virulence proteins such as, Ail (attachment invasion locus, also designated as OmpX), plasminogen activator protease (Pla), and pH 6 antigen (Psa) have been deleted in an effort to generate effective live attenuated vaccine strains (Felek et al., 2010). In a pneumonic plague model, animals infected with a *ompX* mutant of *Y. pestis* CO92 survived for two days longer than those infected with the parent strain (Kolodziejek et al., 2010). Moreover, *Δcaf1* mutants and *ΔpsaA* mutants exhibited decreased virulence in a murine infection model (Weening et al., 2011). In a recent study, a *Δcaf1* mutant of *Y. pestis* CO92 was attenuated for virulence in a mouse model of bubonic plague but not in a pneumonic plague mouse model when compared to the WT CO92 strain (Sha et al., 2011).

7.2 Subunit vaccines based on the F1, LcrV and YscF proteins

The F1 antigen plays important role in preventing phagocytosis by macrophages. In 1952, Baker and colleagues purified the capsular F1 protein. F1 specific antibodies produced in rabbits, agglutinated plague bacilli and passively protected mice and rats following subcutaneous challenge with virulent *Y. pestis* (Baker et al., 1952). Passive transfer of F1-specific antibodies also protected macaques against pneumonic plague (Ehrenkranz and Meyer, 1955). Subsequently, vaccination with recombinant F1 was shown to protect mice against aerosolized *Y. pestis* (Andrews et al., 1996). Despite this apparent success, it is now well established that virulent F1-negative *Y. pestis* strains exist (Winter et al., 1960; Friedlander et al., 1995; Welkos et al.,1995, Davis et al., 1996; Worsham et al., 1995). Thus, vaccines based solely upon F1 antigen will likely fail to protect against all strains of *Y.pestis*.

The multifunctional LcrV protein is important for the virulence of *Y.pestis* (Brubaker et al., 2003; Une and Brubaker, 1984; Viboud and Biliska, 2005; Heesemann et al., 2006; Bacon et al., 1956; Janssen et al., 1963; Lawton et al., 1963, Une et al., 1984). Immunization with purified LcrV protected mice against subcutaneous challenge; protection was also observed following the passive transfer of LcrV-specific antibodies (Une T et al., 1984, Lawton et al., 1963, Une et al., 1984, Sato et al., 1991; Nakajima and Brubaker, 1993; Motin et al., 1994). Immunization with recombinant LcrV was shown to protect mice against aerosol infection with both F1-positive and F1-negative strains of *Y. pestis* (Motin et al., 1994; Price et al., 1989; Leary et al., 1995; Anderson et al., 1996; Anderson et al., 1998). In spite of these important findings, a vaccine based on LcrV alone did not fully protect against pneumonic plague, perhaps due to lack of cross-protective immunity against LcrV variants (Roggenkamp et al., 1997).

YscF, a recently identified vaccine candidate, is located on the cell surface and forms the TTSS channel, which is required for the secretion of Yops and toxins (Allaoui et al., 1995, Haddix and Straley, 1992; Hoiczyk et al., 2001; Marenne et al., 2003). Immunization of mice with YscF resulted in a high anti-YscF titer and provided partial protection against intravenous (i.v.) challenge with *Y. pestis* (Matson et al., 2005; Swietnicki et al., 2005).

Vaccines based on recombinant F1 and LcrV provided better protection than vaccines comprised of either subunit alone (Williamson et al., 1995,1996). F1 and LcrV formulations administered with the adjuvant alum provided protection in mice against pulmonary *Y. pestis* challenge (Williamson et al., 1997; Jones et al., 2000). In a similar study, investigators at the US Army Medical Research Institute of Infectious Diseases (USAMRIID) demonstrated that a formulation consisting of a recombinant F1-LcrV fusion protein (rF1V) and alum protected mice against pulmonary challenge with either F1-positive or negative strains of *Y. pestis* (Anderson et al., 1998, Heath et al., 1998).

Yops have also been investigated as protective antigens. Immunization of mice with recombinant Yops (H, E, N, K, or M) engendered no significant protection against *Y. pestis* infection (Andrews et al., 1999; Leary et al., 1999; Nemeth et al., 1997). However, mice immunized with complexes of YopB, YopD, and YopE (BDE) produced high-titers of antibodies specific for Yop B, D, and E, and were protected against lethal intravenous challenge with $F1^-$ but not $F1^+$ *Y. pestis*. Furthermore, mice passively immunized with anti-BDE serum were also protected from lethal challenge with $F1^-$ *Y. pestis* (Ivanov et al., 2008).

Huang et al. (2009) evaluated a vaccine consisting of a spray-freeze dried powder form of a recombinant F1-V fusion protein in a mouse model. The vaccine engendered an antibody response and provided 70-90% protection against lethal subcutaneous challenge with *Y. pestis*. Ren et al. (2009) developed a vaccine consisting of recombinant F1, and V from *Y.pestis*, and the Protective Antigen from *B. anthracis* (rF1 + rV+ rPA). This formulation protected mice from subcutaneous challenge with 10^7 colony-forming units (CFU) of a virulent *Y. pestis* strain, and fully protected rabbits against subcutaneous challenge with 1.2×10^5 spores of virulent *B. anthracis.*

CpG oligodeoxynucleotide (ODN) has been used as an adjuvant together with F1-V antigen to enhance its immune response in mice. CpG ODNs significantly augmented the antibody response even up to 5 months and increased the efficacy of the vaccine in murine model of bubonic and pneumonic plague (Amemiya et al., 2009).

Immunization with flagellin and with F1-V elicited a robust humoral immune response in mice and two species of nonhuman primates. The flagellin-F1-V formulation fully protected mice against intranasal challenge with *Y. pestis* CO92 (Mizel et al., 2009). Oral immunization with cationic liposome–nucleic acid complexes (CLDC) combined with F1 antigen elicited protective immunity against lethal pneumonic plague in C57BL/6J. This formulation protected mice up to 18 weeks post vaccination. Protection mediated by oral CLDC with F1 antigen depends primarily on CD4+ T cells, with a partial contribution from CD8+ T cells (Jones et al., 2010).

Ramirez and Alejandra (2009) constructed an attenuated *Salmonella* Typhi strain that expressed the F1 antigen of *Y. pestis* (*S.* Typhi (F1)), and evaluated its immunogenicity. Newborn mice primed intranasally with a single dose of *S.* Typhi (F1) exhibited a mucosal and cellular immune response one week post immunization. *S.* Typhi(F1) enhanced the activation and maturation of neonatal $CD11c^+$ dendritic cells, and MHC-II cell surface markers and the production of proinflammatory cytokines. The *S.* Typhi(F1)- based formulation improved the capacity of DC for antigen presentation and T cell stimulation in vitro.

The protective efficacy of the F1 + rV270 (an LcrV variant lacking amino acid residues 271–300) vaccines compared to that of EV76 was evaluated. The F1 + rV270 formulation was tested in both guinea pigs and New Zealand White rabbits by determining the antibody response and protection against subcutaneous challenge with the virulent *Y. pestis* 141 strain (Qi Z et al., 2010).

Xiao et al. (2010) developed an anti-F1-specific human monoclonal antibody (mAb) (m252) and anti-V-specific human mAbs (m253, m254) against the F1 and V antigens, respectively. These monoclonal antibodies were found to be more effective than the corresponding mouse antibodies. Neutralization of TNF-α and IFN-γ interfered with the protective efficacy of F1- or LcrV- specific antibodies against the fully virulent *pgm*-positive *Y. pestis* strain CO92 (Lin et al., 2010). Recently, a recombinant rF1+rV vaccine provided protection in *Cynomolgus macaques* against pneumonic plague following inhalational challenge with a clinical isolate of *Y. pestis* (CO92) (Williamson et al., 2011).

7.3 Plant based vaccines

The use of plant-based oral recombinant vaccines could be an alternative approach for plague immunoprophylaxis. However, F1 and LcrV genes expressed in recombinant plant tissue were relatively less immunogenic due to the lack of signals recognized by the innate immune system through Toll Like receptors. In one such study, Swiss-Webster mice exhibited significant protection following subcutaneous immunization with *Nicotiana tabacum* leaves that expressed a LcrV–F1 (F1-V) translational fusion protein on its surface (Arlen 2008). In a separate study, guinea pigs immunized with a transgenic *Nicotiana benthamiana* tobacco plant expressing the F1-V fusion protein were protected against a subsequent pneumonic plague infection (Del Prete, 2009). However, the amount of recombinant protein produced in plant-based vectors was generally poor. To overcome this problem, the N-terminal of the γ-Zein protein (produced in maize and induces protein body formation) was fused with an F1-V fusion construct, which resulted in up to three times higher accumulation of protein in *Nicotiana tabacum* drived tissues than the F1-V fusion protein alone (Alvarez et al., 2010). Plant-based vaccines have also been evaluated for other Category A agents such as Variola major virus and *B. anthracis* (Rigano et al., 2009). Recently, an F1-V fusion protein expressed in carrot tap roots and lettuce was found to be stable and immunogenic for mice. (Rosales-Mendoza et al., 2010a; Rosales-Mendoza et al., 2010b).

7.4 DNA vaccine straties

DNA vaccines have been developed as an alternative to protein-based vaccines. LcrV- and F1-based DNA vaccines have been developed that contain either all or part of the open reading frames encoding either LcrV, F1, or both. One vaccine containing a portion of *LcrV* that encoded a 127-amino acid peptide, was found to elicit a strong humoral immune response. Furthermore, mice immunized with this vaccine exhibited a 60% survival rate following challenge with *Y.pestis* (Vernazza. et al., 2009). A vaccine consisting of the IL-12 coding sequence and the genes for F1 or LcrV was used to immunize mice intranasally. This formulation enhanced IgA production in the mucosa and showed 80% protection from a subsequent inhalational challenge with *Y.pestis* (Yamanaka et al., 2008)

Recently, a DNA vaccine based on F1 and YscF was constructed by fusion of the gene encoding YscF to the downstream sequence of F1. This strategy enhanced protection resulting from F1 or YscF DNA vaccines alone. This approach suggested a number of ways to develop protective DNA vaccines (Wang et al., 2010). Immunization with the F1-V based DNA vaccine and the adjuvant, lymphotactin (LTN) resulted in high levels of serum IgG and mucosal IgA antibodies (Yamanaka et al., 2010). The LcrV based DNA vaccine elicited a CD8+ immune response against specific epitopes of this antigen (Wang et al., 2011). Immunization of mice with a DNA vaccine consisting of F1 and V and the gene encoding the heat-labile enterotoxin (LT) of *E. coli* as an adjuvant resulted in 40% protection (Rosenzweig et al., 2011).

7.5 Virus vector based vaccines

Live avirulent or attenuated recombinant viruses expressing genes encoding virulence antigens offer several advantages over their bacterial counterparts. Non-enveloped/ naked viruses may be a better vehicle for vaccine development as these viruses can be stored for a long time without losing their infectivity. In one such case, a recombinant vaccinia virus vector was used to express an F1-V fusion protein. The vaccine was orally administered to C57BL/6J mice and was found to protect against an inhalational challenge of ten times the lethal dose of *Y.pestis* KIM/D27. It provided 100% protection up to 45 weeks post-immunization (Bhattacharya et al., 2010). Moreover, a recombinant raccoon pox virus producing F1 antigen elicited significant protection in orally immunized prairie dogs (*Cynomys spp.*) (Rocke et al., 2008). More recently, two recombinant raccoon pox viruses producing the F1 antigen and a 307-amino-acid truncated form of LcrV engendered a better humoral response and protection in both mice and prairie dogs following subcutaneous challenge with virulent *Y. pestis* CO92 (Rocke et al.,2010a, b).

The route of immunization and booster plays an important role in the immune response and subsequent protection. A recombinant Vaccinia virus Ankara vector producing either the full-length F1 or the truncated 307 amino acid peptide form of LcrV was administered intramuscularly (IM). Vaccines consisting of truncated V antigen and full length F1 antigen provided 85% and 50% protection, respectively, against both intranasal and intraperitoneal challenges with *Y. pestis* CO92 (Brewoo et al., 2010). Recently, modified, non-replicating adenovirus vectors were evaluated for the development of antibodies against both the heavy and light chains of a previously identified anti-LcrV protective antibody. Surprisingly, immunized C57BL/6J male mice showed significant levels of IgG that persisted for up to 12 weeks and exhibited 80% protection in mice after intranasal challenge with a 2×10^4-cfu of fully virulent *Y. pestis* CO92 (Sofer-Podesta et al., 2009).

Human vesicular stomatitis virus (VSV) has been evaluated as an effective vector for the development of a novel plague vaccine. VSV was engineered to express LcrV. Immunized female BALB/c mice showed strong humoral responses with an IgG2a bias dichotomy and exhibited 90% protection from an intranasal challenge with *Y. pestis* CO92 (Chattopadhyaya et al., 2008). These finding highlight the importance of the choice of viral-vectors in the development of plague vaccines.

7.6 Synthetic vaccines based on defined B and T cell epitopes

The concept of synthetic peptide vaccines was laid by the pioneering work of Anderer who demonstrated that a peptide from tobacco mosaic virus (TMV) showed immunoreactivity with antiserum against TMV. In addition, a peptide coupled to a carrier induced specific virus precipitating and neutralizing antibodies (Deber et al., 1985). The first step in developing a synthetic peptide vaccine for plague is to identify the relevant antigen(s) determine their amino acid sequence, and identify protective B and T cell epitopes. Sabhnani and Rao (2003) identified the immunodominant epitopes of F1 antigen. The immunogenicity of the B cell (B1, B2, and B3) and T cell (T1, T2) peptides was studied in mice using alhydrogel and liposomes as delivery vehicles. B-T constructs of F1 antigen engendered protection in mice. PLGA (poly (DL-lactide-co-glycolide) microsphere delivery of B-T constructs enhanced protection (Tripathi and Rao, 2006). Later, several B and T cell epitopes of V antigen were identified by direct binding, competitive, and T cell proliferation approaches. V antigen peptides a, g and j were found to be pure B cell epitopes and peptides d and k pure T cell epitopes, whereas other peptides b, f and i showed both B and T cell properties (Khan and Rao, 2008). Furthermore, mice immunized intranasally with B-T conjugates of V antigen peptides entrapped in microspheres resulted in high titers of serum and mucosal IgG and IgA upto 120 day postimmunization. Interestingly, some of the conjugates showed enhanced protection in mice challenged with live bacteria (Uppada and Rao, 2009). Gupta et al. (2009) demonstrated the cell mediated immune response of some of the best B-T conjugates in different strains of mice. Surprisingly, some of the B-T conjugates of F1 and V antigen resulted in good lymphocyte proliferation and cytokine production *in vitro* as determined by ELISPOT assay. FACS analysis of some conjugates showed the presence of IFN-γ and perforin secreting CD4+ cells as compared to CD8+ T cells (Gupta et al. 2011), which demonstrated the importance of CD4+ T cells in conferring immunity in the host.

8. Future perspectives

The development of a fully protective vaccine against plague remains a challenge . A perfect vaccine must protect humans against all three biotypes of *Y.pestis*. None of the formulations of F1 and V based vaccines were fully protective against experimental infections. The ideal vaccine would stimulate robust antibody and cell mediated immune response with respect to serum IgG, IgG sub classes and mucosal IgA along with Th1/ Th2 /Th17 cytokines correlation. These parameters could be exploited for protection studies in humans. Standardized procedures will facilitate human clinical trials to determine vaccine formulations, dosages and schedules that best prime protective responses. Incorporating additional antigens such as YscF into F1/LcrV-based vaccines and modifying existing formulations, on both the DNA and protein level, will be more effective and could lead to fully protective vaccine against all strains of *Y.pestis*. Furthermore, using different ways of immunization with novel delivery vehicles and adjuvants could enhance the immune response and efficacy of different formulations. Currently, we have extended our study by designing MAP (Multiple Antigen Peptide) incorporating the relevant protective epitopes of F1, V and YscF antigen in PLGA nanoparticles using CpG, as an adjuvant to activate Toll Like Receptor 9 (TLR-9) of the innate immune system (Uppada et al. 2011). This preparation gave a better immunogenicity profile than that of single epitope based immunogens.

A better understanding of virulence mechanisms, host pathogen interactions that operate within the body and especially the lungs during infection, could provide some new alternative targets for vaccines and therapeutics. The focus should be on the pneumonic form of disease rather than the bubonic and septicemic forms. Identifying agonists of TLR-2 or TLR-4 is also an important area of research for plague vaccine. Synthetic microbial products that activate the Th1 and Th17 pathways are also beneficial to host immunity. However, given present concerns for bioterrorism, which may involve the release of aerosolized *Y. pestis*, there is now a greater need to explicitly characterize virulence factors that impact pulmonary disease.

9. References

Aepfelbacher M, and Heesemann J (2001). Modulation of Rho GTPases and the actin cytoskeleton by *Yersinia* outer proteins (Yops). Int. J. Med. Microbiol. 291:269–276.

Aepfelbacher M, Zumbihl R, and Heesemann J (2005). Modulation of Rho GTPases and the actin cytoskeleton by YopT of *Yersinia*. Curr. Top. Microbiol. Immunol. 291:167–175.

Allaoui A, Schulte R, Cornelis G R, (1995). Mutational analysis of the *Yersinia enterocolitica virC* operon: characterization of *yscE, F, G, I, J, K* required for Yop secretion and *ysc*H encoding YopR. Mol Microbiol 1995, 18:343-355.

Alvarez ML, Topal E, Martin F, Cardineau GA (2010). Higher accumulation of F1-V fusion recombinant protein in plants after induction of protein body formation. Plant Mol Biol 72:75–89.

Amemiya K, Meyers JL, Rogers TE et al. (2009). CpG oligodeoxynucleotides augment the murine immune response to the *Yersinia pestis* F1-V vaccine in bubonic and pneumonic models of plague. Vaccine 27;16: 2220–2229.

Anderson GW Jr , Heath DG, Bolt CR, Welkos SL, Friedlander AM, (1998). Short- and long-term efficacy of single-dose subunit vaccines against *Yersinia pestis* in mice. Am. J. Trop. Med. Hyg ;58(6): 793–799.

Anderson GW Jr, Leary SE, Williamson ED, et al. (1996). Recombinant V antigen protects mice against pneumonic and bubonic plague caused by F1-capsule-positive and -negative strains of Yersinia pestis. Infect. Immun ; 64(11):4580–4585.

Andersson K, Carballeira N, Magnusson KE, Persson C, Stendahl O, Wolf-Watz H, and Fallman M (1996). YopH of *Yersinia pseudotuberculosis* interrupts early phosphotyrosine signaling associated with phagocytosis. Mol. Microbiol. 20:1057–1069.

Andrews GP, Heath DG, Anderson GW Jr, Welkos SL, Friedlander AM (1996). Fraction 1 capsular antigen (F1) purification from *Yersinia pestis* CO92 and from an *Escherichia coli* recombinant strain and efficacy against lethal plague challenge. Infect. Immun: 64; (6):2180–2187.

Andrews GP, Strachan ST, Benner GE, Sample AK, Anderson GW Jr., Adamovicz JJ, Welkos SL, Pullen JK, and Friedlander AM (1999). Protective efficacy of recombinant *Yersinia* outer proteins against bubonic plague caused by encapsulated and nonencapsulated *Yersinia pestis*. Infect. Immun: 67;1533–1537.

Arlen PA, Singleton M, Adamovicz JJ, Ding Y, Davoodi-Semiromi A, Daniell H (2008) Effective plague vaccination via oral delivery of plant cells expressing F1-V antigens in chloroplasts. Infect Immun: 76;3640–3650.

Bacon GA, Burrows TW (1956). The basis of virulence in *Pasteurella pestis*: an antigen determining virulence. Br. J. Exp. Pathol. 37:481–493.

Bacot AW, and Martin CJ (1914). LXVII. Observations on the mechanism of the transmission of plague by fleas. J. Hyg: 13 (Plague Suppl. 3):423–439.

Bahmanyar M, and Cavanaugh DC (1976). Plague manual. World Health Organization, Geneva, Switzerland.

Baker EE, Sommer H, Foster LE, Meyer E, Meyer KF (1952). Studies on immunization against plague. I. The isolation and characterization of the soluble antigen of *Pasteurella pestis*. J. Immunol: 68;131-145.

Barnes AM, and Quan TJ (1992). Plague, p. 1285-1291. *In* S. L. Gorbach, J. G. Bartlett, and N. R. Blacklow (ed.), Infectious diseases. The W. B. Saunders Co., Philadelphia, Pa.

Becker TM, Poland JD, Quan TJ, White ME, Mann JM, and Barnes AM (1987). Plague meningitis—a retrospective analysis of cases reported in the United States, 1970-1979. West. J. Med. 147:554-557.

Ben-Gurion, R, and Shafferman A (1981). Essential virulence determinants of different *Yersinia* species are carried on a common plasmid. Plasmid: 5 (2); 183-187.

Bhattacharya D, Mecsas J, Hu LT (2010). Development of a vaccinia virus based reservoir-targeted vaccine against *Yersinia pestis*. Vaccine: 28;7683-7689.

Bibikova VA (1977). Contemporary views on the interrelationships between fleas and the pathogens of human and animal diseases. Annu. Rev. Entomol. 22:23-32.

Bioterrorism Overview, Centers for Disease Control and Prevention, 2008-02-12, retrieved 2009-05-22.

Boland A, and Cornelis GR (1998). Role of YopP in suppression of tumor necrosis factor alpha release by macrophages during *Yersinia* infection. Infect. Immun. 66;1878-1884.

Bonacorsi SP, Scavizzi MR, Guiyoule A, Amouroux JH, and Carniel E (1994). Assessment of a fluoroquinolone, three b-lactams, two aminoglycosides, and a cycline in treatment of murine *Yersinia pestis* infection. Antimicrob. Agents Chemother. 38:481-486.

Brewoo JN, Powell TD, Stinchcomb DT, Osorio JE (2010). Efficacy and safety of a modified vaccinia Ankara (MVA) vectored plague vaccine in mice. Vaccine: 28;5891-5899.

Brubaker RR (2003). Interleukin-10 and inhibition of innate immunity to yersiniae: roles of Yops and LcrV (V antigen). Infect. Immun ;71(7):3673-3681.

Brubaker RR (1972). The genus *Yersinia*: biochemistry and genetics of virulence. Curr. Top. Microbiol. Immunol. 57:111-158.

Burroughs AL (1947). Sylvatic plague studies. The vector efficiency of nine species of fleas compared with *Xenopsylla cheopis*. J. Hyg. 45:371-396.

Butler T (1989). The black death past and present. 1. Plague in the 1980s. Trans. R. Soc. Trop. Med. Hyg. 83:458-460.

Cavanaugh DC, Elisberg BL, Llewellyn CH, et al. (1974). Plague immunization. V. Indirect evidence for the efficacy of plague vaccine. J. Infect. Dis; 129(Suppl):S37-S40.

Cavanaugh DC, Randall R (1959).The role of multiplication of *Pasteurella pestis* in mononuclear phagocytes in the pathogenesis of flea-borne plague. J. Immunol; 83:348-363.

Cavanaugh DC (1971). Specific effect of temperature upon transmission of the plague bacillus by the oriental rat flea, *Xenopsylla cheopis*. Am. J. Trop. Med. Hyg. 20:264-272.

Cavanaugh DC, and Williams JE (1980). Plague: some ecological interrelationships, p. 245-256. In R. Traub and H. Starcke (ed.), Fleas. Proceedings of the International Conference on Fleas. A. A. Balkema, Rotterdam, The Netherlands.

Cavanaugh DC, Fortier MK, Robinson DM, Williams JE, and Rust JH Jr. (1979). Application of the ELISA technique to problems in the serologic diagnosis of plague. Bull. Pan Am. Health Org. 13:399–402.

Cavanaugh DC, Wheeler CM, Suyemoto W, Shimada T, and Yamakawa Y (1956). Studies on *Pasteurella pestis* in various flea species. II. Simplified method for the experimental infection of fleas. J. Infect. Dis. 98:107–111.

Centers for Disease Control and Prevention (1994). Human plague-United States, 1993–1994. Morbid. Mortal. Weekly Rep. 43:242–246.

Centers for Disease Control and Prevention (2006). Human plague-four states. MMWR Morb Mortal Wkly Rep.006; 55(34):940-943.

Chase CJ, Ulrich MP, Wasieloski LP Jr, Kondig JP, Garrison J, et al. (2005). Real-time PCR assays targeting a unique chromosomal sequence of *Yersinia pestis*. Clin Chem 51: 1778–1785.

Chattopadhyaya A, Park S, Delmas G, Suresh R, Senina S, Perlin DS, Rose JK (2008). Single-dose, virus-vectored vaccine protection against *Yersinia pestis* challenge: CD4+ cells are required at the time of challenge for optimal protection. Vaccine 26:6329–6337

Conrad, FG, FR LeCocq, and R Krain (1968). A recent epidemic of plague in Vietnam. Arch. Int. Med. 122:193–198.

Cornelis GR (2000). Molecular and cell biology aspects of plague. Proc. Natl. Acad. Sci. USA. 97:8778–8783.

Cornelis GR, Boland A, Boyd AP, Geuijen C, Iriarte M, Neyt C, Sory MP, and Stainier I. (1998). The virulence plasmid of *Yersinia*, an antihost genome.Microbiol. Mol. Biol. Rev. 62:1315–1352.

Craven RB, Maupin GO, Beard ML, Quan TJ, and Barnes AM (1993). Reported cases of human plague infections in the United States, 1970–1991. J. Med. Entomol. 30:758–761.

Crook LD, and. Tempest B. (1992). Plague: a clinical review of 27 cases. Arch. Intern. Med. 152:1253–1256.

Davis KJ, Fritz DL, Pitt ML, et al.(1996). Pathology of experimental pneumonic plague produced by fraction 1-positive and fraction 1-negative *Yersinia pestis* in African green monkeys (*Cercopithecus aethiops*). Arch. Pathol. Lab. Med ;120(2):156–163.

Deber CM, Hruby VJ and Kopple KD (eds) (1985). Peptides: Structure and function. (Rockford:PierceChemical Co.) 23p.

Del Prete G, Santi L, Andrianaivoarimanana V, Amedei A, Domarle O, D' Elios MM, Arntzen CJ, Rahalison L, Mason HS (2009). Plant-derived recombinant F1, V, and F1-V fusion antigens of *Yersinia pestis* activate human cells of the innate and adaptive immune system. Int J Immunopathol Pharmacol 22:133–143.

Doll JM, Zeitz PS, Ettestad P, Bucholtz AL, Davis T, and Gage K (1994). Cat-transmitted fatal pneumonic plague in a person who traveled from Colorado to Arizona. Am. J. Trop. Med. Hyg. 51:109–114.

Du Y, Galyov E, and Forsberg A (1995). Genetic analysis of virulence determinants unique to *Yersinia pestis*. Contrib. Microbiol. Immunol. 13:321–324.

Du Y, Rosqvist R, and Forsberg A (2002). Role of fraction 1 antigen of *Yersinia pestis* in inhibition of phagocytosis. Infect. Immun. 70:1453–1460.

Ehrenkranz NJ, Meyer KF (1955). Studies on immunization against plague. VIII. Study of three immunizing preparations in protecting primates against pneumonic plague. J. Infect. Dis ; 96:138–144.

Felek S, Tsang TM, Krukonis ES (2010). Three *Yersinia pestis* adhesins facilitate Yop delivery to eukaryotic cells and contribute to plague virulence. Infect Immun 78:4134–4150.

Ferber DM, and Brubaker RR (1981). Plasmids in *Yersinia pestis*. Infect. Immun. 31:839–841.

Fields KA, Nilles ML, Cowan C, and Straley SC (1999). Virulence role of V antigen of *Yersinia pestis* at the bacterial surface. Infect. Immun. 67:5395–5408.

Filippov AA, Solodovnikov NS, Kookleva LM, and Protsenko OA (1990). Plasmid content in *Yersinia pestis* strains of different origin. FEMS Microbiol. Lett. 67:45–48.

Finegold MJ (1969). Pneumonic plague in monkeys. An electron microscopic study. Am. J. Pathol ;54 (2):167–185.

Friedlander AM, Welkos SL, Worsham PL, et al. (1995). Relationship between virulence and immunity as revealed in recent studies of the F1 capsule of *Yersinia pestis*. Clin. Infect. Dis ; 21(Suppl 2):S178–S181.

Gage KL, Lance SE, Dennis DT, and Montenieri JA (1992). Human plague in the United States: a review of cases from 1988–1992 with comments on the likelihood of increased plague activity. Border Epidemiol. Bull. 19:1–10.

Galan JE, and Collmer A (1999). Type III secretion machines: bacterial devices for protein delivery into host cells. Science. 284:1322–1328.

Girard G (1963) Immunity in plague. Results of 30 years of work on the *Pasteurella pestis* Ev' (Girard and Robic) strain. Biol Med (Paris);52:631–731.

Gottfried RS (1983). The black death. Natural and human disaster in medieval Europe. The Free Press, New York, N.Y.

Green SP, Hartland EL, Robins-Browne RM, and Phillips WA (1995). Role of YopH in the suppression of tyrosine phosphorylation and respiratory burst activity in murine macrophages infected with *Yersinia enterocolitica*. J. Leukoc. Biol. 57:972–977.

Gupta G, Khan AA & Rao DN (2009). Cell-Mediated Immune Response and Th1/Th2 Cytokine Profile of B-T Constructs of F1 and V Antigen of *Yersinia pestis*. Scandinavian Journal of Immunology 71, 186–198.

Gupta G, et al (2011). Evaluation of CD4+/CD8+ T-cell expression and IFN-γ, perforin secretion for B–T constructs of F1and V antigens of *Yersinia pestis*. Int Immunopharmacol. doi:10.1016/j.intimp.2011.10.012

Haddix PL, Straley SC (1992). Structure and regulation of the *Yersinia pestis yscBCDEF* operon. J Bacteriol 174(14):4820-4828.

Haffkine WM (1897). Remarks on the plague prophylactic fluid. Br. Med. J ;1:1461.

Harris SH (1994). *Factories of Death*. New York, NY: Routledge; 1994:78, 96.

Heath DG, Anderson GW Jr, Mauro JM, et al. (1998). Protection against experimental bubonic and pneumonic plague by a recombinant capsular F1-V antigen fusion protein vaccine. Vaccine ;16(1112): 1131–1137.

Heesemann J, Sing A, Trulzsch K (2006). Yersinia's stratagem: targeting innate and adaptive immune defense. Curr. Opin. Microbiol ; 9 (1) : 55–61.

Higgins JA, Ezzell J, Hinnebusch BJ, Shipley M, Henchal EA, et al. (1998), 5′ nuclease PCR assay to detect *Yersinia pestis*. J Clin Microbiol 36: 2284–2288.

Hinnebusch J, Schwan TG (1993). New method for plague surveillance using polymerase chain reaction to detect *Yersinia pestis* in fleas. J Clin Microbiol 31: 1511–1514.

Hirst LF (1953). *The Conquest of Plague: A Study of the Evolution and Epidemiology*. Oxford, UK: Clarendon Press.

Hoiczyk E, Blobel G (2001). Polymerization of a single protein of the pathogen *Yersinia enterocolitica* into needles punctures eukaryotic cells. Proc Natl Acad Sci U S A, 98(8):4669-4674.

Holt JG, Krieg NR, Sneath PHA, Staley JT, and Williams ST (ed.). (1994). Bergey's manual of determinative bacteriology, 9th ed., p. 175–289. The Williams & Wilkins Co., Baltimore, Md.

Huang XZ, and Lindler LE (2004). The pH 6 antigen is an antiphagocytic factor produced by *Yersinia pestis* independent of Yersinia outer proteins and capsule antigen. Infect. Immun. 72:7212–7219.

Huang J, D'Souza AJ, Alarcon JB, Mikszta JA et al. (2009). Protective Immunity in Mice Achieved with Dry Powder Formulation and Alternative Delivery of Plague F1-V Vaccine. Clin Vacc Immunol:16 719–725

Hull HF, Montes JM, and Mann JM (1987). Septicemic plague in New Mexico. J. Infect. Dis. 155:113–118.

Iqbal SS, Chambers JP, Goode MT, Valdes JJ, Brubaker RR (2000). Detection of *Yersinia pestis* by pesticin fluorogenic probe-coupled PCR. Mol Cell Probes 14: 109–114.

Iriarte M, and GR Cornelis (1998). YopT, a new *Yersinia* Yop effector protein, affects the cytoskeleton of host cells. Mol. Microbiol. 29:915–929.

Iteman I, Guiyoule A, De Almeida AMP, Guilvout I, Baranton G, and Carniel E (1993). Relationship between loss of pigmentation and deletion of the chromosomal iron-regulated *irp2* gene in *Yersinia pestis*: evidence for separate but related events. Infect. Immun. 61:2717–2722.

Ivanov MI, Noel BL, Rampersaud R, Mena P, Benach JL, and Bliska JB (2008). Vaccination of Mice with a Yop Translocon Complex Elicits Antibodies That Are Protective against Infection with F1-*Yersinia pestis*. Infect. Immun. 76;11, 5181–5190.

Janssen WA, Lawton WD, Fukui GM, Surgalla MJ (1963). The pathogenesis of plague. I. A study of the correlation between virulence and relative phagocytosis resistance of some strains of *Pasteurella pestis*. J. Infect. Dis ;113:139–143.

Janssen WA, Surgalla MJ (1969). Plague bacillus: survival within host phagocytes. Science ;163:950–952.

Jones A, Catharine Bosio (2010). Protection against pneumonic plague following oral immunization with a non-replicating vaccine. Vaccine: 16; 28(36):5924-9.

Jones SM, Day F, Stagg AJ, Williamson ED (2000). Protection conferred by a fully recombinant sub-unit vaccine against *Yersinia pestis* in male and female mice of four inbred strains. Vaccine;19(23): 358–366.

Kartman L. (1969). Effect of differences in ambient temperature upon the fate of *Pasteurella pestis* in *Xenopsylla cheopis*. Trans. R. Soc. Trop. Med. Hyg. 63:71–75.

Kawahara K, Tsukano H, Watanabe H, Lindner B, Matsuura M (2002). Modification of the structure and activity of lipid A in *Yersinia pestis* lipopolysaccharide by growth temperature. Infect Immun 70:4092–4098.

Kerschen EJ, Cohen DA, Kaplan AM, and Straley SC (2004). The plague virulence protein YopM targets the innate immune response by causing a global depletion of NK cells. Infect. Immun. 72:4589–4602.

Khan AA, Rao DN (2008). Identifying B and T cell epitopes and studying humoral, mucosal and cellular immune responses of peptides derived from V antigen of *Yersinia pestis*.Vaccine: 26; 316—332.

Kolle W, Otto R (1904). Weitere Untersuchungen uber die Pestimmunitat. Zeitschr. F. Hyg;48:399-428.

Kolodziejek AM, Schnider DR, Rohde HN, Wojtowicz AJ, Bohach GA, Minnich SA, Hovde CJ (2010). Outer membrane protein X (Ail) contributes to *Yersinia pestis* virulence in pneumonic plague and its activity is dependent on LPS core length. Infect Immun;78:5233-5243.

Lathem WW, Crosby SD, Miller VL, Goldman WE (2005). Progression of primary pneumonic plague: a mouse model of infection, pathology, and bacterial transcriptional activity. Proc. Natl Acad. Sci. USA; 102(49):17786-17791.

Lawton WD, Erdman RL, Surgalla MJ (1963). Biosynthesis and purification of V and W antigen in *Pateurella pestis*. J. Immunol; 91:179-184.

Leary SE, Williamson ED, Griffin KF, et al. (1995). Active immunization with recombinant V antigen from *Yersinia pestis* protects mice against plague. Infect. Immun;63(8):2854-2858.

Leary SE, Griffin KF, EE Galyov, J Hewer, ED Williamson, A Holmstrom, A Forsberg, and RW Titball (1999). *Yersinia* outer proteins (YOPS) E, K and N are antigenic but non-protective compared to V antigen, in a murine model of bubonic plague. Microb. Pathog. 26:159-169.

Lederberg J., ed. (2001).*Biological Weapons limiting the threat.*, MIT Press.

Lee VT, Tam C, and Schneewind O (2000). LcrV, a substrate for *Yersinia enterocolitica* type III secretion, is required for toxin targeting into the cytosol of HeLa cells. J. Biol. Chem. 275:36869-36875.

Lien Teh WA (1926). Treatise on Pneumonic Plague. League of Nations Health Organisation; Geneva, Switzerland.

Lindler LE, Fan W, Jahan N (2001). Detection of ciprofloxacin-resistant *Yersinia pestis* by fluorogenic PCR using the LightCycler. J Clin Microbiol 39: 3649-3655.

Lindler LE, and Tall BD (1993). *Yersinia pestis* pH 6 antigen forms fimbriae and is induced by intracellular association with macrophages. Mol. Microbiol. 8:311-324.

Lin JS, et al. (2010).TNF-α and IFN-γ contribute to F1/LcrV-targeted immune defense in mouse models of fully virulent pneumonic plague.Vaccine: 16;29(2):357-62.

Link VB (1955). A History of Plague in the United States of America [Public Health Service Monograph No. 26]. Washington, DC: Government Printing Office, 1955.

Loiez C, Herwegh S, Wallet F, Armand S, Guinet F, et al. (2003). Detection of *Yersinia pestis* in sputum by real-time PCR. J Clin Microbiol 41: 4873-4875.

Lukaszewski RA, Kenny DJ, Taylor R, et al. (2005). Pathogenesis of *Yersinia pestis* infection in BALB/c mice: effects on host macrophages and neutrophils. Infect. Immun;73(11):7142-7150.

Makoveichuk E, Cherepanov P, Lundberg S, Forsberg A and Olivecrona G. (2003). pH6 antigen of *Yersinia pestis* interacts with plasma lipoproteins and cell membranes. J. Lipid Res. 44:320-330.

Marenne MN, Journet L, Mota LJ, Cornelis GR (2003). Genetic analysis of the formation of the Ysc-Yop translocation pore in macrophagesby *Yersinia enterocolitica*: role of LcrV, YscF and YopN. Microb Pathog. 35(6):243-258.

Matson JS, Kelly A Durick, David S Bradley and Matthew L Nilles (2005). Immunization of mice with YscF provides protection from *Yersinia pestis* infections. BMC Microbiology, 5:38.

McDonald C, Vacratsis PO, Bliska JB, and Dixon JE (2003). The yersinia virulence factor YopM forms a novel protein complex with two cellular kinases. J. Biol. Chem. 278:18514–18523.

McDonough KA, Schwan TG, Thomas RE, and Falkow S (1988). Identification of a *Yersinia pestis*-specific DNA probe with potential for use in plague surveillance. J. Clin. Microbiol. 26:2515–2519.

Meyer KF, Cavanaugh DC, Bartelloni PJ, Marshall JD Jr. (1974). Plague immunization. I. Past and present trends. J. Infect. Dis 1974;129 (Suppl):S13–S18.

Meyer KF, Smith G, Foster L, Brookman M, Sung M (1974). Live attenuated *Yersinia pestis* vaccine: virulent in nonhuman primates, harmless to guinea pigs. J. Infect. Dis;129(Suppl):S85–S112.

Meyer KF (1970). Effectiveness of live or killed plague vaccines in man. Bull. World Health Org. 42 (5):653–666.

Meyer KF (1950). Modern therapy of plague. JAMA 144:982–985.

Meyer KF (1961). Pneumonic plague. Bacteriol. Rev. 25:249–261.

Mizel SB, Graff AH et al. (2009). Flagellin-F1-V fusion protein is an effective plague vaccine in mice and two species of nonhuman primates. Clin Vac Immunol: 16;1: 21–28.

Montminy SW, Khan N, McGrath S, Walkowicz MJ, Sharp F, Conlon JE, Fukase K, Kusumoto S, Sweet C, Miyake K, Akira S, Cotter RJ, Goguen JD, Lien E (2006). Virulence factors of *Yersinia pestis* are overcome by a strong lipopolysaccharide response. Nat Immunol 7:1066–1073.

Motin VL, Nakajima R, Smirnov GB, Brubaker RR (1994). Passive immunity to yersiniae mediated by antirecombinant V antigen and protein A-V antigen fusion peptide. Infect. Immun 62(10):4192–4201.

Nakajima R, Brubaker RR (1993). Association between virulence of *Yersinia pestis* and suppression of gamma interferon and tumor necrosis factor alpha. Infect. Immun. ;61(1):23–31.

Nemeth J, and Straley SC (1997). Effect of *Yersinia pestis* YopM on experimental plague. Infect. Immun. 65:924–930.

Norkina OV, Kulichenko AN, Gintsburg AL, Tuchkov IV, Popov Yu A, et al. (1994) Development of a diagnostic test for *Yersinia pestis* by the polymerase chain reaction. J Appl Bacteriol 76: 240–245.

Perry RD, and Fetherston JD (1997). *Yersinia pestis*: etiologic agent of plague. Clin. Microbiol. Rev. 10:35–66.

Peterson JW, Walberg KG, Pawlik J, Bush K, Taormina J, Hardcastle J, Moen S, Thomas J, Lawrence W, Ponce C, Parham T, Chatuev BM, Sower L, Klimpel G, Eaves-Pyles T, Chopra AK (2010). Evaluation of protection afforded by fluoroquinolones against respiratory infections with *Bacillus anthracis*, *Yersinia pestis*, and *Francisella tularensis*. Open Microbiology Journal 4:34–46.

Poland JD, Quan TJ, and AM Barnes (1994). Plague, p. 93–112. *In* G. W. Beran (ed.), Handbook of zoonoses. Section A. Bacterial, rickettsial, chlamydial, and mycotic, 2nd ed. CRC Press, Inc., Ann Arbor, Mich.

Poland JD, and Barnes AM (1979). Plague, p. 515–559. *In* J. H. Steele (ed), CRC handbook series in zoonoses. Section A. Bacterial, rickettsial, and mycotic diseases, vol. I. CRC Press, Inc., Boca Raton, Fla.

Pollitzer R (1954). Plague. W. H. O. Monogr. Ser. 22:1–698.

Price SB, Leung KY, Barve SS, Straley SC (1989). Molecular analysis of *lcrGVH*, the V antigen operon of *Yersinia pestis*. J. Bacteriol ;171:5646–5653.

Price SB, Freeman MD and Yeh KS (1995). Transcriptional analysis of the *Yersinia pestis* pH 6 antigen gene. J. Bacteriol. 177:5997–6000.

Pujol C, Bliska JB (2005). Turning *Yersinia* pathogenesis outside in: subversion of macrophage function by intracellular yersiniae. Clin. Immunol ;114(3):216–226.

Qi Z, Zhou L, Zhang Q (2010). Comparison of mouse, guinea pig and rabbit models for evaluation of plague subunit vaccine F1 + rV270. Vaccine 28 1655–1660.

Ramirez K et. al. (2009). Mucosally delivered *Salmonella typhi* expressing the *Yersinia pestis* F1 antigen elicits mucosal and systemic immunity early in life and primes the neonatal immune system for a vigorous anamnestic response to parenteral F1 boost. J. Immunol. 182; 1211-1222.

Ren J, Dong D, Zhang J, Zhang J, et al. (2009). Protection against anthrax and plague by a combined vaccine in mice and rabbits. Vaccine. 9; 27(52):7436-41

Rigano MM, Manna C, Giulini A, Vitale A, Cardi T (2009). Plants as biofactories for the production of subunit vaccines against biosecurity- related bacteria and viruses. Vaccine 27:3463–3466

Rocke TE, Smith SR, Stinchcom DT, Osorio JE (2008). Immunization of black-tailed prairie dog against plague through consumption of vaccine-laden baits. J Wildl Dis 44:930–937.

Rocke TE, Iams KP, Dawe S, Smith SR, Williamson JL, Heisey DM, Osorio JE (2010a). Further development of raccoon poxvirus vectored vaccines against plague (*Yersinia pestis*). Vaccine 28:338–344.

Rocke TE, Pussini N, Smith SR, Williamson J, Powell B, Osorio JE (2010b). Consumption of baits containing raccoon pox-based plague vaccines protects black-tailed prairie dogs (*Cynomys ludovicianus*). Vector Borne Zoonotic Dis 10:53–58.

Roggenkamp A, Geiger AM, Leitritz L, Kessler A, Heesemann J (1997). Passive immunity to infection with *Yersinia* spp. mediated by anti-recombinant V antigen is dependent on polymorphism of V antigen. Infect. Immun ;65:446–451.

Rosales-Mendoza S, Soria-Guerra RE, Moreno-Fierros L, Alpuche-Solis AG, Martinez-Gonzalez L, Korban SS (2010a). Expression of an immunogenic F1-Vfusion protein in lettuce as a plant-based vaccine against plague. Planta 232:409–416.

Rosales-Mendoza S, Soria-Guerra RE, Moreno-Fierros L, Han Y, Alpuche-Solís AG, Korban SS (2010b). Transgenic carrot tap roots expressing an immunogenic F1-V fusion protein from *Yersinia pestis* are immunogenic in mice. J Plant Physiol 168:174–180.

Rosenzweig JA, Olufisayo Jejelowo, Jian Sha,Tatiana E. Erova, Sheri M. Brackman, Michelle L. Kirtley, Cristina J. van Lier, Ashok K. Chopra(2011).Progress on plague vaccine development. Appl Microbiol Biotechnol DOI 10.1007/s00253-011-3380-6.

Rosqvist R, Forsberg A, Rimpilainen M, Bergman T, Wolf-Watz H (1990). The cytotoxic protein YopE of *Yersinia* obstructs the primary host defense. Mol. Microbiol. 4:657–667.

Russell P, Eley SM, Hibbs SE, et al. (1995). A comparison of Plague vaccine, USP and EV76 vaccine induced protection against *Yersinia pestis* in a murine model. Vaccine ;13:1551–1556.

Sabhnani L, & Rao DN (2003). Developing subunit immunogens using B and T cell epitopes and their constructs derived from the F1 antigen of *Yersinia pestis* using novel delivery vehicles. FEMS Immunol Med Microbiol. 15;38(3):215-29.

Saikaly PE, Barlaz MA, de Los Reyes FL, 3rd (2007). Development of quantitative real-time PCR assays for detection and quantification of surrogate biological warfare agents in building debris and leachate. Appl Environ Microbiol 73: 6557–6565.

Sato K, Nakajima R, Hara F, Une T, Osada Y (1991). Preparation of monoclonal antibody to V antigen from *Yersinia pestis*. Contrib. Microbiol. Immunol;12:225–229.

Sebbane F, Gardner D, Long D, Gowen BB, Hinnebusch BJ (2005). Kinetics of disease progression and host response in a rat model of bubonic plague. Am. J. Pathol ;166(5):1427–1439.

Sha J, Agar SL, Baze WB, Olano JP, Fadl AA, Erova TE, Wang S, Foltz SM, Suarez G, Motin VL, Chauhan S, Klimpel GR, Peterson JW, Chopra AK (2008). Braun lipoprotein (Lpp) contributes to the virulence of yersiniae: potential role of Lpp in inducing bubonic and pneumonic plague. Infect Immun 76:1390–1409.

Sha J, Endsley JJ, Kirtley ML, Foltz SM, Huante MB, Erova TE, Kozlova EV, Popov VL, Yeager LA, Zudina IV, Motin VL, Peterson JW, Chopra AK (2011). Characterization of an F1 deletion mutant of *Yersinia pestis* CO92, pathogenic role of F1 antigen in bubonic and pneumonic plague, and evaluation of the sensitivity and specificity of F1 antigen capture-based dipsticks. J Clin Microbiol 49:1708–1715.

Sing A, Roggenkamp A, Geiger AM, and Heesemann J (2002). *Yersinia enterocolitica* evasion of the host innate immune response by V antigen-induced IL-10 production of macrophages is abrogated in IL-10-deficient mice. J. Immunol. 168:1315–1321.

Sing A, Rost D, Tvardovskaia N, Roggenkamp A, Wiedemann A, Kirschning CJ, Aepfelbacher M, and Heesemann J (2002). Yersinia V-antigen exploits toll-like receptor- 2 and CD14 for interleukin 10–mediated immunosuppression. J. Exp. Med.: 21;196(8):1017-24.

Skottman T, Piiparinen H, Hyytiainen H, Myllys V, Skurnik M, et al. (2007). Simultaneous real-time PCR detection of *Bacillus anthracis, Francisella tularensis* and *Yersinia pestis.* Eur J Clin Microbiol Infect Dis 26: 207–211.

Sofer-Podesta C, Ang J, Hackett NR, Senina S, Perlin D, Crystal RG, Boyer JL (2009). Adenovirus-mediated delivery of an anti-V antigen monoclonal antibody protects mice against a lethal *Yersinia pestis* challenge. Infect Immun 4:1561–1568.

Staskawicz BJ, Mudgett MB, Dangl JL, and Galan JE (2001). Common and contrasting themes of plant and animal diseases. Science. 292:2285–2289.

Sticker G (1908). *Abhandlungen aus der Seuchengeschichte und Seuchenlehre. Band I. Die Geschichte der Pest.* Giessen: A Toepelmann Verlag.

Straley SC, Harmon PA (1984). Growth in mouse peritoneal macrophages of *Yersinia pestis* lacking established virulence determinants. Infect. Immun; 45(3):649–654.

Strong RP (1908). Protective inoculation against plague. J. Med. Res; 18:325–346.

Strong RP (1906). Vaccination against plague. Phillipine J. Sci; 1:181–190.

Sun W, Six D, Kuang X, Roland KL, Raetz CR, Curtiss R III (2011). A live attenuated strain of *Yersinia pestis* KIM as a vaccine against plague. Vaccine 29:2986–2998.

Swietnicki W, Powell BS, Goodin J (2005). *Yersinia pestis* Yop secretion protein F: Purification, characterization, and protective efficacy against bubonic plague. Protein Exp Purif: 42; 166–172

Szaba FM, Kummer LW, Wilhelm LB, Lin JS, Parent MA, Montminy-Paquette SW, Lien E, Johnson LL, Smiley ST (2008). D27-pLpxL, an avirulent strain of *Yersinia pestis,* primes T cells thatprotect against pneumonic plague. Infect Immun 77:4295–4304.

Taylor J (1933). Haffkine's plague vaccine. Indian Med. Res. Memoirs; 27:1–125.

Titball RW, Williamson ED (2004). *Yersinia pestis* (plague) vaccines. Expert Opin. Biol. Ther; 4(6): 965–973.

Tomaso H, Reisinger EC, Al Dahouk S, Frangoulidis D, Rakin A, et al. (2003). Rapid detection of *Yersinia pestis* with multiplex real-time PCR assays using fluorescent hybridisation probes. FEMS Immunol Med Microbiol 38: 117–126.

Tripathi V and Rao DN (2006). Inducing systemic and mucosal immune responses to B-T construct of F1 antigen of *Yersinia pestis* in microsphere delivery. Vaccine. 12; 24(16):3279-89.

Tsukano H, Itoh K, Suzuki S, Watanabe H (1996). Detection and identification of *Yersinia pestis* by polymerase chain reaction (PCR) using multiplex primers. Microbiol Immunol 40: 773–775.

Une T, Brubaker RR (1984). In vivo comparison of avirulent Vwa- and Pgm- or Pstr phenotypes of yersiniae. Infect. Immun; 43(3):895–900.

Une T, Brubaker RR (1984). Roles of V antigen in promoting virulence and immunity in yersiniae. J. Immunol; 133(4):2226–2230.

Uppada JB and DN Rao (2009). Humoral immune responses and protective efficacy of sequential B- and T-cell epitopes of V antigen of *Yersinia pestis* in microparticle delivery by intranasal immunization. Med. Microbiol. Immunnol.198; 4, 247-256.

Uppada JB and Rao DN (2011). Enhanced humoral and mucosal immune responses after intranasal immunization with chimeric multiple antigen peptide of LcrV antigen epitopes of *Yersinia pestis* coupled to palmitate in mice. Vaccine 29 (50):9352-60.

Varma-Basil M, El-Hajj H, Marras SA, Hazbon MH, Mann JM, et al. (2004). Molecular beacons for multiplex detection of four bacterial bioterrorism agents. Clin Chem 50: 1060–1063.

Vernazza C, Lingard B, Flick-Smith HC, Baillie LW, Hill J, Atkins HS (2009). Small protective fragments of the *Yersinia pestis* V antigen. Vaccine 27:2775–2780.

Viboud GI, Bliska JB (2005). *Yersinia* outer proteins: role in modulation of host cell signaling responses and pathogenesis. Annu. Rev. Microbiol; 59:69–89.

Von Reyn CF, Weber NS, Tempest B, Barnes AM, Poland JD, Boyce JM, and Zalma V (1977). Epidemiologic and clinical features of an outbreak of bubonic plague in New Mexico. J. Infect. Dis. 136:489–494.

Wang S, et al. (2011). Involvement of CD8+ T cell-mediated immune responses in LcrV DNA vaccine induced protection against lethal *Yersinia pestis* challenge. Vaccine doi:10.1016/j.vaccine.2010.12.062.

Wang S, Mboudjeka I, Goguen JD, Lu S (2010). Antigen engineering can play a critical role in the protective immunity elicited by *Yersinia pestis* DNA vaccines. Vaccine 28: 2011–2019.

Weening EH, Cathelyn JS, Kaufman G, Lawrenz MB, Price P, Goldman WE, Miller VL (2011). The Dependence of *Yersinia. pestis* capsule for pathogenesis is influenced by mouse background. Infect Immun 79:644–652.

Welkos S, Pitt ML, Martinez M, et al. (2002). Determination of the virulence of the pigmentation-deficient and pigmentation-/plasminogen activator-deficient strains of *Yersinia pestis* in non-human primate and mouse models of pneumonic plague. Vaccine; 20(1718):2206–2214.

Welkos SL, Davis KM, Pitt LM, Worsham PL, Freidlander AM (1995). Studies on the contribution of the F1 capsule-associated plasmid p*Fra* to the virulence of *Yersinia pestis*. Contrib. Microbiol. Immunol; 13:299–305.

Wheelis M. (2002), Biological warfare at the 1346 siege of Caffa, Emerg Infect Dis 8:971-975.

Wigglesworth V B (1984). Insect physiology, p. 54–68, Chapman & Hall, New York.

Williams JE, Gentry MK, Braden CA, Leister F and Yolken RH (1984). Use of an enzyme-linked immunosorbent assay to measure antigenaemia during acute plague. Bull. W. H. O. 62:463–466.

Williamson ED, Eley SM, Griffin KF, et al. (1995). A new improved sub-unit vaccine for plague: the basis of protection. FEMS Immunol. Med. Microbiol; 12(34):223–230.

Williamson ED, Eley SM, Stagg AJ, et al.(1997). A sub-unit vaccine elicits IgG in serum, spleen cell cultures and bronchial washings and protects immunized animals against pneumonic plague. Vaccine;15 (10):1079–1084.

Williamson ED, Sharp GJ, Eley SM, et al.(1996). Local and systemic immune response to a microencapsulated sub-unit vaccine for plague. Vaccine; 14(1718):1613–1619.

Williamson ED,et al. (2011). Recombinant (F1+V) vaccine protects cynomolgus macaques against pneumonic plague. Vaccine; 24; 29(29-30):4771-7.

Winter CC, Cherry WB, Moody MD (1960). An unusual strain of *Pasteurella pestis* isolated from a fatal human case of plague. Bull. W.H.O.; 23:408–409.

World Health Organization (2002). Plaguein Malawi and India. Available at http://www.who.int/csr/don/archive/disease/plague/en/; accessed January 25, 2005.

World Health Organization (2003). Plague in Algeria. Available at http //www.who.int/csr/don /2003_06_24a/ en/; accessed January 25, 2005.

World Health Organization (1970). *Health Aspects of Chemical and Biological Weapons*. Geneva, Switzerland; 1970:98-109.

Woron AM, Nazarian EJ, Egan C, McDonough KA, Cirino NM, et al. (2006). Development and evaluation of a 4-target multiplex real-time polymerase chain reaction assay for the detection and characterization of *Yersinia pestis*. Diagn Microbiol Infect Dis 56: 261–268.

Worsham PL, Stein MP, Welkos SL (1995). Construction of defined F1 negative mutants of virulent *Yersinia pestis*. Contrib. Microbiol. Immunol; 13:325–328.

Xiao X, Zhu Z, Dankmeyer JL, Wormald MM, Fast RL, et al. (2010). Human anti-plague monoclonal antibodies protect mice from *Yersinia pestis* in a bubonic plague model. PLoS ONE 5(10): e13047.

Yamanaka H, Teri Hoyt, Xinghong Yang (2010). A parenteral DNA vaccine protects against pneumonic plague. Vaccine 28 : 3219–3230.

Yamanaka H, Hoyt T, Yang X, Golden S, Bosio CM, Crist K, Becker T, Maddaloni M, Pascual DW (2008). A nasal interleukin-12 DNA vaccine coexpressing *Yersinia pestis* F1-V fusion protein confers protection against pneumonic plague. Infect Immun 76:4564–4573.

Zilinskas RA (2006). The anti-plague system and the Soviet biological warfare program. Crit. Rev. Microbiol; 32(1):47–64.

6

Botulinum Neurotoxins

Robert P. Webb[1], Virginia I. Roxas-Duncan[1] and Leonard A. Smith[2]
[1]*Integrated Toxicology Division,*
US Army Medical Research Institute of Infectious Diseases,
[2]*Senior Research Scientist (ST) for Medical Countermeasures Technology,*
Office of Chief Scientist,
US Army Medical Research Institute of Infectious Diseases, Frederick,
USA

1. Introduction

Botulism is a neuroparalytic disease caused by neurotoxin produced from the bacterium *Clostridium botulinum*. The botulinum neurotoxins (BoNTs) are among the most potent known biological toxins and have an estimated human median lethal dose (LD_{50}) in the nanogram/kilogram range. Botulinum toxins have historically been employed as biological weapons (BW) through state-sponsored programs in Japan, Germany, the United States, Russia and Iraq as well as by independent terrorist organizations. The extreme potency of the toxin, its persistence within affected neurons, the need for protracted intensive care, and the lack of an effective post-intoxication therapeutic intervention make BoNTs a potentially deadly offensive biological weapon.

2. Botulinum neurotoxins as biological weapons

2.1 Historical applications of botulinum toxins in biological warfare

There have been reports of botulinum neurotoxin being used as an offensive weapon since the early 1900s. Anecdotal accounts describe the implementation of crude anaerobic fermenters made by burying canteens filled with water, green beans and slivers of meat to facilitate *C. botulinum* production for use against Mexican federal troops in 1910 (Carrus, 2001). Documented state sponsored programs utilizing BoNT as a potential BW were reported as early as the 1930s when the military medical commander of Unit 731, General Shiro Ishii, confessed to feeding food contaminated with lethal cultures of *C. botulinum* to prisoners of war (Williams & Wallace, 1989). In the early 1940s, the US developed a BoNT-based BW program in response to Allied intelligence reports that Germany was attempting to develop the neurotoxin as an offensive weapon to be used against an invasion force (Franz et al., 1997). The initial efforts of the US program were primarily directed at the isolation and purification of the toxin and the elucidation of the mechanism of pathogenicty of BoNT, then referred to as agent "X" (Cochrane, 1947). In response to the potential threat from Germany, over 1 million doses of a botulinum toxoid vaccine were prepared for Allied troops involved in the D-Day invasion in Normandy (Bryden, 1989). The 1972 Convention on the Prohibition of the Development, Production, and Stockpiling of Bacteriological

(Biological) and Toxin Weapons and on their Destruction signed by President Richard M. Nixon went into effect in March of 1975, effectively terminating the US BW efforts. All of the biological agent stockpiles created in the US offensive program, including botulinum neurotoxins, were destroyed. Despite being signatories on the convention, the Soviet Union continued not only to pursue its biowarfare program, including research on botulinum neurotoxins, but expanded their program during the post-Soviet era (UNSC, 1995; Bozheyeva et al., 1999). Botulinum toxins were reportedly one of several biological agents tested at the Soviet Aralsk-7 site on Vozrozhdeniye (Renaissance) Island in the Aral Sea. The Soviets were also believed to have attempted to use recombinant DNA technology to introduce BoNT genes into alternative strains of bacteria for the purpose of enhancing toxin production (Alibek & Handleman, 1999). Iraq, which also ratified the 1975 convention, reportedly also significantly expanded its biological weapons program (UNSC, 1995). After the Persian Gulf War, Iraq admitted to a United Nations Special Commission inspection team that approximately 4,900 gallons of concentrated botulinum neurotoxins had been produced for use in specially designed bombs, missiles and tank dispersion instruments in 1989 (Zilinskas, 1997). Iraq maintains that no biological weapons were employed during the Persian Gulf War or Operation Iraqi Freedom and that its stockpiles have since been destroyed (Blix, 2004).

The Japanese cult Aum Shrinkyo (now referred to as Aleph) attempted to develop both chemical and biological weapons after its political aspirations were defeated in the 1990 Japanese Diet elections. Formed in 1987 by Shoko Asahara, this group developed rapidly and was reported to have 50,000 members and over US$ 1 billion in financial resources by 1995 (Sugishima, 2003). The Aum executed a deadly sarin nerve gas attack in Matsumoto City on June 27, 1994 which killed seven people. On March 20, 1995 they perpetrated a sarin gas assault on a Tokyo subway which killed 12 people and injured over 1000 individuals. Less than a month later they attempted a cyanide gas release in a restroom of the subway's Shinjuku Station. Senior Aum members obtained soil samples in an attempt to isolate toxin-producing strains of *C. botulinum*. Despite the cult having members with a variety of scientific expertise, they are believed to have experienced difficulty cultivating toxigenic strains of *C. botulinum* and were most likely unable to produce any substantial amount of toxin (Sugishima, 2003; Leitenberg, 1999).

2.2 Domestic threat targets

The possibility of dissemination of toxins such as BoNT through municipal water supplies or centralized agricultural or food distribution hubs has been explored in a number of scenarios. There has never been a confirmed case of waterborne botulism. In 1980, Notermans & Havelaar reported on the stability of BoNT/A, /B and /E when introduced into samples of reservoir surface water, drinking water prepared by sand-filtration, and sterile distilled water. Toxicity was reduced 99% in just over 3 days in the surface water, 9 days in filtered water and relatively stable in sterile distilled water. Treatment with $FeCl_3$, a common coagulant processing step employed in municipal water treatments to remove iron, removed 75-95% of the toxins. Treatment with 1 mg of ozone per liter for 2 min destroyed ≥99% of the toxins and 0.3-0.5 mg/L sodium hypochlorite ablated 99% of the toxicity in 30 seconds. Despite the extreme potency of BoNTs, their application as a bioterrorism weapon by introduction into a water supply in the US would most likely be unsuccessful when conventional municipal water treatment methods are employed (Notermans & Havelaar, 1980; Wannemacher, at al., 1993). Another consideration is that large-capacity reservoirs undergo a relatively slow turn-over rate and so a comparably large inoculum of botulinum toxin would be needed (Burrows et al., 1997). Given the technical difficulties involved in producing such a large amount of toxin, this route seems unlikely. Small-scale (personal-use) water filtration systems utilizing ceramic or membrane filters with a 0.2 to 0.4 μm pore size were found to be insufficient to effectively remove BoNT/B introduced into drinking water. However, a reverse osmosis device was found to remove BoNT levels below the detection limit of the mouse bioassay (Hörman, et al. 2005).

American agriculture has been described as being "concentrated, highly accessible, vertically integrated" and as such, susceptible to the malicious introduction of biological toxins or human pathogens at processing or distribution points that would reach consumers before a significant threat was realized (Parker, 2002). Wein and Liu published a mathematical model to predict the effects of the deliberate introduction of botulinum toxin at various points through the nine-stage milk collection, processing and distribution network in the US, as it is associated with a single processing facility (Wein and Liu 2005). The study has a number of variables such as the amount of toxin employed, the total volume of the milk, the specific effect of the pasteurization process on the toxin and variable delivery time and consumptions rates, but all scenarios support a significant outbreak of up to 100,000 individuals. The report generated considerable controversy but the editors of the publishing journal defended the release, citing its potential contribution to developing defensive counter-measures as well as informing federal and state governments of the putative threat (Alberts, 2005). The devastating potential of an intentional bioterrorism attack using this avenue was illustrated in 1985 when almost 200,000 people were infected with an antibiotic-resistant strain of *Salmonella* caused by an inadvertent contamination at a single northern Illinois dairy processing plant (Ryan, et al., 1987).

The potential susceptibility of centralized food distribution platforms in the US can be illustrated by outbreaks attributed to improper processing of mass distributed consumable products. In September 2006, a total of 6 individuals from 2 US states and 1 Canadian province were admitted to local hospitals with cranial neuropathies and flaccid paralysis necessitating mechanical ventilation (CDC, 2007). All of the individuals tested positive for BoNT/A and one patient eventually died. The outbreaks were traced to a commercially produced carrot juice manufactured in a single plant which was distributed under three different brand labels. The intoxications were attributed to a lapse in refrigeration during transport or storage and a lack of chemical barriers to *C. botulinum* germination during processing. In the summer of 2007, 8 cases of botulism in 3 US states led to a massive recall of canned meat products. The outbreaks were traced to product from a single production line in a single plant that was packaged and distributed under 90 different labels (NCFPD, 2008) and which necessitated the recall of tens of millions of cans of suspect food. While these outbreaks represent unintentional distribution of BoNT, they do reveal the complexity of the food production and distribution network in the US and how it might be compromised by a BW attack using a potent toxin such as BoNT.

3. Microbiology and BoNT toxicity

3.1 The organism and its toxins

Clostridium spp. are gram-positive, spore-forming, obligate anaerobic bacteria that are ubiquitous in soil and both freshwater and marine sediment (Dunbar, 1990) . BoNTs are produced primarily in *C. botulinum* but may also be produced in the closely related *C. butyricum, C. baratii* and *C. argentinense* (Hatheway, 1993). *C. botulinum* strains are classified into four groups (denoted I to IV) based on metabolic activity (Hatheway, 1988) and genetic composition (Collins, 1998; Hill et al., 2007). Group I includes type A strains and proteolytic strains of types B and F; Group II includes type E strains and nonproteolytic strains of types B and F; Group III includes nonproteolytic strains of types C and D; and Group IV includes only strains that produce type G. There are seven immunologically distinct serotypes of BoNTs designated by the letters A through G (BoNT/A to BoNT/G) (Smith & Sugiyama, 1988). BoNT/A, based on animal studies, has a lethal human dose (LD_{50}), assuming 70 kg weight, of approximately 0.09 - 0.15 μg by intravenous administration, 0.7 – 0.9 μg by inhalation, and 70 μg by oral administration (Scott & Suzuki, 1988; Arnon et al., 2001). The toxicity for other serotypes is unknown but all have been shown to uniformly fatal in animals studies. Human botulism is caused primarily by BoNT/A, /B and /E (Arnon et al., 2001), and rarely by BoNT/F (Barash et al., 2005; Gupta et al., 2005). BoNT/C and /D primarily cause botulism in animals. BoNT/G, produced by *C. argentinense*, has been associated with sudden death but not neuroparalytic illness in a few patients in Switzerland (Sonnabend et al., 1981). All seven serotypes can cause inhalational botulism in primates (Middlebrook & Franz, 1997). Recent characterization of an increasing number of unique BoNT subtypes has revealed small to significant variations at the amino acid level (Smith, et al., 2005; Hill, et al. 2007; Smith, et al., 2007). These variations impact binding and protection of neutralizing antibodies (Smith, et al., 2005) and raise concerns that they may prove problematic to the development of prophylactic and therapeutic agents developed against a dissimilar subtype.

BoNTs are produced as a part of a protein complex in which the toxin is non-covalently bound to two or more protein components. This includes the well characterized hemagglutinins (HA) and a nontoxin, nonhemagglutinin (NTNH). The complexes can be distinguished on the basis of their size and serotype association and include the M-(300 kDa in types A-F), L-(500 kDa in serotypes A, B, C, D and G) and LL-(900 kDa in serotype A) forms (Collins & East, 1988). Although neither accessory protein has been implicated in the toxin-mediated blockade of neurotransmitter release, they are believed to protect the toxin against the harsh environment of the gastro-intestinal tract (Simpson, 2004). The neurotoxin is initially produced as a 150-kDa single-chain protoxin that is proteolytically cleaved into an N-terminal 50-kDa light chain (LC) and a C-terminal 100-kDa heavy chain (HC) di-chain that is linked by a single disulfide bond (DasGupta, 1989). The BoNT HC is further delineated into two domains; the N-fragment or translocation domain (Hn) and the C-fragment or receptor-binding domain (Hc). These three domains mediate intoxication of the neuron in a defined tripartite mechanism. The toxin is introduced into the nerve cell by receptor-mediated endocytosis through binding of the Hc domain to specific ectoreceptors on peripheral cholinergic nerve cells (Dong et al., 2006; Rummel et al., 2007). The acidic pH of the endosome initiates a conformation change in the dichain toxin that results in the Hn forming a protein channel that facilitates the translocation of the LC out of the endosomal lumen and into the cytosol. The LC is a zinc-containing endopeptidase that target SNARE (soluble *N*-ethylmaleamide sensitive factor attachment protein receptors) proteins that form the synaptonemal fusion complex in a serotype dependent fashion. The SNARE protein SNAP-25 (synaptosomal-associated protein of 25 kDa) is cleaved at different sites by BoNT/A, /C, and /E, synaptobrevin (also referred to as VAMP; vesicle-associated membrane protein), is cleaved at different sites by BoNT/B, /D, /F, and /G, and syntaxin is cleaved by BoNT/C (Simpson, 2004). Proteolytic cleavage of SNARE proteins prevents the release of acetylcholine across the synaptic cleft of the neuromuscular junction, resulting in a flaccid muscle paralysis which is the primary clinical sign of botulism.

3.2 Epidemiology

Botulism is typically reported in four clinical categories. *Foodborne botulism* is caused by the ingestion of the pre-formed toxin in contaminated food (CDC, 1998). Most outbreaks are associated with home-canned foods in which inadequate processing results in *C. botulinum* spores germinating, reproducing and producing the toxin (Shapiro, et al., 1998). These conditions include an anaerobic environment with temperatures ranging from 4°C to 40°C, a pH range from 4.6 to 7.0, and water activity greater than 0.94 (a_W is intensity with which water associates with various non-aqueous constituents and solids) (Baird-Parker & Freame, 1967; Stringer, et al., 2005). Despite increased educational awareness of the non-permissive conditions for food preparation, foodborne botulism remains a persistent threat. There were, on average, approximately 24 reported cases per year from 1900-2000, but there have been a smaller number of cases (average of 18 year) reported from 2001-2009 (CDC-NBS). In the period from 1950-1996, there were 444 outbreaks in which one or more cases of botulism from a contaminated food source was implicated. Of these outbreaks, 37.6% were caused by type A, 13.7% by type B, 15.1% by type E and 0.7% by type F while 32.9% of the incidents were caused by unidentified serotype(s) (CDC, 1998). Improvements in both differential diagnostic methods and the technology utilized in serotyping have resulted in a decrease in unidentified serotypes. In the United Stated from 1990-2000 BoNT/A was responsible for 50% of all cases of botulism, where types B and E were responsible for 10% and 37% of the intoxications, respectively; only 3.6% of the cases were from an unidentified strain (CDC, 1998).

Infant botulism is a toxicoinfection caused by inhalation or ingestion of clostridial spores that can colonize and produce toxin in the intestinal tract of infants less than 12 months of age (Shapiro, 1998). The ability of the bacteria to thrive and elicit toxin is thought to be attributed in part to a deficiency in protective gastrointesinal bacterial flora and the relatively low levels of inhibitory bile-aid found in children under 12 months (CDC, 1998). This form of the disease was officially recognized in a 1976 report in which two infants presenting with acute infantile hypotonoia and weakness were diagnosed with botulism (Pickett, et al., 1976). This has been the most commonly reported form of the disease in the United States since 1980, with an average of approximately 80-100 cases confirmed annually (Shapiro, 1998). In the US between 1976 and 1996, there were 1442 individual cases of infant botulism reported to the CDC (CDC, 1998). Of these, 46.5% were caused by type A, 51.9% by type B. Interestingly, the incidence of infant botulism in the US has a geographical component with 47.6% of the reported cases occurring in California with Delaware, Hawaii, and Utah also experiencing high incidence (CDC, 1988). The correlation between the increased incidences of infant botulism outbreaks associated with certain geographical locations has not been elucidated.

Wound botulism (WB) results from the growth of *C. botulinum* spores in a contaminated wound with in vivo toxin production. This form of the disease was first reported in 1951 as a relatively rare illness associated with post-operative complications (Davis et al., 1951). Historically, approximately 75% of the wound botulism cases in the US have been reported in California (Weber, et al., 1993) and this represents over 90% of the reported incidences in the world (Benson, 2001). There were 127 cases of wound botulism in California from 1951 to 1998. Of these, 105 were attributed to intravenous drug users and all but one were admitted black-tar heroin users (Benson, 2001). The increased incidence of WB in California has not abated and between 1993 and 2006 an additional 17 cases were identified in intravenous drug users; 16 of which were diagnosed with one or more recurrent episodes (Yuan et al., 2011).

Adult intestinal toxemia botulism is a rare toxicoinfection that occurs in older children and adults with abnormal gastrointestinal tract physiology, such as colitis or intestinal surgical procedures (Freeman et al., 1986; Fenecia et al., 1999). The disease has also been correlated with alteration of protective endogenous microflora by broad-spectrum antibiotics after inflammatory intestinal disease or surgery (Chia et al., 1986).

In addition to the four naturally occurring forms of the disease described previously, there are two additional forms of *inadvertent botulism* that result from the application of the purified toxin. *Iatrogenic botulism* results from the injection of BoNT for either cosmetic or therapeutic purposes. Two adult patients developed symptoms of botulism when given therapeutic doses of BoNT/A drawn from two different production lots (Bakheit, 1997). These cases have since been attributed to either patient sensitivity to the drug or the inadvertent injection of the toxin directly into the vascular capillaries. An adolescent being treated for spastic quadriparesis with Myobloc (botulinum toxin serotype B) developed clinical signs of a systemic BoNT injection (Partikian, 2007). While there are no clear dosing guidelines for BoNT formulations for therapeutic interventions in children, the clinical diagnosis of botulism was again believed to have been the result of inadvertent injection into a blood vessel or diffusion from nearby muscle sites. In November of 2007, four adults were given cosmetic injections of undiluted BoNT/A intended for laboratory research (Chertow et al., 2006). Serial dilutions of two of the individual's serum samples indicated they were given approximately 21 to 43 estimated human lethal doses. All four patients survived but only after prolonged hospitalization with anti-toxin treatment and ventilator support ranging from 40 to 104 days.

Inhalational botulism is intoxication by an inhalational exposure of the aerosolized toxin. The only reported human inhalation incidence occurred in Germany in 1962 during a necropsy when three laboratory workers were exposed to animals subjected to aerosolization of a highly purified, lyophilized BoNT/A (Holzer, 1962). The patients were hospitalized five days postexposure, administered equine antitoxin, and discharged after 9 days. While not a naturally occurring form of the disease, inhalational botulism has implications as a potential weapon of bioterrorism (Middlebrook & Franz 1997; Zilinskas, 1997). An aerosol dispersion of BoNT could create a toxic gas cloud that could encompass a large area and is considered to be a likely scenario for a terrorism attack.

3.3 Clinical symptoms

The clinical presentation of botulism is characterized by distinctive neurological symptoms of the voluntary motor and autonomic cholinergic-associated junctions in the infant, wound and intestinal forms of the disease (CDC, 1998). Foodborne botulism is often accompanied by acute gastrointestinal distress including nausea, abdominal cramps, vomiting and diarrhea that precede the neurological symptoms (Hughes et al, 1981), particularly in types B and E. The initial symptoms of food botulism can manifest anywhere from within a few hours to several days postintoxication. The time to onset of symptoms, the severity and the duration of the disease is largely dictated by the exposure dose and the serotype (Arnon, 2001; Woodruff et al., 1992). Infant botulism may present with constipation, poor feeding, diminished suckling, neck and peripheral weakness, weak crying increased drooling (Corblath, et al., 1993) and ventilatory failure (Arnon, 1992; Long et al., 1985). Wound botulism does not display the gastrointestinal symptoms observed in the foodborne form. Fever, if present, is generally attributed to a wound infection rather than botulism.

The neuroparalytic effects of botulism present as an acute, afebrile, descending, bilateral flaccid paralysis. The initial neurological symptoms generally involve cranial nerves III, IV and VI (Sobel, 2005) and include ocular disorders such as blurred vision, diplopia, ptosis and photophobia (Terranova et al., 1979). This is generally followed by dysfunction of cranial nerves VII and IX which cause, dysphagia, dysphonia and dysarthia. The neurological impairment may then spread to the upper extremities, the trunk and then the lower extremities. Respiratory distress can be caused by a weakened glottis that tends to obstruct the airway during attempted inspiration or from paralytic weakness of the diaphragm and parasternal and intercostas muscles. Fatigue, sore throat, dry mouth, constipation and dizziness have also been reported to be associated with botulinum intoxications (Hughes, 1981). Fatalities are most often the result of respiratory failure or secondary infections typically associated with prolonged mechanical ventilation. Bleck summarized the clinical findings of several published reports of foodborne botulism by symptom and serotype as shown in Table 1 (Bleck, 2000).

The primary neurological disorders associated with botulism are common to the foodborne, intestinal, and wound forms of the disease (Sobel, 2005). The duration and severity of the neuroparalytic effects of the disease can be influenced by both the amount and serotype of the toxin introduced into the system. Insight into the impact of the different serotypes in humans has only recently been investigated and much of the data comes from studies involving the therapeutic applications of BoNTs. Of the three most prevalent serotypes involved in human incidences of botulism, BoNT/A has been shown to have the most persistent action and can last 12-16 weeks when used in therapeutic applications (Eleopra, 2004). Serotype B has also been used in therapeutic applications but only exhibits the comparable efficacy to BoNT/A when used in higher doses (Sloop, et al., 1997; Settler, 2001). Electrophysiological studies conducted in juvenile monkeys using purified BoNT/A (BOTOX, Allergan, Irvine, CA) and BoNT/B (Neurobloc, Elan, Shannon, Ireland) indicated BoNT/A diffusion was more pronounced (Arezzo, 2001). The few studies pertaining to serotype C in humans (Eleopra et al., 1997; Eleopra et al., 1998a, Eleopra et al., 1998b) indicate that it is similar to BoNT/A in terms of the toxicity and duration of activity. A 2004 study evaluated the electrophysical responses to human volunteers injected with low doses

	Type A (%)	Type B (%)	Type E (%)
Neurological symptoms			
Dysphagia	96	97	82
Dry mouth	83	100	93
Diplopia	90	92	39
Dysarthia	100	69	50
Upper extremity weakness	86	64	NA
Lower extremity weakness	76	64	NA
Blurred vision	100	42	91
Dyspnea	91	34	88
Paresthesiae	20	12	NA
Gastrointestinal Symptoms			
Constipation	73	73	52
Nausea	73	57	84
Vomiting	70	50	96
Abdominal cramps	33	46	NA
Diarrhea	35	8	39
Miscellaneous symptoms			
Fatigue	92	69	84
Sore throat	75	39	38
Dizziness	86	30	63
Neurological Findings			
Ptosis	96	55	46
Diminished gag reflex	81	54	NA
Ophthalmoparesis	87	46	NA
Facial paresis	84	48	NA
Tongue weakness	21	31	66
Pupils fixed or dilated	33	56	75
Nystagmus	44	4	NA
Upper extremity weakness	91	62	NA
Lower extremity weakness	82	59	NA
Ataxia	24	13	NA
DTRs diminished or absent	54	29	NA
DTRs hyperactive	12	0	NA
Initial mental status			
Alert	88	93	27
Lethargic	4	4	73
Obtunded	8	4	0

DTRs, deep tendon reflexes; NA, not available.

Table 1. Summary of Symptoms of Patients with Botulism Caused by Serotypes A, B an E· from Springer Scientific Publishing.

of BoNT/A, /B, /C or /F (Eleopra et al., 2004). The results were consistent with other research efforts in that BoNT/B, used in higher doses, and BoNT/C have a similar profile as BoNT/A. As reported in previous studies (Mezaki et al., 1995; Chen et al., 1998), BoNT/F was found to have a shorter duration compared to BoNT/A.

3.4 Diagnosis of botulism

A rapid and accurate identification of botulism is not difficult when the disease is strongly suspected, such as found in the setting of a large outbreak. But because cases of naturally occurring botulism most often occur singularly, the individual diagnosis may prove more challenging. Botulism is thought to be substantially underdiagnosed (CDC, 1988) and with low-level exposure, minor neurological manifestations of the disease may resolve without medical intervention. A differential diagnosis of botulism without concurrent knowledge of a confirmed outbreak can be difficult and other paralytic illnesses may need to be excluded. These include Guillain-Barre syndrome, myasthenia gravis, tick paralysis, and Eaton-Lambert syndrome (Dembek, et al., 2007). Less likely conditions such as tetrodotoxin and shellfish poisoning, aminoglycoside toxicity and a variety of other neurotoxic products and neurological abnormalities may initially present with similar symptoms. However, a thorough medical examination of the patient and their medical history can generally exclude any competing diagnosis. A patient presenting with an acute, bilateral, descending flaccid paralysis that is afebrile and has normal sensorium should suggest a clinical case of botulism.

The most reliable method for the detection of BoNTs and for diagnosing botulism is the mouse bioassay. This test can be performed by the Centers for Disease Control and Prevention (CDC) or state public health laboratories. The assay involves injecting mice with samples collected from patients displaying symptoms of botulism. Mice will typically begin showing signs of botulism within 8 h. The serotype of samples can also be ascertained in this manner by neutralizing the toxin with serotype-specific antibodies prior to injecting the mice (Shapiro et al., 1998). In cases of foodborne or infant botulism, stool samples can also be cultured to look for *C. botulinum*. Samples of the suspected food should also be cultured anaerobically with heat or alcohol treatment to select for spores.

4. Medical countermeasures

4.1 Current medical intervention

Standard therapy for botulism involves administration of botulinum antitoxin in an attempt to prevent neurologic progression of a moderately progressive illness, or to reduce the duration of respiratory failure in individuals with a severe, rapidly progressive illness. This is done in conjuction with careful monitoring of respiratory vital capacity and aggressive ventilatory care for individuals that display respiratory failure. The only specific pharmacological treatment for botulism is administration of equine-derived botulinum antitoxin. On March 12, 2010, a new heptavalent botulinum antitoxin (HBAT, Cangene Corp.) became available through a US CDC-sponsored FDA Investigational New Drug (IND) protocol for the treatment of naturally acquired non-infant botulism (CDC, 2010). This antitoxin replaced the previously FDA-approved equine bivalent botulinum antitoxin AB and an investigational monovalent equine antitoxin E (BAT-AB and BAT-E,

Sanofi Pasteur). HBAT contains equine-derived antibody against all BoNT serotypes: 7,500 U anti-A; 5,500 U anti-B; 5,000 U anti-C; 1,000 U anti-D; 8,500 U anti-E; 5,000 U anti-F; and 1,000 U anti-G per vial. This antitoxin is composed of <2% intact immunoglobulin G (IgG) and ≥90% Fab and F(ab')2 immunoglobulin fragments created by despeciation (CDC, 2010). The recommended adult dosing is one 20 mL vial of HBAT (McLaughlin and Funk, 2010). BabyBIG®, human botulism immune globulin intravenous (BIG-IV), is an FDA-approved drug for the treatment of infant botulism types A and B. Available through the California Infant Botulism Treatment and Prevention Program, BabyBIG® is obtained from the pooled plasma of adults vaccinated with the pentavalent (A-E) botulinum toxoid who displayed high titers of neutralizing antibodies against BoNT/A and /B. Because BabyBIG® is of human origin, it does not carry the risk for anaphylaxis inherent with equine products, nor does BabyBIG® demonstrate a risk for possible lifelong hypersensitivity to equine antigens. BabyBIG® has been shown to significantly shorten the hospitalization period and reduce treatment costs up to $75,000.00 per incident (Thompson et al., 2005; Fox, 2005).

Antitoxin can neutralize toxin molecules that are not yet bound to nerve endings and may limit the progression of the disease and prevent further nerve damage by clearing them from circulation. Thus, the antitoxin should be administered immediately upon a definitive diagnosis of botulism, preferably within 24 h after the onset of symptoms (Tacket et al., 1984; Chang and Ganguly, 2003). Compared to standard care alone, immediate administration of antitoxin has been shown to shorten time on respiratory support, and also reduced the hospitalization period (Shapiro et al., 1997; Tacket et al., 1984). It is not clear how long the toxin can persist in the bloodstream before clearance. Ravichandran reported that BoNT/A had a serum half-life of approximately 4 hours in small animal studies (Ravichandran et al., 2005). This study also suggested that blood does not sequester or modify the toxin in any detectable way. Thus, the blood may act as a reservoir for the toxin until it either enters the target cells or is eliminated from the body. Detectable levels of toxin were observed in one of the four patients in the Florida outbreak 8 days after receiving a massive overdose of an unlicensed preparation of BoNT/A during a cosmetic procedure (Chertow et al., 2006). Under such circumstances, antitoxin administration, even if delayed, may still be effective in limiting the duration of the illness. The use of equine-based antitoxins, but not the human product, has been associated with symptoms of hypersensitivity (including urticaria, serum sickness, and anaphylaxis). Hence, dermal testing is required before antitoxin administration. Due to the risk of adverse reactions, prophylactic antitoxin is not recommended in patients who are exposed to BoNT but have no symptoms. These patients may undergo gastric lavage or induced vomiting in an attempt to eliminate the toxin before absorption (Chan-Tack & Bartlett, 2010).

4.2 Prophylaxis

In the United States, there is currently no FDA-licensed prophylactic product against botulism. Some of the earliest vaccine efforts were initiated during the second World War due to concerns that the toxin might be employed as an offensive biological weapon against the allied forces by Germany. A bivalent A/B toxoid vaccine was produced from 3-day culture autolysates of *C. botulinum* that were chemically neutralized with formaldehyde, filtered and adsorbed onto an alum adjuvant. While the vaccine did elicit the production of neutralizing antibodies, it also displayed a number of localized and systemic reactogenic effects (Reames et al., 1947). An improved product in which the A and B toxins were purified to 10-15% homomgeneity by acid-precipitation of the culture supernatants and adjuvanted onto aluminum phosphate was found to be well-tolerated in humans, displayed only minor localized reactogenic effects and produced significantly improved antibody titers over the previous bivalent toxoid (Fiock et al., 1961). A pentavalent ABCDE toxoid vaccine with 1% thymerosol as a preservative prepared by Parke, Davis and Company was administered to approximately 400 individuals (Fiock et al., 1963). The vaccine displayed minor reactogenic effects and elicted detectable antibody titers to all five serotypes. This product was administered to over 1600 individuals from 1970 to 1981 under an Investigational New Drug (IND) application. The Michigan Department of Public Health produced a pentavalent botulism (ABCDE) toxoid (PBT) using similar procedures as the Parke Davis product, but which contained roughly 50% of the formaldehyde and only 0.01% thymerosol, that has been administered under an IND to at-risk laboratory workers and military personnel. However, the declining immunogenicity, dwindling supplies and local reactogenic effects of the PBT (Rusnak & Smith, 2009; CDC, 2009) have led to recent efforts to create new vaccines.

More contemporary toxoid vaccines have been created by chemical neutralization of the purified toxin (Keller, 2008; Jones, et al., 2008). However, large scale production of these products would require a secure, CDC-licensed facility to both propagate large amounts the bacterium and manipulate the purified toxin. Subsequent efforts have largely relied on the expression of recombinant protein antigens encoding one or more of the BoNT domains.

Codon optimized genes encoding the BoNT (Hc) antigens produced in a *P. pastoris* expression platform have been successfully developed as a recombinant subunit vaccine against serotypes A-F and have been demonstrated to elicit protective immunity in both rodent (Smith, 2009; Rusnak & Smith 2009) and non-human primates (Boles et al., 2006; Morefield, 2008). In February of 2011, the Dynport Vaccine Company announced that phase II clinical trials of a recombinant bivalent Hc vaccine against serotypes A and B (rBV A/B) had been completed and that full licensure would be sought. (CSC, 2011). Recombinant, catalytically inactive BoNT holoproteins made by mutagenesis of key amino acids residues have also been employed as potential vaccine candidates. A recombinant BoNT/C protein with active site mutations $H^{229}G$, $E^{230}T$ and $H^{223}N$ produced in *E. coli* displayed no catalytic activity and elicited protective immunity against the parental toxin when delivered either subcutaneously or orally (Kiyatkin et al., 1997). Pier described the expression of a recombinant BoNT/A gene bearing $R^{363}A$ and $Y^{365}F$ mutations in the LNT01 nontoxigenic strain of *C. botulinum* (Pier et al., 2008). The recombinant protein was unable to cleave SNAP-25 and elicited protective immunity in mice when challenged with BoNT/A. Recombinant BoNT/A with active site mutations $H^{223}A$, $E^{224}A$ and $H^{227}A$ produced in *P. pastoris* was found to be completely non-toxic and provided protective immunity in mice against 1000 MLD_{50} of not only the parental toxin, but against subtypes /A2 and /A3 as well (Webb et al., 2009).

4.3 Post-intoxication interventions

Once the neurotoxic LC is endocytosed within the cytosol of peripheral cholinergic neurons, circulatory antibodies will no longer be effective at neutralizing the catalytic activity and ablating the toxicity. A number of recent research efforts have focused on the development of small-molecule inhibitors to reduce or eliminate the cleavage of SNARE proteins in neurons. The drawbacks associated with the use of peptides as drug candidates (e.g., poor tissue penetration, serum resistance, oral bioavailability, and quick elimination), and the potential usefulness of small molecules as pre- and post-exposure therapeutic agents have led many laboratories to instead pursue small-molecule approaches. To date, research has focused predominantly on developing small-molecule inhibitors that target the BoNT/A LC protease, due to the serotype's persistence and highly toxic nature. A number of BoNT/A small-molecule inhibitors, identified using conventional and novel approaches, have been reported that exhibit varying degrees of inhibitory capacity (Burnett et al., 2003; 2009; Boldt et al., 2006; Park et al., 2006; Tang et al., 2007; Capkova et al., 2007; 2009; Moe et al., 2009; Roxas-Duncan et al., 2009; Burnett et al., 2010). Most of these studies were conducted in vitro using truncated forms of the LC which might not be structurally representative of the intracellular form of BoNT. The inhibitors reported by Roxas-Duncan et al (2009), identified via a hierarchical screening strategy, were evaluated in vitro using both forms of LC (truncated and full-length), and ex vivo using mouse phrenic nerve hemidiaphragm preparations. Despite intensive efforts on small-molecule inhibitor discovery and development, no compound has been identified that would be suitable for preclinical testing. At present, there are only two reports of BoNT/A small-molecule inhibitors that have been tested in vivo. Janda and co-workers described a mouse toxicity bioassay in which two different inhibitors were injected intravenously immediately after an injection of 5-10 i.p. LD_{50} of BoNT/A. One compound, given at a 2.5 mM dose, showed a 36% increase in time to death, while the other, given at a 1 mM dose, resulted in a 16% overall survival rate (Eubanks et al., 2007). In another study, a single dose of three different inhibitors was administered i.p. at 2 mg/kg 30 min prior to a challenge of 5 MLD_{50} of BoNT/A (Pang et al., 2010). The control mice died within 12 hrs. All 3 inhibitors provided 100% protection at 12 hrs and one compound provided 70% and 60% survival rates at 24 and 48 hrs; all three inhibitors provided a 10% overall survival rate with no signs of botulism at 5 days.

Recently, other regions of the LC, in addition to the BoNT active site, generated attention as potential targets for inhibition. Merrino et al., (2006) has focused on a family of bis-imidazole BoNT/A inhibitors targeting the peripheral sites of substrate binding. Silhar et al., (2010) reported on D-chicoric acid, a natural product isolated from Echinacea, that inhibits BoNT/A LC by binding to an exosite.

4.4 Human recombinant monoclonal antibodies

Currently, immunotherapy is deemed as the most effective immediate response to BoNT exposure. However, BabyBig® is exclusively approved for use in infants, and equine antisera can induce serum sickness and anaphylaxis (Arnon et al., 2001; Arnon, 2004). Monoclonal antibody (mAb) combinations (oligoclonal antibodies) may be viable substitutes for polyclonal antisera (Nowakowski et al., 2002; Razai et al., 2005). Construction of scFv phage Ab libraries has enabled the generation of large panels of high-affinity binding monoclonal antibodies. Mouse neutralization studies revealed that effective protection is observed only when combinations of three or more mAbs are used (Nowakowski et al., 2002; Marks, 2004). Under the aegis of the National Institute of Allergy and Infectious

Diseases (NIAID), antibody combinations that effectively protect against multiple BoNT/A, /B, and /E subtypes are currently being produced and tested to support FDA licensure. Antibodies that protect against the four remaining toxin serotypes (BoNT/C, /D, /F, and /G) are also in development.

4.5 Antibodies specific for the catalytic light chain

While a majority of the BoNT immunotherapy research has been focused on antibodies that bind the HC, efforts were also directed to explore the potential for antibodies that bind the enzymatic LC. Using a novel hybridoma method for cloning human antibodies (Adekar et al., 2008; Dessain et al., 2004), a fully human antibody specific for the BoNT/A LC was isolated which potently inhibited BoNT/A in vitro and in vivo, via mechanisms not previously associated with BoNT-neutralizing antibodies (Adekar et al., 2008). In another study, Dong et al. (2010) created a library of non-immune llama single-domain VHH (camelid heavy-chain variable regions) displayed on the surface of the yeast *Saccharomyces cerevisiae*. Library selections against BoNT/A LC yielded 15 yeast-displayed VHHs, eight of which inhibited the cleavage of substrate SNAP-25 by BoNT/A LC. The most potent VHH (Aa1) had a solution K(d) of 1.47×10^{-10} M and an IC_{50} of 4.7×10^{-10} M. X-ray crystal structure of the BoNT/A LC-Aa1 VHH complex revealed that the Aa1 VHH binds the alpha-exosite region of BoNT/A LC. Recently, Tremblay et al. (2010) reported on the selection of small (14 kDa) binding domains specific for the protease of BoNT serotypes A or B from libraries of VHHs or nanobodies cloned from vaccinated alpacas. Several VHHs were demonstrated to exhibit high affinity (K_D near 1 nm) and were potent inhibitors of BoNT/A LC (Ki near 1 nM); a VHH inhibitor of BoNT/A LC was able to protect BoNT/A-mediated SNAP25 cleavage.

4.6 Inhibitors of internalization and translocation

Several compounds that inhibit the acidification process of endosomes by various mechanisms have been evaluated for both toxicity and ability to inhibit BoNT-induced synaptic failure. Lysosomotropic agents ammonium chloride and methylamine hydrochloride have been shown to antagonize the toxin internalization step by delaying the time-to-block of nerve-evoked muscle contractions after exposure to BoNT/A, /B, /C1, and TeNT (Simpson, 1983). However, these amines act by inhibiting the acidification process of endosomes; they do not selectively inactivate the toxins nor irreversibly modify tissue function at concentrations that inhibit the onset of BoNT-induced paralysis. Other candidates that have been examined were uncouplers of oxidative phosphorylation CCCP, FCCP (Adler et al., 1994), and vesicle H^+-ATPase inhibitors including Bafilomycin A, which was shown to antagonize BoNTs A-G (Simpson et al., 1994). Some of these compounds were toxic or had low safety margins, hence they were deemed unsuitable as therapeutic candidates.

Anti-malarial compounds chloroquine and hydroxychloroquine have also been evaluated for potentially inhibiting BoNT-mediated internalization (Simpson, 1982). The efficacy of these agents was found similar to that of ammonium chloride and methylamine hydrochloride; both groups also exhibited a comparable therapeutic window. Deshpande and co-workers (1997) extended the studies on antimalarial agents by examining a large group of 4- and 8-aminoquinolines. Unfortunately, these compounds failed to extend the therapeutic window. The most effective compounds were 4-aminoquinolines and quinacrine that delayed BoNT/A-induced neuromuscular block by more than threefold compared to the control (toxin only) values. Maximum protection was solely achieved when the tissues were exposed to the compounds before or at the same time as the toxin treatment; a delay of >20 min abolished the inhibitory capacity of these compounds.

An additional approach to prevent or reduce BoNT internalization has been attempted by treating nerve-muscle preparations with the protein ionophores nigericin and monensin (Adler et al., 1994; Sheridan, 1996). These ionophores block vesicle acidification by acting as H^+ shunts to neutralize pH gradients, thereby interfering with the delivery of active LC in the cytosol. Though the efficacy of these ionophores was observed to be comparable to other inhibitors of internalization, they were more toxic; high concentrations resulted in a depression of neuromuscular transmission (Adler et al., 1994; Sheridan, 1996).

4.7 Compounds that restore neuronal function

A known potassium channel blocker, 3,4-diaminopyridine (3,4-DAP) was evaluated for its ability to antagonize BoNT-induced depression of tension in rat diaphragm muscles (Adler et al., 1995). BoNT-induced paralysis was nearly completely inhibited after addition of 100 uM of 3,4-DAP, and this effect was sustained even after 4 h of treatment. The antagonistic effects of 3,4-DAP was also demonstrated in vivo, provided its concentration in the plasma is maintained at ~30 μM during the course of intoxication (Adler et al., 2000). However, 3,4-DAP is generally toxic, thus, its high drug concentration requirement prohibits routine therapeutic use (Millard, 2006).

Mastoparan, a phospholipase activator, was evaluated for its ability to attenuate BoNT intoxication. Addition of mastoparan and 80 mM K^+ completely prevented BoNT inhibition of radiolabeled acetylcholine in PC12 cells, but this effect was blocked by either EGTA or the N-type calcium channel blocker ω-conotoxin (Ray et al., 1999). These findings imply that the effects of mastoparan are dependent on Ca^{2+} influx via the neuronal type voltage-sensitive Ca^{2+} channels.

4.8 Drug delivery vehicle research

One significant challenge in the development of BoNT small-molecule therapeutics is the delivery of the compounds to the cytosol of peripheral cholinergic nerve cells (PCNC), which are the sites of BoNT action. In combination with the discovery and development of BoNT small-molecule inhibitors, cell-specific intracellular targeting is critical to increase the therapeutic index and minimize potential systemic toxicity associated with the drug treatment. Several studies have examined the potential of using specific recombinant BoNT domains or a neutralized full-length BoNT holoprotein as drug delivery system. Goodnough et al. observed that BoNT/A and unlabeled rHC were able to compete for binding, implicating specific neuronal targeting (Goodnough et al., 2002). The efficiency of neuron-specific cargo delivery into the cytosol was evaluated by coupling labeled dextran to a recombinant BoNT/A HC using a 3-(2-pyridylthio)-propionyl hydrazide linker (Zhang et al., 2009). A florescent tracking dye was conjugated to the dextran moiety and incubated in mouse cultured mouse spinal cord neurons. The binding of the fluorescent tag and its internalization into the endosomes were observed, but minimal levels were detected in the cytosol. The movement of a small, membrane-permeable dye from the endosome into the cytosol is hypothesized to be due to passive diffusion instead of an active translocation event. Ho et al (2010) reported on a recombinant BoNT/A HC with an amino terminal GFP fusion that was internalized into mouse neurons; however, the GFP cargo was observed to be almost exclusively limited to endocytotic vesicles, with little detectable translocation into the cytosol.

Although the of BoNT heavy chain comprises the domains necessary for binding and internalization into endosomes, recent studies suggest that all or part of the LC is essential to translocate a ligated cargo into the cytosol.

Recombinant BoNT/D fusion proteins bearing amino terminal GFP, luciferase, dihydrofolate reductase or BoNT/A LC protein were found to promote translocation of cargo proteins into the cytosol in an enzymatically active form (Bade et al., 2004). A recombinant neutralized BoNT/A bearing an $E^{224}A$ $E^{262}A$ double mutation, labeled with Alexa-488, has been shown to specifically bind and internalize into human SH-SY5Y neuroblastoma cells (Sing et al., 2010). Additionally, this protein was found to marginally bind to the surface of human rhabdomyosarcoma cells with a toxicity limit of 1 µg in mice. No additional information is available regarding the drug conjugation study on this protein. Moreover, recombinant versions of full-length BoNT/A holotoxin devoid of catalytic activity were recently developed (Pier et al., 2008; Webb et al., 2009; Yang et al., 2008) which could be potentially used to deliver conjugated therapeutic cargoes.

5. Emergency preparedness and public response

The 2007 anthrax attacks in the United States illustrated the need to develop a comprehensive preparedness plan for identifying and managing healthcare resources in the event of a biological attack. Anthrax, plague, botulinum toxins, smallpox, tularemia, and viral hemorrhagic fever viruses have been identified as having a significant potential for use in a bioterrorism attack because they can be easily disseminated or transmitted, have high morbidity or mortality rates and would cause widespread social disruption (Rotz et al., 2002). A bioterrorism attack involving dissemination of BoNT by existing food or water distribution networks is theoretically possible but this route is associated with significant logistical difficulties (Franz, et al., 1997; Zilinskas, 1999) and most experts believe that an aerosol dispersion poses the greatest threat (Arnon, 2002). Because botulism is a relatively rare disease, clinicians and the healthcare infrastructure in general have limited experience in diagnosis of any form of the disease. A 2005 study reported that of 631 physicians participating in a mock bioterrosim event, slightly less than half provided an accurate diagnosis and plan of management for botulism (Cosgrove, 2005). In the event of a biological attack with BoNT, a rapid and accurate diagnosis of the agent by physicians and clinical laboratories would be crucial to an equally rapid response and mobilization of equipment and biological agents for management. Health care providers who suspect botulism should immediately call their state health department's emergency 24-hour emergency telephone number. The state health department will contact the CDC to report suspected botulism cases, arrange for a clinical consultation by telephone and, if indicated, request release of botulinum antitoxin. State health departments should call the CDC 24-hour telephone number at 770-488-7100. The call will be taken by the CDC Emergency

Operations Center, which will page the Foodborne and Diarrheal Diseases Branch medical officer on call. The CDC established the Laboratory Response Network (LRN) in 1999; a national network of about 150 federal, state, local and military labs that can respond to biological and chemical terrorism, and other public health emergencies (CDC-EPR). The LRN hierarchy also includes *reference labs* that can perform tests to detect and confirm the presence of a threat agent to ensure a rapid local response in the event of a bioterrorism incident without having to rely on confirmation from CDC labs. *Sentinel labs* are comprised of thousands of hospital-based labs that have direct contact with patients. These labs might well be the first facility to spot a suspicious specimen and refer it to the appropriate reference lab (Sentinel, ASM).

The ability of the government and healthcare infrastructure to respond to a bioterroism attack using BoNT in a densely populated urban environment would largely dictated be by the ventilator and antitoxin supplies and how quickly they could be mobilized to the outbreak area. Approximately 120,000 of the 200,000 doses of the HBAT contracted by the Biomedical Advanced Research and Development Authority (BARDA) have been delivered for use in the US national strategic stockpile and the remaining 80,000 doses are scheduled for delivery by 2014. A 2010 study estimated that there are approximately 63,066 full-featured mechanical ventilators in the US, 46.4% of which were capable of ventilating pediatric and neonatal patients (Rubinson et al, 2010). Additionally, there was an estimated 82,775 additional positive pressure ventilators (PPV) that could be brought on-line in response to an acute respiratory failure (ARF) surge event. This study may represent a conservative estimate as it only accounted for survey responders and it did not consider the various units rented by hospitals, those facilities who failed to respond to the survey or those at nursing facilities or schools.

6. Conclusion

BoNT has been investigated as a BW by a number of different state-sponsored initiatives and terrorist organizations and is considered a biological threat to both our military and the public. Effective medical countermeasures against BoNT intoxication are limited. Currently, the only available treatment other than supportive care is a new investigational botulinum heptavalent equine-based antitoxin. However, antitoxin cannot intervene in the pathogenesis of the disease once the toxin enters the nerve cell, and cannot support all those infected in the event of a biological terrorist attack. Hence, there is a critical need for postintoxication therapy that can be administered rapidly and effectively to a large infected population. Because small molecules provide an opportunity to treat botulism both before and after cellular intoxication has occurred, considerable research efforts have been devoted to the development of these types of inhibitors. A number of strong contributions to the field have been made, yet no small molecule inhibitor was identified that possesses the appropriate characteristics (safety, efficacy, solubility) required to be a pharmaceutical intervention.

Research studies addressing these obstacles are underway. Continuing efforts will be facilitated particularly by the availability of structural information and by knowledge of the mechanism of the BoNT LC-mediated proteolysis of SNARE proteins. Additionally, potential novel strategies to therapeutic development, e.g., host-directed therapeutics, and targeting pathways involved in the cellular response to BoNT intoxication, are being explored. An understanding of these mechanisms may provide insight into the design and development of innovative and effective therapeutic strategies to counteract BoNT intoxications.

7. References

Adekar S.P., Jones, R.M. & Elias, M.D., et al. (2008). Hybridoma populations enriched for affinity-matured human IgGs yield high-affinity antibodies specific for botulinum neurotoxins. *J Immunol Methods,* Vol.333, No.1-2, pp. 156–166, ISSN 0022-1759

Adler, M., Deshpande, S.S. & Sheridan, R.E., (1994). Evaluation of captopril and other potentially therapeutic compounds in antagonizing botulinum toxin-induced muscle paralysis, In: *Therapy with Botulinum Toxin*; Jankovic, J., & Hallett, M. (Eds). pp. 63–70, Marcel Dekker Inc., ISBN 0824788249, New York, NY, USA

Adler, M., Scovill, J. & Parker, G., et al. (1995). Antagonism of botulinum toxin-induced muscle weakness by 3,4-diaminopyridine in rat phrenic nerve-hemidiaphragm preparations. *Toxicon,* Vol.33, No.4, pp. 527-537, ISSN 0041-0101

Adler, M., Capacio, B. & Deshpande, S.S. (2000) Antagonism of botulinum toxin A-mediated muscle paralysis by 3, 4-diaminopyridine delivered via osmotic minipumps. *Toxicon,* Vol.38, No.10, pp. 1381-1388, ISSN 0041-0101

Alberts, B. (2005). Modeling attacks on the food supply. *PNAS,* Vol.102, No.8, pp. 9737-9738, ISSN 0027-8424

Alibek, K. & Handleman, S. (1999). *Biohazard.* Dell Publishing, ISBN, 0385334966, New York, New NY.

Arezzo, J.C., Litwak, M.S. & Caputao, F.A., et al. (2000). Spread of paralytic activity of Neurobloc™ (botulinum toxin type B) and Botox® (botulinum toxin type A) in juvenile monkeys: an electrophysiological model. *Eur J Neurol,* Vol.8, No.S4, pp. 26 ISSN 1351-5101

Arnon, S. (1998) Infant botulism, In: *Textbook of pediatric infectious diseases,* Feigen, R. And Cherry, J. (Ed), 4th ed. W. B. Saunders, pp. 1570-1577, ISBN 0721664482 Philadelphia, PA, USA.

Arnon, S. (1999) Botulism as an intestinal toxaemia, In: *Infections of the gastrointestinal tract,* M.J. Baser, Guerrant, R.L. & P.D. Smith, et al. (Ed.), pp. 257-271, Raven Press, ISBN: 0781702267, New York, NY, USA.

Arnon, S.S., Schechter, R. & Inglesby, T., et al. (2001). Botulinum toxin as a biological weapon. Medical and public health management. *JAMA,* Vol.285, No.1, pp. 1059-1070, ISSN 0098-7484

Arnon SS. (2004). Infant Botulism. In: *Textbook of Pediatric Infectious Diseases,* Feigin, R.D., Cherry, J., & Demmler, G.J. (Eds) pp. 1758–1766, Saunders, ISBN 0721693296. Philadelphia, PA, USA

Bade, S., Rummel, A. & Reisinger, C., et al. (2004). Botulinum neurotoxin type D enables cytosolic delivery of enzymatically active cargo proteins to neurons via unfolded translocation intermediates. *J Neurochem,* Vol.91, No.6, pp. 1461-1472, ISSN 0022-3042

Bakheit, A.M., Ward, C.D. & McClellan D.L. (1997) Generalised botulism-like syndrome after intramuscular injections of botulinum toxin type A: a report of two cases. *J Neurology, Neurosurgery and Psychiatry*, Vol.62, No.2, pp. 198, ISN 0022-3050

Baird-Parker, A.C. & Freame, B. (1967). Combined effect of water activity, pH and temperature on the growth of *Clostridium botulinum* from spore and vegetative cell inocula. *J Appl Bact*, Vol.30, No.2, pp. 420-429, ISSN 0021-8847

Barash, J.R., Tang, T.W.H., & Arnon S.S. (2005). First case of infant botulism caused by *Clostridium baratii* type F in California. *J Clin Microbiol*, Vol.43, No.8, pp. 4280–4282, ISSN 0095-1137

BB-IND 61 Protocol CDC IBR#392, version 8.0. IND protocol: Use of penatavalent (ABCDE) botulinum toxin aluminum phosphate adsorbed (PBT) for workers at risk of occupational exposure to botulinum neurotoxins. Spnsored by: Centers for Disease Control and Prevention, Atlanta, GA. October 6, 2009.

Bleck, T.P. (2009). Botulism as a potential agent of bioterrorism, In: *Bioterrorism and Infectious Agents: A New Dilemma for the 21st Century*, Fong, I.W. & Alibek, K. (Eds), pp.193-202, Springer, ISBN 1441912657, Ney York, NY, USA

Blix, H. (2004) *Disarming Iraq*. (1st ed.), Pantheon, ISBN 0375423028, New York, NY, USA.

Benson, S.B., Passaro, D. & McGee, J., et al. (2000) Wound botulism in California, 1951-1998: Recent epidemic in heroin injectors. *Clin Infec Dis*, Vol.31, No.4, pp.1018-1024, ISN 1058-4838

Boles, J., West, M. & Montgomery, V.A., et al. (2006). Recombinant C fragment from botulinum neurotoxin B serotype (rBoNTB(Hc)) immune responses and protection in the rhesus monkey. *Toxicon*, Vol.47, No.9 pp.877-884, ISSN 0041-0101

Boldt, G.E., Eubanks L.M. & Janda K.D. (2006). Identification of a botulinum neurotoxin A protease inhibitor displaying efficacy in a cellular model. *Chem Commun* (Cambridge) Vol.29, pp.3063-3065, ISSN 1359-7345

Bozheyeva, G., Kunakbayev, Y. & Yeleukenov, D. (1999). Former soviet biological weapons facilities in Kazakhstan: past, present and future. Occasional paper No.1. Monterey, CA. Center for Nonproliferation Studies, Monterey Institute for International Studies, pp. 1-20

Burnett, J.C., Schmidt, J. & Stafford, R.G., et al. (2003). Novel small-molecule inhibitors of botulinum neurotoxin A metalloprotease activity. *Biochem Biophys Res Commun*, Vol.310, No.1, pp. 84-93, ISSN 0006-291X

Burnett, J.C., Wang. C., & Nuss, J.E., et al. (2009). Pharmacophore-guided lead optimization: the rational design of a non-zinc coordinating, submicromolar inhibitor of the botulinum neurotoxin serotype A metalloprotease. *Bioorg Med Chem Lett*, Vol.19, No.19, pp. 5811-5813, ISSN 0960-894X

Burnett, J.C., Li, B. & Pai, R., et al. (2010). Analysis of botulinum neurotoxin serotype A metalloprotease inhibitors: analogs of a chemotype for therapeutic development in the context of a three-zone pharmacophore. Open Access Bioinformatics 2: 11-18. DOI 10.2147/OAB.S7251

Burrows, W.D., Valcik, J.A. & Seitzinger, A. (1997). Natural and terrorst threats to drinking water supplies. In, Proceedsing of the 23rd environmental symposium, 7-10 April 1997, New Orleans, LA, American Defense Preparedness Association

Carrus, S. (2001) Bioterroism and biocrimes. The illicit use of biological agents since 1900. Center for counterproliferation research, National Defense University, pp.90, ISBN 1410100235, Washington, D.C., USA

CDC. (1998). Botulism in the United States, 1899-1996. Handbook for epidemiologists, clinicians, and laboratory workers. Atlanta, GA: Centers for Disease Control and Prevention. Available at http://www.cdc.gov/ncidod/dbmd/diseaseinfo/files/botulism.PDF

CDC. Emergency preparedness and response (EPR). Facts about the laboratory response network. Accessed 08/01/2011, http://www.bt.cdc.gov/lrn/factsheet.asp

CDC. (2010). Investigational heptavalent botulinum antitoxin (HBAT) to replace licensed botulinum antitoxin AB and investigational botulinum antitoxin E. MMWR 59: 229.

CDC. National Botulism Surveillance (NBS), accessed 08-23-2011, available from http://www.cdc.gov/nationalsurveillance/botulism_surveillance.html

CDC (2006). Botulism associated with commercial carrot juice - Georgia and Florida, September 2006. MMWR weekly, October 13, 2006/55(40), pp. 1098-1099.

CDC. (2007). Botulism Associated with Commercial Carrot Juice --- Georgia and Florida, September 2006, 08/24/2011, Available from: http://www.cdc.gov/mmwr/preview/mmwrhtml/mm5540a5.htm

CDC. (2008). Public Health Preparedness: Mobilizing State by State http://www.bt.cdc.gov/publications/feb08phprep/

Capková, K., Yoneda, Y. & Dickerson, T., et al. (2007). Synthesis and structure-activity relationships of second-generation hydroxamate botulinum neurotoxin A protease inhibitors. *Bioorg Med Chem Lett*, Vol.17, No.23, pp. 6463-6466, ISSN 0960-894X

Capková, K., Hixon, M.S. & Pellett, S. et al. (2009). Benzylidene cyclopentenediones: First irreversible inhibitors against botulinum neurotoxin A's zinc endopeptidase. *Bioorg Med Chem Lett,* Vol.20, No.1, pp. 206-208, ISSN 0960-894X

Chang, G.Y., & Ganguly, G. (2003). Early antitoxin treatment in wound botulism results in better outcome. *Eur Neurol,* Vol.49, No.3, pp. 151-153, ISSN 0014-3022

Chan-tack, K.M., & Bartlett J. (2010). Botulism. http://emedicine.medscape.com/article/213311-overview

Chia, J., Clark, J. & Ryan, C. (1986). Botulism in an adult associated with food-borne intestinal infection with *Clostridium botulinum*. *NEJM*, Vol.6, No.4, pp. 239-241, ISSN 0028-4793

Chen, R., Karp, B.I. & Hallett, M. (1998). Botulinum toxin type F for treatment of dystonia: Long-term experience. *Neurology*, Vol.51, No.5, pp. 1494-1496, ISSN 0028-3878

Chertow, S., Tan, E.T. & Maslanka, S.E. et al. (2006). Botulism in 4 adults following cosmetic injections with an unlicensed, highly concentrated botulinum preparation. *JAMA*, Vol.296, No.20, pp.2476-2479, ISSN 0098-7484

Cochrane, R.C. (1947). Biological warfare research in the United States, In: History of chemical warfare service in world war II (01 July 1940-15 August 1945). Vol.2, historical sections, plans, training and intelligence division, office of the chief chemical corps, US department of the army, 1947. Unclassified. Archived at the US Army Medical Research Institute for Infectious Diseases, Fort Detrick, MD.

Collins, M.D. & East A.K. (1998). Phylogeny and taxonomy of the food-borne pathogen *Clostridium botulinum* and its neurotoxins. *J App Micro*, Vol.84, No.1, pp. 5-17, ISSN 1364-5072

Cornblath, D.R., Sladky, J.T. & Sumner, A.J. (1998). Clinical electrophysiology of infantile botulism. *Muscle Nerve*, Vol.6, No.6, pp. 448-452, ISSN 0148-639X

Cosgrove, S.E., Perl, T.M. & Song, X., et al. (2005) Ability of physicians to diagnose and manage illness due to category A bioagents. *Arch Int Med*, Vol.165, No.17, pp. 2002-2006, ISSN 0003-9926

CSC Press Release. (2011). CSCs DynPort Vaccine Company Completes Vaccinations and Study Visits in Phase 2 Botulinum Vaccine Clinical Trial, Febraury 11, 2011, http://www.csc.com/dvc/press_releases/60409-cscs_dynport_vaccine_company_completes_vaccinations_and_study_visits_in_phase_2_botulinum_vaccine_clinical_trial, accessed 08/01/2011

Davis, J.B., Mattman, L.H. & Wiley, M. (1951). *Clostridium botulinum* in fatal wound infection. *JAMA*, Vol.146, No.7, pp. 646-648, ISSN 0098-7484

DasGupta, B. (1989). The structure of botulinum neurotoxins, In: *Botulinum Neurotoxin and Tetanus Toxin*, pp. 53-67, Academic Press, Inc., ISBN 0306444127, New York, NY, USA

Dembek, Z.F., Smith, L.A. & Rusnak, J.M. (2007). Botulinum toxin: Cause, effects, diagnosis, clinical and laboratory identification, and treatment modalities. *Dis Med Pub Health Prep*, Vol.1, No.2, pp. 122-134, ISSN 1935-7893

Deshpande, S.S., Sheridan, R.E. & Adler, M. (1995). A study of zinc-dependent metalloendopeptidase inhibitors as pharmacological antagonists in botulinum neurotoxin poisoning. *Toxicon*, Vol.33, No.4, pp. 551-557, ISSN 0041-0101

Deshpande, S.S., Sheridan, R.E. & Adler, M. (1997). Efficacy of certain quinolines as pharmacological antagonists in botulinum neurotoxin poisoning. *Toxicon*, Vol.35, No.3, pp. 433-435, ISSN 0041-0101

Dessain, S.K., Adekar, S.P. & Stevens, J.B., et al. (2004). High efficiency creation of human monoclonal antibody-producing hybridomas. *J Immunol Methods*, Vol.291, No.1-2, pp. 109–122, ISSN 0022-1759

Dong, M., Yeh, F. & Tepp, W. H., et al. (2006). SV2 Is the Protein Receptor for Botulinum Neurotoxin A. *Science*, Vol.312, No.5773 , pp. 592-596, ISSN 0036-8075

Dunbar, E.M. (1990). Botulism, *J Infect*, Vol.20, No.1, pp. 1-3, ISSN 0163-4453

Eleopra, R., Tugnoli, V. & Rosetto, O., et al. (1997). Botulinum neurotoxin serotype C: a novel effective botulinum therapy in humans. *Neurosci Letters*, Vol.224, No.2, pp.91-94, ISSN 0304-3940

Eleopra, R., Tugnoli, V. & Rosetto, O., et al. (1998a). Different time courses of recovery after poisoning with botulinum neurotoxin serotypes A and E in humans. *Neurosci Letters*, Vol.256, No.3, ISSN 0304-3940, pp. 135-138

Eleopra, R., Tugnoli, V. & De Grandis, D., et al. (1998b). Botulinum toxin serotype C treatment in subjects affected by focal dystonia and resistant to toxin serotype A. *Neurology*, Vol.50, No.S4, pp. A72, ISSN 0028-3878

Eleopra, R., Tugnoli, V, & Rocco, Q., et al. (2004). Different types of botulinum toxins in humans. *Movement Disorders*, Vol.19, No.S8, pp. S53-S59, ISSN 0885-3185

Eubanks, L. M., Hixson, M. S., W. & Jin, W., (2007). An in vitro and in vivo disconnect uncovered through high-throughput identification of botulinum neurotoxin A antagonists. *PNAS*, Vol.104, No.8, pp. 2602-2607, ISSN 0027-8424

Feneica, L., Franciosa, G. & Pourshaban, M. (1999). Intestinal toxemia botulism in two young people, caused by *Clostridium botulinum* type E. *Clin Inf Dis*, Vol.29, No.6, pp. 1381-1387, ISSN 1058-4838

Fiock, M.A., Device, L.F. & Gearinger, et al. (1962). Studies on immunity to toxins of Clostridium botulinum VIII. Immunological reponses of man to purified bivalent botulinum toxoid. *J Immun*, Vol.88, No.3, ISSN 0022-1767

Fiock, M.A., Cardell, A. & Gearinger, N.F. (1963) Studies on immunity to toxins of Clostridium botulinum IX. Immunological response of man to purified pentavlent ABCDE botulinum toxoid. *J Immunology*, Vol.90, No. 5, pp.697-702, ISNN 0022-1767

Fox, C.K., Keet, C.A., & Strober, J.B. (2005). Recent advances in pediatric botulism. *Pediatr Neurol*, Vol.32, No.3, pp. 149-154, ISSN 0887-8994

Franz, D., Parrott, C. & Takafuji, E. (1997). The U.S. Biological Warfare and Biological Defense Programs. In: *Textbook of Military Medicine, Part I: Warfare, Weaponry, and Then Casualty: Medical Aspects of Chemical and Biological Warfare*, Slidell, F., Takafuji, E. & Franz, D (Eds.) Borden Institute, Walter Reed Washington, DC, USA.

Franz, D.R., Jahrling, P.B. & Friedlander, A.M., et al. (1997). Clinical recognition and management of patients exposed to biological warfare agents. *JAMA*, Vol.278, No.5, pp. 399-411, ISSN 0098-7484

Freedman, M., Armstrong, R.M. & Killian, J.M. (1986) Botulism in a patient with jejunoileal bypass. *Ann Neurol*, Vol.20, No.5, pp. 641-643, ISSN 0364-5134,

Gupta, A., Sumner, C.J. & Castor M, et al. (2005). Adult botulism type F in the United States, 1981-2002. *Neurology*, Vol.65, No.11, pp. 1694-700, ISSN 0028-3878

Goodnough, M.C., Oyler, G. & Fishman, P.S., et al. (2002). Development of a delivery vehicle for intracellular transport of botulinum neurotoxin antagonists. *FEBS Lett*, Vol.513, No.2-3, pp. 163-168, ISSN 0014-5793

Hatheway, C.L. (1988). Botulism, In: *Laboratory Diagnosis of Infectious Diseases Principles and Practice*, Balows A., Hausler, J.W.J. & Ohashi, M. et al. (Eds), pp. 111–133, ISBN 0387967559, Springer Scientific, New York, NY, USA

Hatheway C.L. (1993). *Clostridium botulinum* and other clostridia that produce botulinum neurotoxin, In: *Clostridium botulinum: Ecology and control in foods*. Hauschild A.H.W. & Dodds K.L. (Eds), pp. 3-20, Marcel Dekker, Inc., ISBN 082478748X, New York, NY, USA.

Hill K.K., Smith T.J. & Helma C.H., et al. (2007). Genetic diversity among botulinum neurotoxin-producing clostridial strains. *J Bact*, Vol.189, No.3, pp 818-832, ISSN 0021-9193

Ho, M., Chang, L.H., & Pires-Alves, M., et al. (2010). Recombinant botulinum neurotoxin A heavy chain-based delivery vehicles for neuronal cell targeting. *Prot Eng Des Sel*, Vol.24, No.3, pp 247-253, ISSN 1741-0126

Holzer, E. (1962) Botulism caused by inhalation. *Medizinische Klinik*, Vol.31, pp.1735-740, ISSN 0723-5003

Hörman, A., Nevas, M., & Lindström, M., et al. (2005). Elimination of botulinum neurotoxin (BoNT) type B from drinking water by small-scale (personal use) water purification devices and detection of BoNT in water samples. *App Env Micro*, Vol.71, No.4, pp. 1941-1945, ISSN 1098-5336

Hughes, J.M., Blumenthal, J.R. & Merson, M.D., et al. (1981) Clinical features of types A and B food-borne botulism. *Ann Int Med*, Vol.95, No.4, pp. 442-445, ISSN 0003-4819

Jones, R.G.A, Liu, Y. & Rigsby, P. (2008). An improved method for development of toxoid vaccines and antitoxins. *J Immun Meth*, Vol.137, No.1, pp. 42-48, ISSN 0022-1759

Keller, J.E. (2008). Characterization of new formalin-detoxified botulinum neurotoxin toxoids. *Clin Vacc Imm*, Vol.15, No.9, pp.1374-1379, ISSN 1556-6811

Kyatkin, N., Maksymowych, & Simpson, L.A. (1997). Induction of an immune response by oral administration of recombinant botulinum toxin. *Inf Imm*, Vol.65, No.11, pp. 4586–4591, ISSN 0019-9567

Leitenberg, M. (1999). Aum Shinrikyo's efforts to produce biological weapons: A case study in the serial propagation of misinformation. *Terrorism and Political Violence*, Vol.11, No.4, pp. 152-158, ISSN 0954-6553

Long, S.S., Gajewski, J.L. & Brown, L.W., et al. (1985). Clinical, laboratory and environmental features of environmental botulism in southeastern Pennsylvania. *Pediatrics*, Vol.75, No.5, pp. 935-941, ISSN 0031-4005

Marks, J.D. (2004). Deciphering antibody properties that lead to potent botulinum neurotoxin neutralization. *Mov Disord,* Vol.19, No.S8, pp. S101–108, 0885-3185

Mezaki, T., Kaji, R. & Kohara, N., et al. (1995). Comparison of Therapeutic Efficacies of Type A and F Botulinum Toxins for Blepharospasm: A double-blind, controlled study. *Neurology*, Vol.45, No.3, pp. 506-508, ISSN 0028-3878

Merino, I., Thompson, J.D. & Millard CB, et al. (2006). Bis-imidazoles as molecular probes for peripheral sites of the zinc endopeptidase of botulinum neurotoxin serotype A. *Bioorg Med Chem*, Vol.14, No.10, pp. 3583-3591, ISSN 0968-0896

Middlebrook, J.L., & Franz, D.R. (1997). Botulinum toxins. In: *Textbook of Military Medicine, Part I: Warfare, Weaponry, and Then Casualty: Medical Aspects of Chemical and Biological Warfar*e, Sidell, F.R., Takafuji, E.T., & Franz, D.R., (Eds.) pp. 643-54. Borden Institute, Walter Reed Army Medical, Center Washington, DC, USA.

Millard, C. (2006). Medical defense against toxin weapons: review and perspective. In: *Infectious disease: biological weapons defense: infectious diseases and counterterrorism*, Lindler, L.E., Lebeda F.J. & Korch G.W. (Eds.), pp. 255-276, Humana Press, Inc., ISBN 1588291847, Totowa, NJ, USA

McLaughlin J, Funk B. 2010. New recommendations for use of heptavalent botulinum antitoxin (HBAT). State of AK Bull 5:1. http://www.epi.Alaska.gov

Moe, S.T., Thompson, A.B., & Smith, G.M. et al. (2009). Botulinum neurotoxin serotype A inhibitors: Small-molecule mercaptoacetamide analogs. *Bioorgan Med Chem*, Vol.17, No.8, pp. 3072-3079, ISSN 0968-0896

Moorefield, G.L., Tamariello, R., & Purcell, B. et al. (2008). An alternative approach to combination vaccines: intradermal administration of isolated components for control of anthrax, botulism, plague and staphylococcal toxic shock. *J Immune Based Ther Vacc*, Vol.6, No.5, pp. 1-11, ISSN 1476-8518

Nowakowski, A., Wang, C. & Powers, D.B. et al. (2002). Potent neutralization of botulinum neurotoxin by recombinant oligoclonal antibody. *PNAS*, Vol.99, No.17, pp. 11346–11350, ISSN 0027-8424

Notermans, S. & Havelaar, A.H. (1980). Removal and inactivation of botulinum toxins during production of drinking water from surface water. *Antonie van Leeuwenhoek*, Vol.46, No.5, pp. 511-514, ISSN 0003-6072

Pang, Y.P., Davis, J., & Wang, S., et al. (2010). Small molecules showing significant protection of mice against botulinum neurotoxin serotype A. *PLoS ONE*, Vol. 5, No. 4, pp. e10129, ISSN 1932-6203

Park, J.G., Sill, P.C. & Makiyi, E.F. et al. (2006). Serotype-selective, small-molecule inhibitors of the zinc endopeptidase of botulinum neurotoxin serotype A. *Bioorg Med Chem*, Vol.14, No.2, pp. 395–408, ISSN 0968-0896

Parker, H.S. (2002) *Agricultural Bioterrorism: A federal strategy to meet the threat*. McNair paper 65, Institute for National Strategic Studies, ISSN 1071-7552, Washington D.C., USA

Partikan, A., & Mitchell, W.G. (2007). Iatrogenic botulism in a child with spastic quadriparesis. *J Child Neur*, Vol.16, No.22, pp. 1235-1237, 0883-0738

Pickett, J., Berg, B. & Chaplin, E. et al. (1976). Syndrome of botulism in infancy: clinical and electrophysiological study. *NEJM*, Vol.295, No.14, pp.770-772, ISSN 0028-4793

Pier, C.L., Tepp, W.H., & Bradshaw, M., et al. (2008). Recombinant holotoxoid vaccine against botulism. *Infect Immun*, Vol.76, No.1, pp. 437-42, ISSN 0019-9567

Ravichandran, E., Gong, Y. & Fetwah, H. et al. (2005). An initial assessment of the systemic pharmacokinetics of botulinum toxin. *J Pharm Exp Ther*, Vol.318, No.3, pp. 1343-1351, ISSN 0022-3565

Ray, P., Ishida, H. & Millard, C.B., et al. (1999). Phospholipase A2 and arachidonic acid-mediated mechanism of neuroexocytosis: a possible target of botulinum neurotoxin A other than SNAP-25. *J Appl Toxicol*, Vol.19, No.S1, pp. S27-28, ISSN 0260-437X

Razai, A., Garcia-Rodriguez, C. & Lou, J. et al. (2005). Molecular evolution of antibody affinity for sensitive detection of botulinum neurotoxin type A. *J Mol Biol*, Vol.351, No.1, pp. 158–169, ISSN 0022-2836

Reames, H.R., Kadull, P.J. & Housewright, R.D. (1946). Studies on botulinum toxoids types A and B III. Immunization of man. *J of Immun*, Vol.55, No.4, pp. 309-324, ISSN 0022-1767

Rotz, L.D., Khan, A.S. & Lillibridge, S.R., et al. (2002) Public health assessment of potential biological terrorism agents. *Emerg Inf Dis*, Vol.8, No.2, pp. 225-230, ISSN 1080-6040

Roxas-Duncan, V., Enyedy, I. & Montgomery, V.A., et al (2009). Identification and biochemical characterization of small-molecule inhibitors of *Clostridium botulinum* neurotoxin serotype A. *Antimicrob Agents Chem*, Vol.53, No.8, pp. 3478-3486, ISSN 0066-4804

Rubinson, L., Vaughn, F. & Nelson, S. (2010). Mechanical ventilators in US acute care hospitals. *Dis Med Pub Health Prep*, Vol.4, No.3, pp. 199-206. ISSN 1935-7893

Rummel, A., Eichner, T. & Weil, T. et al. (2007). Identification of the protein receptor binding site of botulinum neurotoxins B and G proves the double-receptor concept. *PNAS*, Vol.104, No.1, pp 359-364, ISSN 0027-8424

Rusnak, J.M. & Smith, L.A. (2009). Botulinum neurotoxin vaccines. Past history and recent developments. *Human vaccines*, Vol.5, No.12, pp. 794-805, ISSN 1554-8600

Ryan, C.A., Nickels, M.K. & Hargrett, N.T. et al. (1987). Massive outbreak of antimicrobial resistant salmonellosis traced to pasteurized milk. *JAMA*, Vol.285, No.2, pp.3269-3274, ISSN 0098-7484

Sheridan R.E. (1996). Protonophore antagonism of botulinum toxin in mouse muscle. *Toxicon*, Vol.34, No.8, pp. 849-855, ISSN 0041-0101

Scott, A.B., & Suzuki, D. (1988). Systemic toxicity of botulinum toxin by intramuscular injection in the monkey. *Mov Dis*, Vol.3, No.4, pp.333–335, ISSN 0885-3185

Sentinel laboratory guidelines for suspected agents of bioterrorism. Botulinum toxin. *ASM*, accessed 08/01/2011, http://www.asm.org/index.php/policy/sentinel-level-clinical-microbiology-laboratory-guidelines.html

Settler, P.E. (2001). Pharmacology of botulinum type B. *Eur J Neurol*, Vol.8, No.S4, pp. 9-12, ISSN 1351-5101

Shapiro, R.L., Hatheway, C. & Becher, J. et al. (1997). Botulism surveillance and emergency response. A public health strategy for a global challenge. *JAMA*, Vol.278, No.5 pp. 433-435, ISSN 0098-7484

Shapiro, R.L., Hatheway, C. & Swerdlow, M.D. (1998). Botulism in the United States: A clinical and epidemiological review. *Ann Int Med*, Vol.129, No.3, pp. 221-228, ISSN 0003-4819

Silhar, P., Capkova, K. & Salzameda, N.T. (2010). Botulinum neurotoxin A protease: Discovery of natural product exosite inhibitors. *J Am Chem Soc*, Vol.132, No.9, pp. 2868-2869, ISSN 0002-7863

Sing, B.R., Thirunanvukkarasu, N., & Ghosal, K., et al. (2010). Clostridial neurotoxins as a drug delivery vehicle targeting nervous system *Biochimie*, Vol.92, No.9, pp. 1252-1259, ISSN 0300-9084

Simpson L.L. (1982). The interaction between aminoquinoloines and presynaptically acting neurotoxins. *J Pharmacol Exp Ther*, Vol.222, No.1, pp. 43-48, ISSN 0022-3565

Simpson L.L. 1983. Ammonium chloride and methylamine hydrochloride antagonize clostridial neurotoxins. *J Pharmacol Exp Ther*, Vol.225, No.3, pp. 546-552, ISSN 0022-3565

Simpson L.L. (2004). Identification of the major steps in botulinum toxin action. *Ann Rev Pharmacol Toxicol*, Vol.44, pp. 167-193, ISSN 0362-1642

Sloop, R.R., Cole, B.A. & Esculin, R.O. (1997). Human responses to botulism injection: type B compared to type A. *Neurology*, Vol.49, No.1, ISSN 0028-3878, pp. 189-194

Smith, L.A. (2009). Botulism and vaccines for its prevention. *Vaccine*, Vol.27, No.S4, pp. D33-D39, ISSN 0264-410X

Smith L.D.S. & Sugiyama, H. (1988). *Botulism: The Organism, its Toxins, the Disease*, (2nd ed.), Charles C. Thomas, ISBN 0398054460, Springfield, IL, USA

Smith, T.J., Lou, J. & Geren, I.N. et al. (2005). Sequence variation within botulinum neurotoxin serotypes impacts antibody binding and neutralization. *Infec and Imm*, Vol.73, No.9, ISSN 0019-9567, pp. 5450-5457

Smith, T.J., Hill, K.K. & Foley, B.T. et al. (2007). Analysis of the neurotoxin complex genes in *Clostridium botulinum* A1-A4 and B1 strains: BoNT/A3, /Ba4 and /B1 clusters are located within plasmids. *PLosS One*, Vol.2, No.12, pp.1-10, ISSN 1544-9173

Stringer, S.C., Webb, M.D. & George, S.M. et al. (2005). Heterogeneityof times required for germination and outgrowth from single spores of nonproteolytic *Clostridium botulinum*. *App Env Micro*, Vol.71, No.9, ISSN 0099-2240, pp.4998-5003

Sonnabend, O., Heinzle, R. & Sigrist, T., et al. (1981). Isolation of *Clostridium botulinum* type G and identification of type G botulinal toxin in humans: report of five sudden unexpected deaths. *J. Infect. Dis.*, Vol.143, No.1, ISSN 0022-1899, pp. 22–27

Sugishima, M. (2003). Aum Shinrikyo and the Japanese law on biotrerrorism. *Prehospital and disaster medicine*, Vol.18, No.3, pp.179-183, ISSN 1049-023X

Tacket, C.O., Shandera, W.X., & Mann, J.M., (1984). Equine antitoxin use and other factors that predict outcome in type A foodborne botulism. *Am J Med*, Vol. 76, No. 5, pp. 794-798, ISSN 0002-9343.

Tang J.J., Park, G., & Millard, C.B. et al. (2007). Computer-aided lead optimization: improved small-molecule inhibitor of the zinc endopeptidase of botulinum neurotoxin serotype A. *PLoS ONE*, Vol.2, No.8, pp. 2:e761, ISSN 1932-6203

Terranova, W., Palumbo, J.N. & Breman, J. G. (1979). Ocular findings in botulism type B. *JAMA*, Vol.241, No.5, pp. 475-477, ISSN 0098-7484

Tremblay, J.M., Kuo, C.L. & Abeijon, C. et al. (2010). Camelid single domain antibodies (VHHs) as neuronal cell intrabody binding agents and inhibitors of *Clostridium botulinum* neurotoxin (BoNT) proteases. *Toxicon*, Vol.56, No.6, pp. 990-998, ISSN 0041-0101

United Nations Security Council. (1995). Tenth report of the executive chairman of the special commissions established by the secretary-general pursuant to paragraph 9(b)(I) of security council resolution 687 (1991) and paragraph 3 of resolution 699 (1991) on the activities of the special commission. New York, pp.S/1995/1038.

Varma, J.K., Katsitadze, G., & Moiscrafishvili, M. et al. (2004). Signs and symptoms predictive of death in patients with foodborne botulism-Republic of Georgia, 1980-2002. *Clin Infect Dis*, Vol.39, No.33, pp.357-362, ISSN 1058-4838

Wannemacher, R.W., Dinterman, R.E., & Thompson, W.L. et al. (1993) Treatment for removal of biotoxins from drinking water. Technical report 9120. U.S. Army Biomedical Research and Development Laboratory, Fort Detrick, Frederick, Md.

Wein, L.M. & Liu, Y. (2005) Analyzing a bioterror attack on the food supply: The case of botulinum toxin in milk. *PNAS*, Vol.102, No.28, pp. 9984-9899, ISSN, 0027-8424

Webb, R.P., Smith, T.J. & Wright, P. et al. (2009). Production of catalytically inactive BoNT/A1 holoprotein and comparison with BoNT/A1 subunit vaccines against toxin subtypes A1, A2, and A3. *Vaccine*, Vol.27, No.33, pp. 4490-4497, ISSN 0264-410X

Woodruff, B.A., Griffin, P.M. & McCroskey L.M. (1992). Clinical and laboratory comparison of botulism from toxin types A, B, and E in the United States, 1975-1988. *J Infect Dis*, Vol.166, No.6, pp. 1281-12866, ISSN 0022-1899

Williams, P. & Wallace, D. (1989). *Unit 731: Japan's Secret Biological Warfare in World War II*. The Free Press, ISBN 0029353017, New York, NY, USA.

Yang, Y., Lindo, P. & Riding, S. et al. (2008). Expression, purification and comparative characterization of enzymatically deactivated recombinant botulinum neurotoxin type A. *Botulinum* Vol.1, No.2, pp. 219-241, ISSN 1754-7318

Yuan, J., Inami, G., & Mohle-Boetani, J. (2011) Recurrent wound botulism among injection drug users in California. *Clin Infec Dis*, Vol.52, No.7, pp. 862-866, ISSN 1058-4838

Zhang, P., Ray, R., & Sing, B.R., et al. (2009) An efficient drug delivery vehicle for botulism countermeasure. *BMC Pharm*, Vol.9, No.12, pp. 1-9, ISSN 1471-2210

Zilinkas, R.A. (1997). Iraq's biological weapons: the past as future? *JAMA*, Vol.278, No.5, pp. 418-424, ISSN 0098-7484

7

Ricin Perspective in Bioterrorism

Virginia I. Roxas-Duncan[1] and Leonard A. Smith[2]
[1]*Integrated Toxicology Division,*
U.S. Army Medical Research Institute of Infectious Diseases,
[2]*Senior Research Scientist (ST) for Medical Countermeasures Technology,*
Office of Chief Scientist, U.S. Army Medical Research Institute of Infectious Diseases,
USA

1. Introduction

Ricin is one of the most toxic and easily produced plant toxins. It is derived from the castor plant, *Ricinus communis* (Fig. 1), a shrub native to Africa but currently is being cultivated in many areas of the world for its co mmercial products, primarily castor oil. The seeds of *R. communis*, commonly called beans (although not a true bean) (Fig. 2), are oblong, brown, and have a thick mottled shell sometimes used to make decorative necklaces and bracelets. Castor seeds contain 40 to 60% vegetable oil that is rich in triglycerides, mainly ricinolein (McKeon et al., 1999). Castor oil is used in a number of products. For many years, purified castor oil has been ingested as a human nutritional supplement, emetic, or purgative worldwide (Scarpa and Guerci, 1982; Caupin, 1997; Olsnes, 2004). In addition to castor oil production, castor plants are also being grown for aesthetic (ornamental garden bush) and ecological values. It is used extensively as a decorative plant in parks and other public areas. Ecologically, despite the ricin being poisonous to humans and many animals, *R. communis* is the host plant of insects including moths and butterflies, and is also used as a food plant by some Lepidopteran larvae and birds.

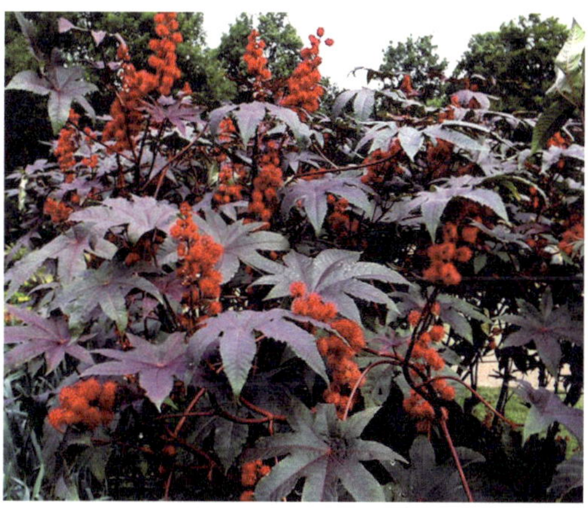

Fig. 1. Castor plant, *Ricinus communis*, a large shrub having large palmate leaves and spiny capsules containing seeds that are the source of castor oil and ricin (Adapted from http://dtirp.dtra.mil/images/RicinusCommunis.jpg)

Castor seeds contain large amounts of ricin, which is also present in lower concentrations throughout the plant. Ricin content significantly varies among cultivars/accessions and may range from 0.1 to 4% of the weight of the seed (Auld et al., 2003; Baldoni et al., 2011; Pinkerton et al., 1999). Ricin is one of the most potent poisons in the plant kingdom (Lee & Wang, 2005). Because of the wide availability of its source plants, ease of production, stability, and lethal potency, ricin toxin is considered to be a bioterrorism threat. Ricin is the most common biological agent used in biocrimes, and has also been reported as one of the most prevalent agents involved in WMD (weapons of mass destructions) investigations (FBI, n.d.). Recent attempted uses of ricin by various extremists and radical groups have heightened concerns regarding ricin's potential for urban terrorism.

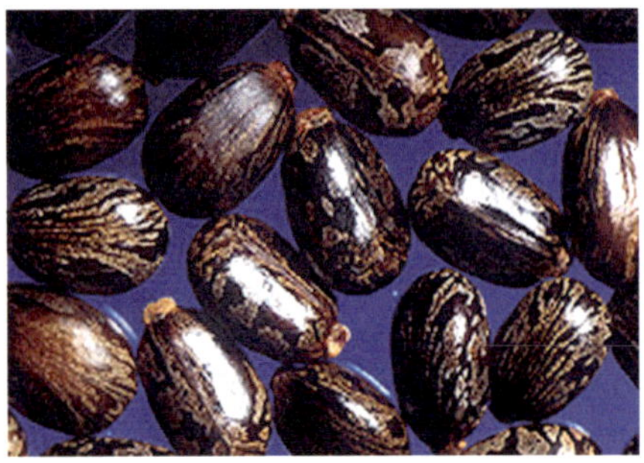

Fig. 2. Castor seeds (Adapted from
http://www.ars.usda.gov/is/AR/archive/jan01/plant0101.htm)

2. History, biological warfare and terrorism

The castor plant belongs to the genus *Ricinus* of the Euphorbiaceae or spurge family (Atsmon, 1985). *R. communis* is indigenous to the southeastern Mediterranean region, eastern Africa, and India, but is now widespread throughout temperate and subtropical regions (McKeon et al., 2000; Phillips & Rix, 1999). The gourd mentioned in the Book of Jonah (Jon 4:6-9; Old Testament), bears the Hebrew name kikayon, and is presumed to be the kiki of the Egyptians, the castor-oil plant (Easton's Bible Dictionary, n.d.). It is commonly known as "Palm of Christ" or *Palma Christi*, that derives from castor oil's ability to heal wounds and cure ailments. Castor seeds have been found in Egyptian tombs dating back to 4000 BC, and were used in folk medicines against a wide variety of diseases. The plant has been cultivated for its commercial products, primarily castor oil, for at least 4000 years (Olsnes, 2004). Castor oil was used in rituals of sacrifice to please the gods in early civilizations. In Ancient Egypt and in Europe, it has been used for lighting, body ointments, improving hair growth and texture, and medicinal purposes, where it was regarded as a folk medicine. In India, castor oil has been documented since 2000 BC and was mainly used in lamps and in local medicine as a laxative, purgative, cathartic and other ethnomedical systems. In China, castor seed and its oil have been prescribed for centuries in local medicine for internal use. In Italy, castor oil was used as an instrument of coercion by the Squadristi, the Fascists armed squads of dictator Benito Mussolini; this idea originated from Gabriele D' Annunzio, a controversial nationalist, poet and war veteran (MacDonald, 1999). Political dissidents and regime opponents were forced to ingest the oil in large amounts, triggering severe diarrhea and dehydration that oftentimes led to death (New World Encyclopedia, n.d.).

In recent centuries, however, natural castor oil was at first identified as a laxative and as a lubricant for the wheels of wagons and carts, as well as aircrafts during World War I (WWI). Today, castor oil (extracted minus the ricin) has a wide variety of commercial applications (International Castor Oil Association, ICOA, 1992). It is used for medicinal purposes both internally, as a strong and effective purgative or cathartic, and externally to treat corns, among other purposes (Sims & Frey, 2005). Castor oil and its derivatives also have numerous industrial merits, being used in a wide variety of products, such as the basic ingredient in racing motor oil for high-performance engines, a fuel additive for two-cycle engines, a primary raw material in the production of nylons and other resins and fibers, and a component in paint and varnish, insulation, fabric coatings, soap, ink, plastics, hydraulic fluids, lubricants, guns, insecticidal oils, cosmetics, and antifungal compounds (Brugsch, 1960; Caupin, 1997; McKeon et al., 1999; Sims & Frey, 2005). Because of its economic benefits and myriads of uses, castor seeds are currently being produced in more than 30 countries in the world. In 2008, world's production of castor oil totaled to 1,605,362 metric tons (MT) (Food and Agricultural Organization of the United Nations Statistical Database, FAOSTAT, 2011); the leading producers include India (1,171,000 MT), China (190,000 MT), and Brazil (122,140 MT). After oil extraction and inactivation of ricin, the defatted waste "mash" (also called castor bean meal) is used as animal feed while the seed husks are used as high nitrogen fertilizer (Kole, 2011).

Ricin toxin was discovered in 1888 by Hermann Stillmark, a student at the Dorpat University in Estonia (Stillmark, 1888, as cited in Franz and Jaax, 1997). During Stillmark's extensive research, he also observed that ricin caused agglutination of erythrocytes and precipitation of serum proteins (Olsnes, 2004). Olsnes and Phil (1972) demonstrated that ricin inhibited protein synthesis, and suggested that the effects resulted from restricted elongation of nascent polypeptide chain. Subsequent studies revealed that the molecular target of the toxin was the 60S ribosomal subunit (Olsnes and Phil, 1982).

In the last decade, immunotoxins using the ricin A-chain chemically-linked to monoclonal antibodies have been used as an alternative in therapies against cancer, AIDS and other illnesses (Engert et al., 1997; Schnell et al., 2003; Youn et al., 2005). Ricin-based immunotoxins, some of which contained deglycosylated ricin A chain conjugated to either the anti-CD22 antibody RFB4 (Amlot et al., 1993; Sausville et al., 1995), or its Fab fragment (Vitetta et al., 1991) have also been shown to provide enhanced therapeutic efficacy and resulted in improved antitumor activity (Li et al., 2005; Kreitman et al., 2005; Vitetta, 2006). However, the U.S. Food and Drug Administration (FDA) has placed a hold on the clinical testing of RTA-based immunotoxins because they caused vascular leak syndrome (VLS) in humans.

2.1 Biological warfare and terrorism

2.1.1 History of ricin as a biological weapon

During WWI, ricin was investigated as a potential offensive biological weapon. Two methods of weaponizing the toxin were explored, i.e., bullets and shrapnel coated with ricin, or a 'dust cloud' of toxin inhaled into the lungs (Smart, 1997). Nonetheless, the thermal instability of ricin constrained its initial use in exploding shells, and ethical and treaty issues limited its use as a poison or blinding agents (Hunt et al., 1918, as cited in Millard &

LeClaire, 2007). WWI ended before the toxin could be weaponized and tested. During WWII, ricin was produced in hundreds of kilograms and armed into W bombs (ricin-containing bombs), but apparently was never used in battle (Franz & Jaax, 1997). Although its toxicity made it marginally better over existing agents, ricin was surpassed by the even more potent biological agents of the time. Interest in ricin continued for a short period after WWII, but soon subsided when the U.S. Army Chemical Corps began a program to weaponize sarin. During the Cold War, the Soviet Union also studied ricin as a possible biological weapons agent. Ken Alibek, a former top official involved in Russia's biological weapons program who defected to the U.S. in 1991, claimed that Russia developed ricin toxin as a weapon, and that the ricin toxin used against the Bulgarian dissident Georgi Markov, as well Vladimir Kostov (another Bulgarian exile in Paris), was concocted in Russian laboratories (Maman & Yehezkelli, 2005). During 1989, approximately 10 L of concentrated ricin solution was reportedly manufactured at Salman Park just south of Baghdad, some of which were used in animal testing and as payload in artillery shells (Zilinskas, 1997). More recently, ricin has been used by terrorist organizations (CDC, 2008). In 2002, a report emerged that Ansar al-Islam, a Sunni Islamic group allegedly linked to Osama Bin Laden's al-Qaeda organization, had been testing biological weapons including ricin at a small facility in northern Iraq (BBC News, 20 August 2002). A news item documented evidence of the manufacture of ricin and botulinum toxin in Iraq (Mendenhall, 2003). Syria was also believed to have produced unknown quantities of the toxin. Iran allegedly procured 120 tons of castor beans in 1992, presumably for ricin production (Croddy & Wirtz, 2005). Ricin was also found in Afghanistan after the collapse of the Taliban Government in 2001 (GlobalSecurity.org, n.d.; Barceloux, 2008).

Ricin is currently monitored as a Schedule 1 toxic chemical under the Convention on the Prohibition of the Development, Production, Stockpiling and Use of Chemical Weapons and on Their Destruction (CWC). Also, the intentional use of ricin or related toxins as weapons is prohibited under the 1972 Convention on the Prohibition of the Development, Production and Stockpiling of Bacteriological (Biological) and Toxin Weapons and on Their Destruction (BTWC) (Millard & Le Claire, 2007; Poli, 2007). The possession or transfer of ricin, abrin, or genes encoding functional forms of these toxins is also regulated in the U.S. by the Centers for Disease Control and Prevention (CDC) Select Agents and Toxins Program.

Although ricin's potential use as a military weapon was investigated, its utility over conventional weaponry remains disputed. Despite its toxicity, ricin is less potent than other agents such as botulinum neurotoxin or anthrax. Kortepeter & Parker (1999) estimated that eight metric tons of ricin would have to be aerosolized over a 100 km^2 area to achieve about 50% casualty, whereas only kilogram quantities of anthrax spores would cause the same effect. Furthermore, dispersal of ricin on a wide scale is logistically impractical. Thus, while ricin is easy to produce, it is not as likely to cause as many casualties as other agents (Schep et al., 2009). However, it has been the agent of choice in numerous biocrimes (see below).

2.1.2 Ricin as a terrorist weapon

Ricin has been classified by the CDC as a Category B agent. Category B agents are moderately easy to disseminate, can cause morbidity and low mortality, and include *Coxiella burnetii*, *Brucella* spp, *Burkholderia mallei*, *B. pseudomallei*, alphaviruses (VEE, EEE, WEE),

Rickettsia prowazekii, toxins (e.g., ricin, Staphylococcal enterotoxin B, epsilon toxin of *Clostridium perfringens*), *Chlamydia psittaci*, food safety threats (e.g., *Salmonella* spp., *Escherichia coli* O157:H7, *Shigella*), and water safety threats (e.g. *Vibrio cholerae, Cryptosporidium parvum*) (Rotz et al., 2002). Though ricin is not considered an effective weapon of mass destruction, its potential as a weapon of terror cannot be discounted. Further, ricin's notoriety is likely driven by the ready availability of castor beans, press coverage, and popularization on the internet. In the U.S. for example, the use of ricin as a biological agent in bioterrorism and homicides is of particular concern especially after the events of September 11, 2001. Worldwide, numerous cases involving the possession, experimentation, or planned misuse of ricin by bioterrorists and extremist groups have been investigated or prosecuted by law enforcement agencies (Franz and Jaax, 1997; James Martin Center for Nonproliferation Studies (CNS), 2004; Research International, Inc. (RII), 2011). The following incidents have reportedly involved the use and/or possession of ricin.

- On September 7, 1978 while waiting at a bus stop in London, a Bulgarian dissident, Georgi Markov, felt a jab in the back of his right thigh and saw a man picking up an umbrella (Crompton & Gall, 1980). Markov, a 49-year-old novelist and playwriter had published and broadcasted anticommunist views. An assassin reportedly injected a small pellet of ricin (believed to have been supplied by the KGB), into Markov's right thigh using a weapon in the shape of an umbrella (Maman & Yehezkelli, 2005). He subsequently developed severe gastroenteritis, high fever, and died 3 days later (discussed in detail later in this chapter). At autopsy, a small 1.53-mm metallic sphere that had 2 tiny holes and could hold a volume of 0.28 mm^3, was found at the wound site. No specific isolation of any poison was possible. Because of the small volume and rapid demise of the patient, ricin was believed to be the only capable inciting agent. The coroner recreated the scenario by injecting a pig with a somewhat greater dose than Markov had received (Crompton & Gall, 1980). With an illness similar to Markov's, the animal died 26 hours later. Thereafter the coroner was satisfied that Markov had been unlawfully killed by a tiny pellet containing 0.2 to 0.5 mg dose of ricin (Musshoff & Madea, 2009). The KGB denied any involvement although high-profile defectors Oleg Kalugin and Oleg Gordievsky have since confirmed the KGB's involvement (Pearce, 2011).
- In 1981, exposed CIA double agent Boris Korczak was reportedly shot with a ricin-laced pellet (Carus, 2002). He survived this assassination attempt which was thought to be the work of the KGB.
- In 1982, William A. Chanslor, a Texas attorney was sentenced to jail for 3 years and fined $5,000 for plotting to kill his 39-year-old wife with ricin. He claimed that he wanted the ricin to assist his wife, paralyzed from the waist down due to a stroke, in committing suicide (Time Magazine, 16 August 1982).
- In 1983, two brothers were arrested by the Federal Bureau of Investigation (FBI) for producing an ounce of pure ricin (RII, 2011).
- In 1983 and 1985, Montgomery Todd Meeks, a high school senior was tried and convicted of attempted murder and solicitation to murder in connection with a plot to kill his father using ricin (Trager, 1985, as cited in Carus (2002). He claimed that the act was motivated by his father's abuse (RII, 2011).
- In 1991, four members of the Minnesota Patriots Council, a radical tax-protesting militia organization, acquired castor beans and planned to use ricin to assassinate local deputy

sheriffs, U.S. Marshals, and IRS agents. Despite having no specific expertise in biological warfare, they extracted about 0.7 g of 5% ricin, which was enough to kill about 100 people. Two members were convicted in 1994, and the other two in 1995 under the Biological Weapons Anti-Terrorism Act (BWATA) law (RII, 2011).

- On April 21, 1992, the Washington Post published an article regarding the unsuccessful attempt to poison the famous Soviet dissident Alexander Solzhenitsyn with the same lethal chemical (thought to be ricin) used to kill Bulgarian dissident Georgi Markov in London in 1978 (Remnick, 21 April 1992).
- In December 1995, Thomas Lewis Lavy, an electrician from Valdez, Alaska was arrested in Onia, Arkansas for possession of ricin (Kifner, 2005). In April 1993, he was caught while trying to smuggle 130 g of ricin and other materials from Alaska into Canada, and was then charged under BWATA with possession of a biological toxin with intent to kill. Lavy killed himself in his prison cell several days after his arrest (RII, 2011).
- In 1995, a federal case was brought against Dr. Ray W. Mettetal, Jr., a neurologist at Rockingham Memorial Hospital in Harrisonburg, Virginia, after ricin was discovered in his possession and also of providing false information (Carus, 2002).
- In 1995, Deborah Green, a non-practicing oncologist from Prairie Village, Kansas, attempted to murder her husband, Michael Farrar, a cardiologist, with ricin (Musick, 25 May 2000; Carus 2002). Green had purchased the castor beans through a special order from a garden center in Kansas City, Missouri, and placed them in Farrar's food. It is unclear if she extracted the ricin or merely added the beans to the food. Later, Farrar had to undergo multiple heart and brain surgeries related to the poisoning (CNS, 2004).
- In 1997, a man was indicted under the provisions of BWATA for possessing ricin and nicotine sulfate. He pled guilty to manufacturing ricin and was sentenced to more than 12 years in prison (Cordesman, 2002).
- On August 25, 1998, Dwayne Lee Kuehl was arrested in Escanaba, Michigan, for producing ricin with intent to use it against an Escanaba city housing inspector (RII 2011).
- In November 1999, FBI agents apprehended James Kenneth Gluck in Tampa, Florida, for threatening to kill court officials in Jefferson County, Colorado with ricin (The New York Times, 08 November 1999).
- In August 2001, the FSB (Russian Federal Security Service) told the Itar-Tass news service it had intercepted a recorded conversation between two Chechen field commanders (Brigadier General Rizvan Chitigov and field commander Hizir Alhazurov) about instructions on the homemade production of poisons against Russian troops (RII, 2011). Russian authorities reportedly raided Chitigov's home and seized materials, including instructions on how to produce ricin from castor beans, a small chemical laboratory, three homemade explosives, two land mines, and 30 grenades (Gad, 2007).
- In June 2002, Ken Olson, an Agilent software engineer, was convicted of ricin possession (Tizon, 2004). He was given a 13-year, 9-month sentence in April 2004.
- In August 2002, the Sunni miltant group Ansar al-Islam was reported to be involved in testing biological agents including ricin on barnyard animals and perhaps even an unwitting human subject (BBC News, 20 August 2002).

- In December 2002, six terrorist suspects were arrested in Manchester, England. Their apartment was serving as a "ricin laboratory." Among them was a 27-year-old chemist who was producing the toxin (CDC, 2003a).
- In January 2003, authorities discovered traces of ricin in the apartment of six Algerians in Wood Green, northern London (Hopkins & Branigan, 08 January 2003). They also discovered castor beans and equipment for crushing the beans. Those arrested are believed to be part of a terrorist cell known as the "Chechen network" which may have ties to the Algerian group behind the millennium bomb plots in the U.S. All but one of the suspects was acquitted of charges in April, 2005 (Research International, 2011).
- In October 2003, an envelope with a threatening note and a sealed container that had ricin in it was discovered at a mail processing and distribution facility in Greenville, South Carolina. The note threatened to poison water supplies if demands were not met (CDC, 2003b).
- In February 2004, traces of ricin were discovered on an automatic mail sorter in the mailroom of the Dirksen Senate Office building in Washington, D.C which handled mail addressed to Senate Majority Leader Bill Frist (CNN.com, 04 February 2004).
- In January 2005, the FBI arrested an Ocala, Florida man after agents found ricin and other products in the home he lives in with his mother (CNN.com, 14 January 2005).
- On October 3, 2006, a survivalist from Phoenix, Arizona was sentenced to 7 years in prison for attempting to manufacture ricin (Martens, 2006).
- In 2007, traces of ricin had been found at Limerick Prison (Lally, 2007). The ricin was smuggled into Ireland from the U.S. in a contact lens case, to be used in an assassination plot. An arrest was made before the ricin could be used (RII, 2011).
- In November 2008, Roger Von Bergendorff was fined and sentenced to 3.5 years in prison for having ricin and unregistered firearm silencers. In February 2008, Bergendorff was living in a motel room in Las Vegas, Nevada when he was taken to a hospital in critical condition. Authorities recovered castor beans, a weapons cache, a copy of "The Anarchist Cookbook" with a page about ricin marked, and 4 crude grams of ricin in his room. Investigators also found respirators, gloves and chemicals that could be used in the production of ricin in one of Bergendorff's storage units in Utah (Powers, 18 November 2008).
- In June 2009, a father and son, Ian and Nicky Davison were arrested after the discovery of ricin at a house in County Durham (BBC News, 06 June 2009). Ian Davidson was sentenced to 10 years in May 2010 for preparing acts of terrorism, three counts of possessing material useful to commit acts of terrorism and possessing a prohibited weapon; his son was given 2 years youth detention for possessing material useful to commit acts of terrorism (Wainwright, 2010).In January 2011, The FBI has arrested the owner of a Coventry Township, Ohio home for unlawful possession of ricin (Sharma, 29 January 2011).
- In June 2011, Michael Crooker, a former Agawam man, was sentenced to 15 years in federal prison for illegally possessing ricin and threatening a prosecutor (Associated Press, AP, 22 June 2011). In another report during the same period, a British citizen, Asim Kauser, was brought to court on charges including possessing instructions for producing ricin (Global Security Network, GSN, 17 June 2011).

The above events clearly demonstrate that ricin is readily available or accessible, relatively easy to produce, and seemingly, a biological weapon of choice by extremist groups and individuals. Hence, it should be seriously considered as a potential bioterrorism threat agent.

3. Description of the agent

3.1 Overview of ribosome-inactivating proteins

Ricin belongs to a diverse family of ribosome-inactivating proteins (RIPs) that include numerous other toxins from a wide variety of plants, as well as potent bacterial Shiga and Shiga-like toxins (Endo et al., 1988). RIPs possess N-glycosidase activity that depurinates a highly conserved adenine residue within the specific 14 nucleotide region (also known as α-sarcin/ricin loop) of the 28S ribosomal RNA (rRNA) subunit of 60S ribosome (Endo et al., 1987; Endo & Tsurugi, 1987). There are three types of RIPs. Type 1 RIPs are monomeric N-glycosidase enzymes of approximately 30 kDA molecular mass, and are frequently found in higher plants, e.g., pokeweed antiviral protein, trichosanthin, saporin, and luffin (Nielsen & Boston, 2001). In general, type I RIPs are not cytotoxic because they lack the means of entering the cell (B chain) to inactivate ribosomes (Lord et al., 1994).

Type 2 RIPs are glycosylated heterodimers possessing an N-glycosidase enzyme (denoted A chain) linked through a disulfide bond to a galactose-binding lectin (denoted B-chain) that facilitates endocytosis (Lord et al., 1994; Stirpe & Battelli, 2006). Type 2 RIPs include potent toxins such as ricin, abrin (isolated from the seeds of rosary pea, *Abrus precatorius*), modeccin (from the fruits and roots of *Adenia digitata*), volkensin (from the roots of *A. volkensii*), and viscumins (from mistletoe, *Viscum album*; Lord et al., 1994). Some type 2 RIPs possess an aberrant or non-functional B-chain, hence are relatively nontoxic. These include nigrin b from the elderberry plant (*Sambucus nigra*), lectins from winter aconite (*Eranthis hyemalis*), and ebulin lectins from dwarf elder (*S. ebulus*).

Type 3 RIPs are the least common class and resemble type I plant RIPs in catalytic activity and overall net charge (Nielsen & Boston, 2001). They are synthesized as inactive precursor molecules with a polypeptide insert in the active site region of the A chain domain (Chaudhry et al., 1994).

3.1.2 Biochemistry of ricin

Ricin is the most well-characterized member of the type 2 RIPs. It consists of two glycoprotein subunits, designated A chain (RTA) and B chain (RTB), of approximately equal molecular mass (~32 kDa) linked by a single disulfide bond (Fig. 3). The ricin toxin is stored in the matrix of the castor seed, together with a 120 kDa lectin called *R. communis* agglutinin I (RCA). RCA is composed of two ricin-like dimers. Although the nucleotide sequences of ricin and RCA are similar, these proteins are products of distinct genes (Kole, 2011); it has been suggested that the ricin gene evolved first and then duplicated to give rise to the RCA gene (Ready et al., 1984). Compared with ricin, RCA is virtually nontoxic (Olsnes et al., 1974) but is a powerful red blood cell agglutinin (Hegde & Podder, 1992).

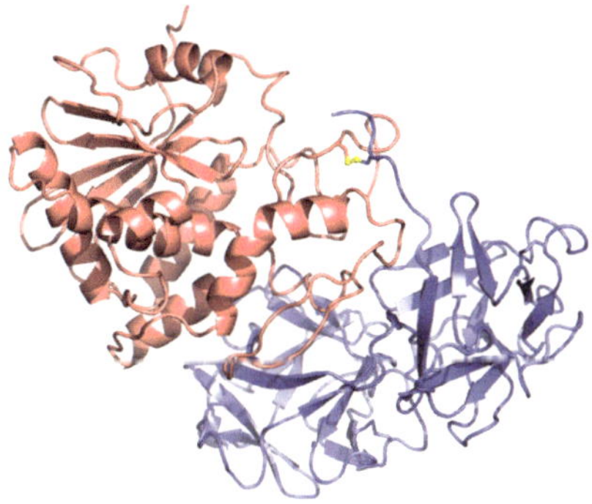

Fig. 3. Three-dimensional representation of ricin. The A chain (RTA) is depicted in red, the B chain (RTB) in blue, and the disulfide bond in yellow. (Image courtesy of Dr. Mark A. Olson, Integrated Toxicology Division, USAMRIID, Fort Detrick, MD).

3.1.2.1 Primary structure of ricin/RCA

The ricin protein's coding region consists of a 24 amino acid N-terminal signal sequence preceding a 266 amino acid RTA. The RTB has 262 amino acids. A 12-amino acid linker joins the two chains. The nontranslated mRNA regions of ricin and RCA are identical (Roberts, et al., 1985; Lamb et al., 1985). The signal peptide preceding the RTA in both lectins and the linker peptide joining the RTA and RTB are also alike in size and amino acid sequence. Overall, the RCA and RTA chains are 93% homologous (18 amino acid variants) while the corresponding B chains differ in 41 amino acids, and are 84% homologous (Lamb et al., 1985).

3.1.2.2 Ricin secondary structure

The carboxyl-terminal end of the RTA folds into a domain that interacts between the two domains of the B chain (Montfort et al., 1987). A disulfide bond is formed at amino acid 259 of the RTA and amino acid 4 of the RTB (Robertus, 1988; 1991; Lord et al., 1994). Thirty percent of the RTA protein is helical (Fig. 4). The RTA folds into three somewhat arbitrary domains. The active site cleft of the RTA is located at the interface between all three domains. A conformational change occurs in the active site when the RTA is released from the RTB.

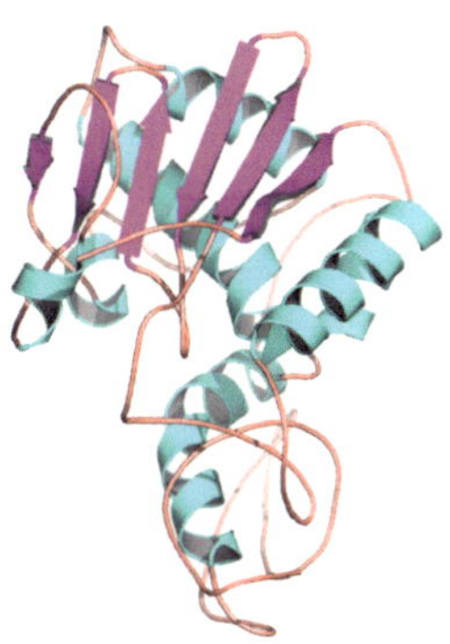

Fig. 4. Ribbon representation of RTA. The RTA has three structural domains and exhibits a substantial amount of secondary structure. Color schemes: cyan = helix; magenta = strands; red = coil regions. (Image courtesy of Dr. Mark A. Olson, Integrated Toxicology Division, USAMRIID, Fort Detrick, MD).

3.2 Pathogenesis

Ricin is a toxalbumin, a biological toxin whose mechanism of action is inhibition of protein synthesis in eukaryotic cells which results in cell death (CDC, 2006a). The dimeric A-B chain structure is crucial to cellular internalization and subsequent toxicity. Cell entry by ricin involves a series of steps, summarized as follows: 1) the RTB portion of the ricin molecule binds to cell surface glycolipids or glycoproteins possessing 1,4-linked galactose residues; 2) once bound to the cell surface, the toxin is internalized by endocytosis and routed to the cytosol. The presence of the B-chain facilitates transport of the A-chain into the cytosol; 3) toxin entry into early endosomes; 4) ricin vesicular transport from early endosomes to the trans-Golgi network; 5) retrograde vesicular transport through the Golgi network to reach the endoplasmic reticulum; 6) reduction of the disulfide bond connecting RTA and RTB; 7) partial unfolding of the RTA to render it translocationally competent to cross the endoplasmic reticulum (Endo et al., 1987; Olsnes & Koslov, 2001; Lord et al., 1994; 2003). Transport to the cytosol is the rate-limiting step during the decline in protein synthesis (Hudson and Neville, 1987).

Once transported from the ER to the cytoplasm, the RTA can interact with the ribosome, which acts as a suicidal chaperone stimulating proper refolding and resumption of catalytic activity (Lord et al., 2003). Ricin has a Michaelis constant (K_M) of 0.1 µmol/L for ribosomes and an enzymatic constant (K_{cat}) of 1,500/min. It depurinates a specific adenosine residue (A4324) near the 3′ end of 28S ribosomal RNA subunit in the 60S ribosome subunit (Robertus, 1991). This halts the binding of elongation factor-2, which then results in the inhibition of protein synthesis in eukaryotic cells (Endo et al., 1987). Catalytic studies showed that single ricin molecule in the cytosol can inactivate over 1500 ribosomes per minute and eventually kills the cell (Olsnes et al.,1975; Cawley and Houston, 1979).

Ricin is more active against animal than plant or bacterial ribosomes (Cawley and Houston, 1979). Ribosomes which lack the specific 28S subunit containing the GAGA tetranucleotide sequence are generally not susceptible to the toxin.

3.3 Toxicity

Ricin's toxicity is dependent on a number of factors including route of exposure (inhalation, parenteral (injection), ingestion, dermal contact, or ocular contact), amount of toxin administered, and animal species.

3.3.1 Route of administration

Ricin is extremely toxic by inhalation, and least potent by the oral route. In mice, the approximate dose that is lethal to 50% of the exposed population (LD_{50}) and time to death are, respectively, 3-5 µg/kg (Franz and Jaax, 1997) and 60 hours by inhalation (Kortepeter et al., 2001a), 20 mg/kg and 85 hours by ingestion (Franz and Jaax, 1997), 5 µg/kg and 90 hours by intravenous injection (Franz and Jaax, 1997), and 24 µg/kg and 100 hours by subcutaneous injection (Franz and Jaax, 1997). Low oral toxicity is possibly due to poor toxin absorption and partial degradation in the gut. Higher toxicities by other routes may be related to accessibility of target-cell populations and the availability of toxin receptors among cell types. Skin testing in mice showed no dermal toxicity, indicating poor absorption across the skin (Wannemacher & Anderson, 2005).

3.3.2 Amount of toxin administered

Ingestion and mastication of 3-6 castor beans is the estimated fatal dose in adults; the fatal dose in children is not known, but is likely less (CDC, 2006a). Most cases of castor bean ingestion do not result in poisoning, because: a) it is difficult for ricin to be released from ingested castor beans; b) ricin release requires mastication, and the degree of mastication is likely to be important in determining the extent of poisoning; and c) ricin is not as well absorbed through the gastrointestinal tract when compared to injection or inhalation (CDC, 2006a).

3.3.3 Animal species

The lethality of ricin by different routes in several animal species was summarized by Millard & LeClaire (2007). By ingestion, the hens were the least sensitive to the toxin (LD_{50} = 14 g/kg), and the horses were the most sensitive (LD_{50} = 0.1 g/kg). By injection, rabbits had an LD_{50} = 0.1 µg/kg (i.m.), and 0.5 µg/kg (i.v.), while guinea pigs had <1.1 µg/kg (i.v.) and 0.8 µg/kg (i.m.) (Millard & LeClaire, 2007).

3.4 Human toxicity

Limited information is available regarding human toxicity. Based on animal experiments and accidental human exposures, the approximate LD_{50} and time to death for humans are, respectively, 3 µg/kg and 36-72 hours by inhalation, 30 µg/kg and 6-8 days by ingestion, 3 µg/kg and 36-72 hours by intravenous injection, and 500 µg and 3-6 days by subcutaneous injection (based on Georgi Markov's assassination) (Franz & Jaax, 1997; Maman & Yehezkelli, 2005; Mirarchi, 2010).

The vulnerability of certain populations (e.g., children, pregnant women, the elderly, those with immunosuppression, or underlying respiratory or gastrointestinal tract disease) to the health effects of ricin exposure is unknown; however, persons with pre-existing tissue irritation or damage may sustain further injury upon ricin exposure (CDC, 2006a).

3.5 Transmission

Ricin may adhere to skin, nonetheless, person-to-person transmission through casual contact has not been reported. Ricin is transmitted by the airborne route through release of the toxin in the form of a powder, or a mist, or reaerosolization of ricin into the air from disturbed surfaces (CDC, 2006a). However, to be effective, the toxin would need to be dispersed in particles smaller than 5 microns (CDC, 2006a).

4. Clinical symptoms, signs and pathology

The clinical signs, symptoms, and pathological manifestations of ricin toxicity vary with the dose and route of exposure, as detailed below. For symptomatic patients, the clinical course presents with the rapid onset of nausea, vomiting, and abdominal pain. Gastrointestinal bleeding, anuria, diarrhea, cramps, and vascular collapse can also occur (Challoner & McCarron, 1990). Most symptoms develop less than 6 hours after ingestion, although the lag time from ingestion of castor seeds to onset of symptoms has ranged from 15 minutes to almost 10 hours. Progression to death occurs within 36 to 72 hours of exposure, depending on the route of exposure and the dose received (CDC, 2008).

4.1 Injection

In humans, subcutaneous or intramuscular injection of high doses of ricin results in severe local lymphoid necrosis, gastrointestinal hemorrhage, liver necrosis, diffuse nephritis, and diffuse splenitis. Ricin injection leads to necrosis at the injection site, which may predispose one to secondary infection (Passeron et al., 2004). Crompton & Gall (1980) summarized the clinical signs and symptoms for the Bulgarian dissident Georgi Markov, whose well-publicized assassination was attributed to intramuscular injection of ricin (~500 µg), as follows: there was an immediate local pain, followed by general weakness within about 5 hours. This was followed by elevated temperature, nausea, and vomiting 15 to 24 hours later. Thirty-six hours after the incident, the patient was admitted to the hospital feeling very ill. He exhibited fever, tachycardia, normal blood pressure, swollen and sore lymph nodes in the affected groin, and and a 6-cm diameter area of induration and inflammation was observed at the injection site on his thigh. Over the next 48 hours, he became suddenly hypotensive and tachycardic; developed GI hemorrhage, hypovolemic shock, and renal failure. His white blood count was 26,300/mm^3. Early on the third day after the attack, he became anuric and began vomiting blood. An electrocardiogram demonstrated complete atrioventricular conduction block. He died shortly thereafter; at the time of death, his white blood count was 33,200/mm^3. The autopsy revealed pulmonary edema that was thought to have been secondary to Markov's cardiac failure, hemorrhagic necrosis of the small bowel, and hemorrhages in lymph nodes near the injection site, myocardium, testicles, and pancreas (Crompton and Gall, 1980).

A case of a 20-year-old male who allegedly committed suicide by injecting (s.c.) castor bean extract was reported to show severe weakness, nausea, dizziness, headache, chest, back, and abdominal pain 36 hours after the injection (Targosz et al., 2002). This patient subsequently developed a bleeding diathesis, liver failure, and renal failure. He succumbed to cardiac arrest. Postmortem examination revealed hemorrhagic foci in the brain, myocardium, and the pleura (Targosz et al., 2002).

A 36-year-old chemist who allegedly injected (i.m.) himself with an unknown amount of ricin prepared from homogenized castor seeds reportedly experienced headache and rigors 10 hours after exposure. He then developed anorexia, nausea, sinus tachycardia, lymphadenopathy at the injection sites, and erythematous areas around the puncture wounds (Fine et al., 1992).

In a clinical study involving cancer patients, intravenous administration of 40 low doses (18–20 µg/m^2 of estimated body surface area) of ricin was well tolerated (Fodstad et al., 1984). Flu-like symptoms with fatigue and muscular pain were common, and sometimes nausea and vomiting occurred. The symptoms began 4 to 6 hours after administration and lasted for 1 to 2 days. Phase I/II clinical trials of two experimental immunotoxins containing deglycosylated RTA (RFT5.dgA and Ki-4.dgA) administered i.v. to Hodgkins' lymphoma patients revealed maximum tolerated doses (MTDs) of 15 and 5 mg/m^2 of estimated body surface area for RFT5.dgA and Ki-4.dgA, respectively (Schnell et al., 2003).

4.2 Oral intoxication

Ricin is less toxic by oral ingestion than by other routes (Rauber & Heard, 1985), probably due to poor absorption of the toxin and possibly partial enzymatic degradation in the digestive tract. The effects of oral intoxication vary among individuals, are dose dependent, and have different signs and symptoms. Rauber & Heard (1985) reviewed 751 cases of castor bean ingestion and reported 14 fatalities (1.9% death rate). The number of beans ingested by patients who died greatly varied. For instance, of the two lethal cases of oral intoxication documented since 1930, one involved a 24-year-old man who ate 15 to 20 beans, and the other was a 15-year-old boy who had 10 to 12 beans. All of the described serious, or fatal cases of castor bean ingestion have the same general clinical history: rapid (less than a few hours) onset of nausea, vomiting, and abdominal pain followed by diarrhea, hemorrhage from the anus, anuria, cramps, dilation of the pupils, fever, thirst, sore throat, headache, vascular collapse, and shock. Death occurred on the third day or later. The most common autopsy findings in oral intoxication were multifocal ulcerations and hemorrhages of gastric and small-intestinal mucosa, which may be quite severe; lymphoid necrosis in the mesenteric lymph nodes, gut-associated lymphoid tissue (GALT), and spleen; Kupffer cell and liver necrosis; diffuse nephritis; and diffuse splenitis (Rauber & Heard, 1985; Bradberry et al., 2003).

4.3 Inhalation

There are no documented cases of aerosol exposure to ricin in humans. Lesions induced by oral and parenteral exposure are consistent with those from animal studies, suggesting that the same would hold true for aerosol exposures. An allergic syndrome has been reported in workers exposed to castor bean dust in or around castor oil-processing plants (Brugsch, 1960). The clinical picture is characterized by the sudden onset of congestion of the nose and throat, itchiness of the eyes, urticaria, and tightness of the chest. In more severe cases, wheezing can last for several hours, and may lead to bronchial asthma. Affected individuals respond to symptomatic therapy and removal from the exposure source.

5. Diagnosis

Ricin poisoning can be diagnosed based on clinical and epidemiological information, e.g., ingestion of castor beans, or occurrence of multiple cases during a short period, suggesting a common-source etiology (Wortmann, 2004). Ricin intoxication should be suspected if clinicians are presented with a number of patients having acute lung injury. A covert dispersion of aerosolized ricin is expected to be diagnosed, post factum, only after clinical symptoms occur (Kortepeter et al., 2001b). One common problem encountered in patients treated with ricin immunotoxins is the VLS, in which fluids leak from blood vessels leading to hypoalbumina, weight gain and pulmonary edema (Ghetie & Vitetta, 1994a). In patients who may be targets of an assassination attempt, ricin injection should be considered if there are signs of rapid onset of symptoms similar to VLS. Ricin ingestion should be suspected if patients with gastrointestinal hemorrhage and hypotension have eaten from the same food source.

Because ricin is immunogenic, acute as well as convalescent sera should be obtained from patients 2 weeks after exposure for measurement of antibody response (Franz & Jaax, 1997). Immunoassay (for blood or other body fluids) or immunohistochemistry techniques (for direct analysis of tissues) may be useful for confirming ricin intoxication (Poli et al., 2007). However, identification of the toxin in body fluids or tissues is challenging because ricin is bound very quickly, and is also metabolized before excretion (Ramsden et al., 1989).

Currently, two types of laboratory testing are available for suspected ricin exposures. For environmental cases (determined by the CDC for suspected exposures from the environment, or by the FDA for suspected exposures from food or medication), ricin can be detected qualitatively by time-resolved fluorescence immunoassay (TRFIA), and polymerase chain reaction (PCR) in specimens (e.g., filters, swabs, or wipes). For biologic samples, selected specimens can be assessed for urinary ricinine, a marker of ricin exposure, using HPLC-ESI-MS (CDC, 2006b).

The differential diagnoses of aerosol exposure to ricin include staphylococcal enterotoxin B (SEB), community-acquired pneumonia, inhalational anthrax, Q fever, tularemia, plague, and exposure to pyrolysis by-products of organofluorine polymers, or other chemical warfare agents such as phosgene (Eitzen et al., 1998). For ingested ricin, differential diagnoses include enteric pathogens, enterotoxins, and other toxins, including caustic agents, mushroom species, hydrocarbons, and pharmaceuticals such as salicylates and colchicine. Several factors discriminate ricin intoxication from other agents, such as: 1) clinical progression despite antibiotics (as opposed to infectious agents); 2) lack of mediastinitis (as seen with pulmonary anthrax); 3) progressive decline in clinical status (patients exposed to SEB tend to stabilize), and a slower progression than patients exposed to phosgene (Eitzen et al., 1998; Kortepeter et al., 2001a; 2001b).

5.1 Prognosis and cause of death

Death from ricin exposure could occur within 36 to 72 hours (CDC, 2008). If death has not occurred within 3-5 days, the patient usually survives. A mortality rate of 1.9% (14 of 751 patients) was reported after castor bean ingestion (Rauber & Heard, 1985). Even with little or no effective supportive care, the death rate in symptomatic patients has been approximately 6%. No information is available regarding human mortality rate after ricin inhalation.

The exact cause of death from ricin poisoning possibly varies with route of exposure. Ricin ingestion results in ulceration and hemorrhage of the stomach and small intestine mucosa, necrosis of the mesenteric lymphatics, liver necrosis, nephritis, and splenitis (Poli et al., 2007). Injection of the toxin may lead to severe local lymphoid necrosis, gastrointestinal hemorrhage, liver necrosis, diffuse nephritis, and diffuse splenitis. Intravenous administration of ricin in rats resulted in diffuse damage to Kupffer cells within 4 hours, followed by endothelial cell damage, formation of thrombi in the liver vasculature, and finally, hepatocellular necrosis (Bingen et al., 1987; Derenzini et al., 1976). In mice, rats, and primates, high doses by inhalation apparently produce lethal pulmonary damage, probably due to hypoxemia resulting from massive pulmonary edema and alveolar flooding (Poli et al., 2007).

6. Medical management

Currently, there is no FDA-approved therapeutic for ricin exposure. Countermeasures that have demonstrated capability to disrupt the ricin intoxication process include vaccines and antibody therapy. Both rely on the ability of antibody to prevent the binding of ricin to cell receptors. To ensure maximum protection, the vaccine must be given before exposure, and sufficient antibody must be produced. Similarly, administration of preformed antibodies affords maximum protection if antibody is present before exposure.

Treatment is largely symptomatic and basically supportive to minimize the effects of the poisoning. Because ricin acts rapidly and irreversibly (directly on lung parenchyma after inhalation or is distributed rapidly to vital organs after parenteral exposure), postexposure therapy is more challenging than with slowly processed, peripherally acting agents that can be treated with antibiotics (Franz & Jaax, 1997).

6.1 Vaccination and passive protection

Inhalational exposure is best countered with active vaccination or prophylactic administration of aerosolized specific antibody (Franz and Jaax, 1997). However, there is currently no licensed vaccine available. Development of a ricin vaccine previously focused on either a deglycosylated ricin A chain or formalin-inactivated toxoid (Hewetson et al., 1996). Both vaccines confer protection against aerosolized ricin. Nevertheless, ricin is not completely inactivated by formalin and may retain some of its enzymatic activity (albeit approximately 1,000-fold lower than native ricin). Deglycosylated ricin A chain may lead to local or systemic VLS.

Recent research has focused on developing recombinant RTA subunit vaccines devoid of cytotoxicity and other potential deleterious activities. Several ricin vaccines candidates that are based on engineered RTA molecules have shown protection with different animal models, but demonstration of their human protection proved to be more challenging (Vitetta et al., 2005). USAMRIID has engineered a recombinant ricin vaccine 1-33/44-198 (rRTA 1-33/44-198) (RV*Ec*), with increased protein stability over the parent RTA subunit and devoid of enzymatic (N-glycosidase) activity (Olson et al., 2004), lacking vascular leak activity (Porter et al., 2011) described in RTA-based immunotoxins, and fully protected vaccinated animals against supralethal aerosol challenges (McHugh et al., 2004; Carra et al., 2007). A cGLP pre-clinical toxicity study of RV*Ec* in New Zealand white rabbits demonstrated that no treatment-related or toxicologically significant effects were observed with RV*Ec* during this study (McClain et al., 2011). A phase I clinical study is ongoing at USAMRIID to evaluate the safety and immunogenicity of RV*Ec* in humans (USAMRIID, 13 April 2011; AP, 13 April 2011).

A recombinant protein RTA vaccine, RiVax, has been developed based on mutations of both the enzymatic and a reported VLS-inducing site (Smallshaw et al., 2002). RiVax elicited protective immunity in mice, and had sufficient pre-clinical safety data (Smallshaw et al., 2005). Results from the initial Phase I human trial showed that RiVax appeared to be immunological and well tolerated in humans (Vitetta et al., 2006). However, while such results were encouraging, vaccine formulation and stability remain problematic. Hence, a lyophilized formulation that retained immunogenicity when stored at 4°C was developed (Smallshaw & Vitetta, 2010; Marconescu et al., 2010).

Passive protection with aerosolized anti-ricin immunoglobulin (IgG) has also been evaluated as prophylaxis before aerosol challenge. Administration of nebulized anti-ricin IgG effectively protected against lung lesions and lethality in mice when challenged with an aerosol exposure to ricin (Poli et al., 1996). Extrapolation of these data to clearance rates of IgG from the airways of rabbits suggests that anti-ricin–specific antibodies may provide protection for up to 2 to 3 days or longer. These findings imply that inhaling protective antibody from a portable nebulizer just before an attack might provide some protection in nonimmune individuals (Poli et al., 1996). However, the window of opportunity for treatment by intravenous administration or inhalation of specific antibody after exposure is probably minimal at best.

Recent pre-clinical studies have shown the powerful protection afforded by neutralizing monoclonal antibodies (administered singly or in combination) against a lethal dose challenge of ricin, demonstrating proof of concept for passive immunotherapy for the treatment of ricin poisoning or for preexposure prophylaxis (Neal, 2010; 2011; Prigent, 2011).

6.2 Supportive and specific therapy

Supportive medical care depends on the route of exposure and clinical manifestations. For oral intoxication, supportive therapy includes intravenous fluid, electrolyte replacement, monitoring of liver and renal functions, gastric emptying/lavage, syrup of ipecac, cathartics, and, activated charcoal (Ellenhorn, 1997; Franz & Jaax, 1997). Patients who have ingested beans and presented asymptomatic should remain under observation for 4-6 hours after ingestion. For inhalational intoxication, respiratory support is given as needed. Aerosol-exposed patient may require the use of positive-pressure ventilator therapy, fluid and electrolyte replacement, antiinflammatory agents, and analgesics (Kortepeter et al., 2001b). Dermal exposures require supportive treatment. Percutaneous exposures would necessitate judicious use of intravenous fluids and monitoring for symptoms associated with VLS, including hypotension, edema, and pulmonary edema (Poli et al., 2007). Supportive care includes correction of coagulopathies, respiratory support, and monitoring for liver and renal failure .

Several research groups have engaged in the development of RTA active site inhibitors or RTB receptor antagonists as clinical antidotes against ricin poisoning, or as therapeutic adjuncts to vaccination. Small molecules that exhibited modest IC_{50} values (Bai et al., 2010; Wahome et al., 2010; Pang et al., 2011), including a compound that showed *in vivo* efficacy (Stechmann et al., 2010) have been described. An effective and essentially irreversible RTA inhibitor is thought to be practically useful as a pretreatment for military forces or civilian first-responders (Millard & LeClaire, 2007).

7. Medical therapy of ricin

In addition to studies pertaining to the natural toxicity of the protein, ricin has also been used extensively in the design of therapeutic immunotoxins. In such, ricin, RTA, or a related toxin is chemically or genetically linked to a binding ligand such as an antibody or growth factor that recognizes cancer cells, then it may be taken up by the cancer cells and ultimately kill them (Frankel, 1988). Immunotoxins using RTA or blocked ricin, have been evaluated in phase I clinical trials for control of several cancers (Ghetie & Vitetta, 1994b; Lynch et al., 1997; Schnell et al., 2003; Vitetta, 2006).

8. Summary

Ricin is a potent toxin derived from the seeds of the castor plant, *R. communis*. Because of its potency, stability, worldwide availability, and relative ease of production, ricin is considered a significant biological warfare or terrorism threat. Ricin was developed as an aerosol biological weapon by the U.S. and its allies during WWII, although it was never used in battle. As a biological or chemical weapon, ricin has not been considered as very powerful in comparison with other agents such as botulinum neurotoxin or anthrax. However, its effectiveness as a discrete weapon of terror-targeted assassinations, biocrimes, or small-scale operations does raise potential concern. Ricin's popularity as well as its track record in actually being exploited by extremists groups and individuals highlight the need to be vigilant of its latent misuse. Clinical manifestations of ricin poisoning vary depending on the routes of exposure. Diagnosis is based upon both epidemiological and clinical parameters. Laboratory confirmation of clinical samples is possible by immunoassay but complicated by pharmacokinetic factors. Currently, there is no U.S. FDA-approved drug or vaccine against ricin poisoning. Treatment is purely supportive. Prophylaxis will be best accomplished by vaccination. Ricin vaccine candidates are currently in advanced development in laboratory and clinical trials.

9. Acknowledgment and disclaimer

This work was supported by Defense Threat Reduction Agency, JSTO-CBD Project Numbers CBM.VAXBT.03.10.RD.P.011 and CBCALL12-VAXBT4-1-0385. We are grateful to Dr. Mark A. Olson for providing the three-dimensional images of ricin, and Lorraine Farinick for assistance with graphics.

The opinions or assertions contained herein are the private views of the authors and are not necessarily the official views of the U.S. Army or the Department of Defense.

10. References

Amlot, P.L., Stone, M.J., Cunningham D, et al. (1993). A Phase I Study of an Anti-CD22-deglycosylated Ricin A Chain Immunotoxin in the Treatment of B-cell Lymphomas Resistant to Conventional Therapy. *Blood*, Vol. 82, pp. 2624-2633, ISSN 0006-497

AP. (13 April 2011). Army Starts Clinical Trials on Ricin Vaccine, In: Army Times, 20072011. Available from http://www.armytimes.com/news/2011/04/ap-army-medical-research-ricin-041311/

AP. (22 June 2011). Former Agawam Man Sentenced for Ricin, Prosecutor Threat, In: *Gazettenet.com*, 04.08.2011. Available from http://www.gazettenet.com/2011/06/22/former-agawam-man-sentenced-for-ricin-prosecutor-threat

Atsmon, D. 1985. Castor. In: *Oil Crops of the World*, G. Robbelen, R.K. Downey & A. Ashri (Eds), pp. 438-447, McGraw Hill Pub. Co., ISBN 0070530815, New York

Audi J, Belson M, Patel M, Schier, J. Osterloh, J. (2005). Ricin Poisoning: A Comprehensive Review. *JAMA*, Vol. 294, pp. 2342-2351, ISSN 0098-7484

Auld, D.L., Pinkerton, S.D., Boroda, E., et al. (2003). Registration of TTU-LRC Castor Germplasm with Reduced Levels of Ricin and RCA_{120}. *Crop Science*, Vol. 43, p.746-747, Online ISSN 1435-0653; Print ISSN 0011-183X

Bai, Y., Watt, B., Wahome, P.G., et al. (2010). Identification of New Classes of Ricin Toxin Inhibitors by Virtual Screening. *Toxicon*, Vol. 56, pp. 526-534, ISSN 0041-0101

Baldoni, A.B., De Carvalho, M.H., Sousa, N.L., et al. (2011).Variability of ricin content in mature seeds of castor bean. *Pesq Agropec Bras*, Vol. 46 (7), Available from http://www.scielo.br/scielo.php?pid=S0100-04X2011000700015&script=sci_arttext

Balint, G.A. (1974). Ricin: the Toxic Protein of Castor Oil Seeds. *Toxicology*, Vol. 2, pp. 77-102, ISSN 0300-483X

Barceloux, D. (2008). Castor Bean and Ricin, In: *Medical Toxicology of Natural Substances: Foods, Fungi, Medicinal Herbs, Plants, and Venomous Animals, pp.* 718-726. John Wiley and Sons, ISBN 047172761X, 9780471727613, Hoboken, New Jersey

Bingen, A., Creppy, E.E., Gut, J.P., et al. (1987). The Kupffer Cell is the First Target in Ricin-induced Hepatitis. *J Submicrosc Cytol*, Vol.19, pp. 247–256

BBC News (20 August 2002). U.S. Knew of bioterror Tests in Iraq, In: *BBC News*, 07.08.2011. Available from http://news.bbc.co.uk/2/hi/americas/2204321.stm

BBC News (06 June 2009). Pair Questioned over Ricin Find, In: *BBC News*, 07.08.2011. Available from http://news.bbc.co.uk/1/hi/8086701.stm

Bradberry, S.M., Dickens, K.J., Rice, P., et al. (2003). Ricin Poisoning. *Toxicol Rev*, Vol. 22, pp. 65-70, ISSN 1176-2551

Brugsch, H.G. (1960). Toxic Hazards: the Castor Bean. *N Engl J Med*, Vol. 62, pp. 1039-1040, ISSN 0028-4793

Carus, W.S. (2002). Bioterrorism and Biocrimes: The Illicit Use of Biological Agents since the 1900, Center for Counterproliferation Research, National Defense University, ISBN 9781410100238, Available from http://books.google.com/books?id=1jEP8Ve4zwgC

Carra, J.H., Wannemacher, R.W., Tammariello, R.F., et al. (2007). Improved Formulation of a Recombinant Ricin A-chain Vaccine Increases Its Stability and Effective Antigenicity. *Vaccine*, Vol. 25, pp. 4149–4158, ISSN 0264-410X

Caupin, H.J. (1997). Products from Castor Oil: Past, Present, and Future, In: *Lipid Technologies and Applications*, F.D. Gunstone and F.B. Padley (Eds.), pp. 787-795, Marcel Dekker, Inc., ISBN 0-8247-9838-4, New York

Cawley, D.B. & Houston, L.L. (1979). Effect of Sulfhydryl Reagents and Protease Inhibitors on Sodium Dodecyl Sulfate-heat Induced Dissociation of *Ricinus communis* Agglutinin. *Biochem Biophys Acta, Vol.* 81, pp. 51-62, ISSN 0006-3002

CDC. (2003a). Recognition, Management and Surveillance of Ricin-Associated Illness [Web cast script], December 30, 2003, 07082011. Available from http://www2.cdc.gov/phtn/webcast/ricin/RicinScript.rev.07-14-04.htm

CDC. (2003b). Investigation of a Ricin-containing Envelope at a Postal Facility: South Carolina. *MMWR*, Vol. 52(46), pp. 1129-1131 ISSN 01492195, 1545861X

CDC. (2006a). Ricin: Epidemiological Overview for Clinicians. 22.06.2011. Available from http://www.bt.cdc.gov/agent/ricin/clinicians/epidemiology.asp

CDC. (2006b). Laboratory Testing for Ricin. 19.09.2011. Available from http://www.bt.cdc.gov/agent/ricin/labtesting.asp

CDC. (2008). Facts about Ricin (Updated March 5, 2008). Available from http://www.bt.cdc.gov/agent/ricin/facts.asp

Chaudhry, B., Mu¨ller-Uri, F., Cameron-Mills, V., et al. (1994). The Barley 60 kDa Jasmonate-induced Protein (JIP60) is a Novel Ribosome-inactivating protein. *The Plant Journal*, Vol. 6, pp. 815–24, ISSN (electronic) 1365-313X

Challoner, K.R. & McCarron, M.M. (1990). Castor Bean Intoxication: Review of Reported Cases. *Ann Emerg Med*, Vol.19, pp. 1177-1183, ISSN 0196-0644

CNN.com (04 February 2004). Frist: Ricin Confirmed, But No Illness Reported, In: *Cable News Network (CNN.com)*. 04.08.2011. Available from http://articles.cnn.com/2004-02-03/us/senate.hazardous_1_deadly-toxin-ricin-deadly-poison-mailroom?_s=PM: US

CNN.com. (14 January 2005). Florida Man Faces Bioweapon Charge, In: *CNN.com*. 5.08.2011. Available from http://articles.cnn.com/2005-01-13/us/ricin.arrest_1_ricin-steven-michael-ekberg-castor-beans?_s=PM:US

CNS. (2004). Combating the Spread of Weapons of Mass Destruction, In: *James Martin Center for Nonproliferation Studies*, 07.08.2011, Available from http://cns.miis.edu/ stories/pdfs/080229_ricin.pdf

Cordesman, A.H. (2002). *Terrorism, Asymmetric Warfare and Weapons of Mass Destruction: Defending the U.S. Homeland*, p. 28, Greenwood Publishing Group, ISBN 0275974278, Washington, DC

Croddy, E. & Wirtz, J.J. (2005). *Weapons of Mass Destruction: An Encyclopedia of Worldwide Policy, Technology, and History*, Vol. 2, p. 241, ABC-CLIO, ISBN 1851094903 (hardback); ISBN 1-85109-495-4 (e-book), Santa Barbara, California

Crompton, R. & Gall, D. (1980). Georgi Markov: Death in a Pellet. *Med Leg J*. Vol. 48, pp. 51–62

Derenzini, M., Bonetti, E., Marionozzi, V., et al. (1976). Toxic Effects of Ricin: Studies on the Pathogenesis of Liver Lesions. *Virchows Arch B Cell Pathol*, Vol. 20, pp. 15–28, ISSN 0340-6075

Easton's Bible Dictionary. (n.d.). 22.06.2011. Available from http://www.sacred-texts.com/bib/ebd/ebd153.htm#005

Eitzen, E., Pavlin, J., Cieslak, T, et al. (1998). Medical Management of Biological Casualties Handbook, 3rd ed, 101-106. USAMRIID, Fort Detrick, MD

Ellenhorn, M.J. (1997). *Ellenhorn's Medical Toxicology: Diagnosis and Treatment of Human Poisoning*, 2nd ed, pp. 1847–1849, Williams & Wilkins, ISBN-13: 9780683303872 ISBN-10: 0683303872, Baltimore, Maryland

Endo, Y. & Tsurugi, K. (1987). RNA N-glycosidase Activity of Ricin A-chain. Mechanism of Action of the Toxic Lectin Ricin on Eukaryotic Ribosomes. *J Biol Chem*, 262, pp. 8128–8130, ISSN 0021-9258

Endo Y, Mitsui K, Motizuki M, Tsurugi K. (1987). The Mechanism of Action of Ricin and Related Toxic Lectins on Eukaryotic Ribosomes. The Site and the Characteristics of the Modification in 28 S Ribosomal RNA Caused by the Toxins. *J Biol Chem* Vol. 262, pp. 5908–5912, ISSN 0021-9258

Endo, Y., Tsurugi, K. Yutsuodo, T., et al. (1988). Site of Action of a Vero Toxin (VT2) from *Escherichia coli* O157:H7 and of Shiga Toxin on Eukaryotic Rbosomes. RNA N-glycosidase Activity of the toxins. *Eur J Biochem, Vol.* 171, pp. 45-50, ISSN 0014-2956

Engert, A., Diehl, V., Schnell, R., et al. (1997). A Phase I Study of an Anti-CD25 Ricin- A chain Immunotoxins (RFT5-SMPT-dgA) in Patients with Refractory Hodgkin's Lymphoma. *Blood* Vol. 89, pp. 403-410, ISSN 0006-497

FAOSTAT (2011). 24.07.2011. Available from http://faostat.fao.org/site/339/default.aspx

Fine, D.R., Shepherd, H.A., Griffiths, G.D. & Green, M. (1992) Sub-lethal Poisoning bySelf-injection with Ricin. *Med Sci Law*, Vol. 32, pp. 70–72

Fodstad, O., Kvalheim, G., Godal, A., et al. (1984). Phase I Study of the Plant Protein Ricin. *Cancer Res*, Vol. 44, pp. 862–865

Frankel, A. (1988). Immunotoxins, *Volume 37 of Cancer Treatment and Research*, 565 p. Kluwer Academic Publisher, ISBN 0898389844, 9780898389845, Norwell, Massachusetts

FBI (n.d.). Terrorism 2002-2005, In: *U.S. Dept. of Justice, Federal Bureau of Investigation, Reports and Publications*, 22.07.2011. Available from http://www.fbi.gov/stats-services/publications/terrorism-2002-2005

Franz, D.R. & Jaax, N.K. (1997). Ricin Toxin, In: *Medical Aspects of Chemical and Biological Warfare*, Sidell F.R., Takafuji, E.T. & Franz, D.R. (Eds), 631-642, Walter Reed Army Medical Center, Borden Institute, ISBN-10 9997320913, Washington, DC

Gad, S.C. (2007). *Handbook of Pharmaceutical Biotechnology, Vol. 2. Of Pharmaceutical Development Series*, p. 1598, John Wiley and Sons, Inc., ISBN 0471213861, 9780471213864, Hoboken, NJ

Ghetie, M.A. & Vitetta, E. (1994a). Recent Developments in Immunotoxin Therapy. *Current Opinion in Immunology*, Vol. 6, pp. 707-714, ISSN 0952-7915

Ghetie, V. & Vitetta, E. (1994b). Immunotoxins in the Therapy of Cancer: From Bench to Clinic. *Pharmacol Ther* Vol. 63, pp. 209-231, ISSN 0163-7258

GSN. (17 June 2011). U.K. Man Charged with Possessing Ricin Recipe, In: *Global Security Newswire*, 07.08.2011. Available from http://gsn.nti.org/gsn/ nw_20110617 _5703.php

GlobalSecurity.org. (n.d.). Weapons of Mass Destruction (WMD): Ricin, In: *GlobalSecurity.org*, 02.08.2011. Available from http://www.globalsecurity.org/wmd/intro/ bio_ricin.htm

Hegde, R., Podder, S.K. (1992). Studies on the Variants of the Protein Toxins Ricin and Abrin. *Eur Jour Biochem*, Vol. 204, No. 1, pp. 155-164, ISSN 0014-2956

Hewetson J., Rivera V., Lemley P., et al. (1996). A Formalinized Toxoid for Protection of Mice from Inhaled Ricin. *Vacc Res*, Vol. 4, pp. 179–187

Hopkins, N. & Branigan, T. (08 January 2003). Poison Find Sparks Terror Alert, In: *The Guardian*, 07.08.2011. Available from http://www.guardian.co.uk/uk/2003/ jan/08/terrorism.alqaida

Hudson T. & Neville, D.M., Jr. (1987). Temporal Separation of Protein Toxin Translocation from Processing Events. *J Biol Chem*, Vol. 262, pp. 16484–16494, ISSN 0021-9258

ICOA. (1992). The Chemistry of Castor Oil and Its Derivatives and Their Applications. Westfield, New Jersey

Kifner, J. (2005). Man Arrested In Poison Case Kills Himself In Jail Cell, In: *The New York Times*, 01.08.2011. Available from http://www.nytimes.com/1995/12/24/us/man-arrested-in-poison-case-kills-himself-in-jail-cell.html?pagewanted=2&src=pm.

Kole, C. (2011). Wild Crop Relatives - Genomic and Breeding Resources: Oilseeds, C. Kole, (Ed.), p. 295, Springer, ISBN 9783642148705, Available from http://books.google.com/books?id=zWp--NMP3hAC

Kortepeter, M.G., Christopher, G., Cieslak, T., et al. (2001a). *USAMRIID's Medical Management of Biological Casualties Handbook*, 4th ed. USAMRIID, Fort Detrick, MD, pp. 130–137

Kortepeter, M.G., Cieslak, T.J., & Eitzen, E.M. (2001b). Bioterrorism. *J Environ Health*, Vol. 63(6), pp. 21-24, ISSN 0022-0892

Kortepeter, M.G. & Parker G.W. (1999). Potential biological weapons threats. *Emerg Infect Dis*, Vol. 5, pp. 523–527, ISSN 1080-6059

Kreitman, R.J., Squires, D.R., Stetler-Stevenson, et al. (2005). Phase I trial recombinant immunotoxin RFB4(dsFv)-PE38 (BL22) in patients with B-cell malignancies. *J Clin Onco*, Vol. 23, pp. 6719-6729, ISSN 0277-5379

Lally, C. (2007). Prison alert over ricin traces find, In: *The Irish Times*, 06.08.2011. Available from http://www.highbeam.com/doc/1P2-24880932.html

Lamb, F.I., Roberts, L.M., Lord, J.M. (1985). Nucleotide sequence of cloned cDNA coding for preproricin. *European Journal of Biochemistry*, Vol. 148, pp. 265–70.

Lee, M.D. & Wang, R.Y. (2005). Toxalbumins, In: *Critical Care Toxicology*, J. Brent, K.L. Wallace, K.H. Burkhart, S.D. Phillips, J.W. Donovan (Eds.), 1345-1349, Elsevier Mosby, ISBN 0815143877, Philadelphia

Li, Z., Yu, T., Zhao, P. & Ma, J. (2005). Immunotoxins and Cancer Therapy. *Cell Mol Immunol*, Vol. 2, pp. 106-112

Lord, J.M., Roberts, L.M. & Robertus, J.D. (1994). Ricin: structure, mode of action, and some current applications. *FASEB J*, Vol. 8, pp. 201-208, ISSN 0892-6638

Lord, M.J., Jolliffe, N.A., Marsden, C.J., et al. (2003). Ricin: Mechanisms of Cytotoxicity. *Toxicol Rev*, Vol. 22, pp. 53–64, ISSN 1176-2551

Lynch, T. J. Jr., Lampert, J.M., Coral, F., et al. (1997). Immunotoxin Therapy of Small-cell lung cancer: A Phase I Study of N901-Blocked Ricin. *J Clin Oncol*, Vol. 15, pp. 723-734, ISSN 0277-5379

MacDonald, H. (1999). *Mussolini and Italian Fascism*, pp. 15-17, Nelson Thornes, ISBN 9780748733866, Retrieved from http://books.google.com/books?id=221 W9vKkWrcC

Maman, M., & Yehezkelli, Y. (2005). Ricin: a Possible, Non-infectious Biological Weapon, In: *Bioterrorism and Infectious Agents*, S. Fong and K. Alibek, (Eds.), 205-216, Springer Science and Business Media, ISBN-10 0-387-28294-7, New York, NY

Marconescu, P.S., Smallshaw, J.E., Pop, L.M., et al. (2010). Intradermal administration of RiVax protects mice from mucosal and systemic ricin intoxication. *Vaccine*, Vol. 28, pp. 5315-5322, ISSN: 0264-410X

Martens, B. (2006). Owner of Northwoods Cabin Sentenced for Attempted Production of Ricin. WSAW.com, Oct 3, 2006. Available from http://www.wsaw.com/home/headlines/4294797.html

McHugh, C.A., Tammariello, R.F., Millard, C.B., Carra, J.H. (2004). Improved stability of a protein vaccine through elimination of a partially unfolded state. *Protein Sci* 13, pp. 2736–2743 ISSN 0961-8368

McKeon, T.A., Lin, J.T. and Stafford, A.E. (1999). Biosynthesis of ricinoleate in castor oil. *Adv Exp Med Biol*, Vol. 464, pp. 37–47, ISSN 0065-2598

McKeon, T.A., Chen, G.Q. & Lin, J.T. (2000). Biochemical aspects of castor oil biosynthesis. *Biochem Soc Trans.* 28, pp. 972–974, ISSN 0300-5127

McLain, D.E., Horn, T.L., Detrisac, C.J., et al. (2011). Progress in biological threat agent vaccine development: a repeat-dose toxicity study of a recombinant ricin toxin A-chain (rRTA) 1-33/44-198 vaccine (RVEc) in male and female New Zealand white rabbits. *Int J Toxicol*, Vol. 30, pp. 143-152 ISSN 1091-5818

Mendenhall, P. (2003). Positive test for terror toxins in Iraq. Evidence of ricin, botulinum at Islamic militants' camp. MSNBC.com, April 4, 2003. 07.08.2011. Available from http://www.msnbc.msn.com/id/3070394/ns/world_news/t/positive-test-terror-toxins-iraq/

Millard, C.B. & LeClaire, R.D. (2007). Ricin and Related Toxins: Review and Perspective. In: *Chemical Warfare Agents: Chemistry, Pharmacology, Toxicology, and Therapeutics, 2nd ed.* J.A. Romano Jr. & B.J. Lukey, (Eds.), 423-467. CRC Press, Taylor & Francis Group, ISBN 978-1-4200-4661-8, Boca Raton, FL.

Mirarchi, F.L. (2010). CBRNE - Ricin, In: *Medscape Reference*, 10082011. Available from http://emedicine.medscape.com/article/830795-overview#showall

Montfort, W., Villafranca, J.E., Monzingo, A.F., et al. (1987). The three-dimensional structure of ricin at 2.8 Å proteins are targeted by different mechanisms. *J Biol Chem*, Vol. 262, pp. 5398–403, ISSN 0021-9258

Muldoon, D.F. & Stohs, S.J (1994). Modulation of ricin toxicity in mice by biologically active substances. *J Appl Toxicol*, Vol. 14, pp.81-86, ISSN 0260-437X

Musick, J. (25 May 2000). Debora Green Back in Court. In: *Pitch News*, 19.08.2011. Available from http://www.pitch.com/kansascity/debora-green-back-in-court/Content?oid=2160233

Musshoff, F. & Madea, B. (2009). Ricin Poisoning and Forensic Toxicolog. *Drug Test Anal*, Vol. *1*, pp. 184–191, ISSN (printed) 1942-7603; ISSN (electronic) 1942-7611

Neal, L.M., O'Hara,J., Brey, R.N. 3rd, et al. (2010). A monoclonal immunoglobulin G antibody directed against an immunodominant linear epitope on the ricin A chain confers systemic and mucosal immunity to ricin. *Infect Immun*, Vol. 78, pp. 552-61, ISSN 0019-9567

Neal, L.M., McCarthy, E.A., Morris, C.R., et al. (2011). Vaccine-induced intestinal immunity to ricin toxin in the absence of secretory IgA. *Vaccine*, Vol. 29(4), pp. 681-689, ISSN 0264-410X

New World Encyclopedia (n.d.). 22.06.2011. Available from http://www.newworldencyclopedia.org/entry/Castor_oil_plant

Nielsen, K. and Boston, R.S. (2001) Ribosome-inactivating proteins: a plant perspective. *Annu Rev Plant Physiol Plant Mol Biol*, Vol. 52, pp. 785–816

Olsnes, S. (2004). The history of ricin, abrin and related toxins. *Toxicon,* Vol. 44, pp. 361-370. ISSN 0041-0101

Olsnes, S. & Pihl, A. (1972). Ricin - a potent inhibitor of protein synthesis. *FEBS Lett,* Vol. 20, pp. 327-329, ISSN 0014-5793

Olsnes, S., Saltvedt, E. & Pihl, A. (1974). Isolation and comparison of galactose-binding lectins from *Abrus precatorius* and *Ricinus communis. J Biol Chem,* Vol. 249, pp. 803-810, ISSN 0021-9258; Online ISSN 1083-351X.

Olsnes, S., Refsnes, K., Christensen, T.B. & Pihl, A. (1975). Studies on the structure and properties of the lectins from *Abrus precatorius* and *Ricinus communis. Biochim Biophys Acta,* Vol. 405, pp. 1-10, ISSN 0006-3002

Olsnes, S. & Pihl, A. (1982). Toxic lectins and related proteins. In. *Molecular Actions of Toxins and Viruses.* P. Cohen & S. van Heyningen, (Eds.), Elsevier Press, ISBN-10 0444804005, New York, NY.

Olsnes, S. & Kozlov, J.V. (2001). Ricin. *Toxicon* Vol. 39, pp. 1723-1728 ISSN 0041-0101

Olsnes, S. (2004). The history of ricin, abrin and related toxins. *Toxicon,* Vol. 44, pp. 361-370, ISSN 0041-0101

Olson, M.A., Carra, J.H., Roxas-Duncan, V., et al. (2004). Finding a new vaccine in the ricin protein fold. *Protein Eng Des Sel,* Vol. 17, pp. 391-397, ISSN 1741 -0126

Pang, Y.P, Park, J.G, Wang, S., et al. (2011). Small-Molecule Inhibitor Leads of Ribosome-Inactivating Proteins Developed Using the Doorstop Approach. *PLoS ONE* 6(3): e17883. doi:10.1371/journal.pone.0017883.

Passeron, T., Mantoux, F., Lacour, J.P, et al. (2004). Infectious and toxic cellulitis due to suicide attempt by subcutaneous injection of ricin. *Brit J Dermatol,* pp. 150-154, ISSN 0007-0963

Pearce, J. (2011). *Solzhenitsyn: A Soul in Exile,* Ignatius Press, ISBN 9781586174965, Available from http://books.google.com/books?id=lgPwzq0M9lkC

Poli, M.A., Rivera, V.R., Pitt, M.L., et. al. (1996). Aerosolized specific antibody protects mice from lung injury associated with aerosolized ricin exposure. *Toxicon,* Vol. 34:1037-1044, ISSN 0041-0101

Poli, M.A., Roy, C., Huebner, K.D., et al. (2007). Ricin. In. *Medical Aspects of Biological Warfare, rev ed.,* Z.F. Dembek (Ed.), pp. 323-335, Borden Institute, Walter Reed Medical Center, ISBN 978-0160797316, Washington, DC

Porter, A., Phillips, G., Smith, L., et al. (2011). Evaluation of a ricin vaccine candidate (RVEC) for human toxicity using an in vitro vascular leak assay. *Toxicon,* Vol. 58(1), pp. 68-75 ISSN 0041-0101

Powers, A. (18 November 2008). Man with ricin is sentenced, In: *Los Angeles Times.* 07.08.2011. Available from http://articles.latimes.com/2008/nov/18/nation/na-ricin18

Phillips, R. & Rix, M. (1999). *Annuals and Biennials,* Macmillan, ISBN 0333748891. London.

Pinkerton, S.D, Rolfe, R., Auld, D.L., et al. (1999). Selection of Castor for Divergent Concentrations of Ricin and *Ricinus communis* agglutinin. *Crop Science,* Vol. 39, pp. 353-357, Online ISSN 1435-0653; Print ISSN 0011-183X

Prigent, J., Panigai, L., Lamourette, P., et al. (2011). Neutralising Antibodies against Ricin Toxin. *PLoS ONE* 6(5): e20166. doi:10.1371/journal.pone.0020166, ISSN 1932-6203

Ramsden, C.S, Drayson, M.T., Bell, E.B. (1989). The toxicity, distribution, and excretion of ricin holotoxin in rats. *Toxicology*, Vol. 55, pp. 161–171, ISSN 0300-483X

Rauber, A. & Heard, J. (1985). Castor bean toxicity re-examined: a new perspective. *Vet Hum Toxicol* 27: 490-502, ISSN 0145-6296

Remnick, D. (21 April 1992). KGB plot to assassinate Solzhenitzen reported; Russian Tabloid Says 1971 Attempt Left Dissident Burned, In: *The Washington Post, p. D2*, 22072011, Available from http://www.highbeam.com/doc/1P2-1001929.html

Research International, Inc. (RII). (2011). A Ricin Primer. 07.08.2011. Available from http://www.resrchintl.com/Ricin_Primer.html

Roberts, L.M., Lamb, F.I., Pappin, D., et al. (1985). The primary sequence of *Ricinus communis* agglutinin. *J Biol Chem*, Vol. 260, pp. 15682-15686, ISSN 0021-9258; Online ISSN 1083-351X

Robertus J. (1988). Toxin Structure, In: *Immunotoxins*, A. Frankel (Ed.), 11–24, Kluwer Academic Publishers, ISBN 0-89838-984-4, Boston, Massachusetts

Robertus, J.D. (1991). The structure and action of ricin, a cytotoxic N-glycosidase. *Semin Cell Biol*, Vol. 2, pp. 23-30, ISSN 1043-4682

Rotz, L.D., Khan, A.S., Scott, R. *et al.* (2002). Public Health Assessment of Potential Biological Terrorism Agents. *Emerging Infectious Disease*, Vol. 8, pp. 225-230.

Sausville, E.A., Headlee, D., Stetler- Stevenson, M., et al. (1995). Continuous infusion of the anti-CD22 immunotoxin IgG-RFB4-SMPT-dgA in patients with B-cell lymphoma: A phase I study. *Blood*, Vol. 85, pp. 3457-3465, ISSN 0006-497

Scarpa, A. & Guerci, A. (1982). Various Uses of the Castor Oil Plant (*Ricinus communis*): A review. *J. Ethnopharm*, Vol.5, pp. 117-137, ISSN 0378-8741

Schep, L.J., Temple, W.A., Butt, G.A., Beasley, M.D. (2009). Ricin as a Weapon of Mass Terror - Separating Fact from Fiction. *Environ Int, Vol.* 35 (8), pp. 1267–1271. doi:10.1016/j.envint.2009.08.004. PMID 19767104

Schnell, R., Borchmann, P., Staak, J.O.et al., (2003). Clinical Evaluation of Ricin A-chain Immunotoxins in Patients with Hodgkin's Lymphoma. *Ann Oncol, Vol.* 14, pp. 729-736, ISSN Online1569-8041; ISSN Print 0923-7534

Sharma, P. (29 January 2011). Man Arrested after Ricin Found in House, In: *TOPNEWS*, 07.08.2011. Available from http://topnews.us/content/233593-man-arrested-after-ricin-found-house.

Sims, J., and R.J. Frey. (2005). Castor Oil, In: *The Gale Encyclopedia of Alternative Medicine, J.* Longe (Ed.), Thomson/Gale, ISBN 0787693960, Farmington Hills, Michigan

Smallshaw, J.E., Firan, A., Fulmer, J.R., Ruback, S.L., Ghetie, V., Vitetta, E.S. (2002). A Novel Recombinant Vaccine Which Protects Mice against Ricin Intoxication. *Vaccine*, Vol. 20, pp. 3422–3427, ISSN 0264-410X

Smallshaw, J.E., Richardson, J.A., Pincus, S., et al. (2005). Preclinical Toxicity and Efficacy Testing of RiVax, a Recombinant Protein Vaccine against Ricin. *Vaccine*, Vol. 23, pp. 4775-4784

Smart, J.K. (1997). History of Chemical and Biological Warfare: an American Perspective. In: *Medical Aspects of Chemical and Biological Warfare, Part I: Warfare, Weaponry, and the Casualty*, R. Zajtchuk (Ed), pp. 9–86, Borden Institute, Washington, DC, Department of the Army, Office of the Surgeon General

Stechmann B, Bai SK, Gobbo E, Lopez R, Merer M, et al. (2010). Inhibition of Retrograde Transport Protects Mice from Lethal Ricin Challenge. *Cell*, Vol. 141, pp. 231-242, ISSN: 0092-8674

Stirpe,F. & Batelli, M.G. (2006). Ribosome-inactivating Proteins: Progress and Problems. *Cell Mol Life Sci*, Vol. 63(16), pp. 1850-1866

Targosz, D., Winnik, L., Szkolnicka, B. (2002). Suicidal Poisoning with Castor Bean (*Ricinus communis*) Extract Injected Subcutaneously – Case Report. *J Toxicol Clin Toxicol*, Vol. 40, p. 398, ISSN 0731-3810

The New York Times. (08 November 1999). National News Briefs; Material for Poison Gas Found in Suspect's Home. 22072011. Available at http://www.nytimes.com/1999/11/08/us/national-news-briefs-material-for-poison-gas-found-in-suspect-s-home.html

TIME Magazine. (16 August 1982). Law: Poison Plot, 07.08.2011. Available from http://www.time.com/time/magazine/article/0,9171,950736-1,00.html

Tizon, T.A. (2004). Post-9/11 Hysteria Blamed in Poison Case. Man Accused of Plotting against Wife Convicted under Anti-terrorist Law, In: *The Baltimore Sun*, April 20, 2004. 07.08.2011. Available from http://articles.baltimoresun.com/2004-04-20/news/0404200117_1_olsen-possession-hysteria

Thompson, W. L., Scovill, J. P. & Pace, J. G. (1995). Drugs that Show Protective Effects from Ricin Toxicity in *In Vitro* Protein Synthesis Assays. *Natural Toxins*, 3: 369–377. doi: 10.1002/nt.2620030508

USAMRIID. (13 April 2011). USAMRIID Begins Clinical Trial of New Vaccine to Protect Against Ricin Toxin. 07072011. Available from http://www.usamriid.army.mil/press%20releases/Ricin%20News%20Release%2013%20Apr%202011.pdf

Vitetta, E.S., Stone, M., Amlot, P., et al. (1991). Phase I Immunotoxin Trial in Patients with B-cell lymphoma. *Cancer Res*, Vol. 51, pp. 4052-4058, ISSN Online 1538-7445; ISSN Print 0008-5472

Vitetta, E.S., Smallshaw, J.E., Coleman, E., et al. (2005). A Pilot Clinical Trial of a Recombinant Ricin Vaccine in Normal Humans. *PNAS*, Vol. 103, pp. 2268-2273, ISSN (printed): 0027-8424. ISSN (electronic)

Vitetta, E. (2006). Biomedical and Biodefense Uses for Ricin. *An ActionBioscience.org original interview*. 08.08.2011. Available from http://www.actionbioscience. org/newfrontiers/vitetta.html#primer

Wahome, P., Bai, Y., Neal, L., et al. (2010). Identification of Small-molecule Inhibitors of Ricin and Shiga Toxin using a Cell-based High Throughput Screen. *Toxicon, Vol.* 56, pp. 313-323, ISSN 0041-0101

Wainwright, M. (2010). Neo-Nazi Ian Davison Jailed for 10 years for Making Chemical Weapon. *The Guardian*, 14 May 2010, amended 17 May 2010. 07.08.2011. Available from http://www.guardian.co.uk/uk/2010/may/14/neo-nazi-ian-davison-jailed-chemical-weapon.

Wannemacher, R. & Anderson, J. (2005). Inhalation Ricin: Aerosol Procedures, Animal Toxicology, and Therapy, In: *Inhalation Toxicology*, 2nd ed., H. Salem (Ed.), CRC Press, 973–979, ISBN 0849340497, Boca Raton, Florida

Watson, W.A., Litovitz, T.L., Rodgers, G.C., et al. (2003). 2002 Annual Report of the American Association of Poison Control Centers Toxic Exposure Surveillance System. *Am J Emerg Med*, Vol. 21, pp. 353–421.

Wortmann, G. (2004). Ricin Toxin, In: *Physician's Guide to Terrorist Attack*, M.J. Roy (Ed.), 175-179, Human Press Inc., ISBN 1592596630, Totowa, New Jersey

Youn Y.S., Na, D.H., Yoo, S.D., et al. (2005). Carbohydrate-specifically Polyethylene Glycol-modified Ricin A-chain with Improved Therapeutic Potential. *Int J Biochem Cell Biol*, Vol. 37, pp. 1525-1533, ISSN: 1357-2725

Zilinskas, RA 1997. Iraq's Biological Weapons: The Past or Future. *JAMA,* Vol. 278, pp. 418-424, ISSN 0098-7484

8

Spatio-Temporal Disease Surveillance

Ross Sparks, Sarah Bolt and Chris Okugami
CSIRO Mathematics, Informatics and Statistics, Sydney, Australia

1. Introduction

Concern over bio-terrorism has led to a demand for automated methods for the surveillance of disease counts with the ability to rapidly detect outbreaks of disease. While traditional statistical process control methods such as control charts have been found to have early detection properties when monitoring univariate disease counts, these are often inadequate for detecting bio-terrorism events.

There are two principal impediments in statistical process control methods for the detection of bio-terrorism events: firstly, these methods aggregate over space by examining total counts and thus ignore the spatial dimension of the task and secondly they fail to adjust for the usual (seasonal) behaviour of diseases (e.g., Steiner *et al.*, 2011 where the focus is early detection of the start of influenza outbreak). If disease outbreaks were expected to be spread relatively uniformly in space, then the former reason is unimportant. However, since bio-terrorism attacks are likely to be introduced to specifically targeted locations, then the resulting disease instances are likely to cluster in space. Consequently, monitoring total counts is likely to reduce the signal-to-noise ratio of this outbreak by aggregating over regions where there is no outbreak. Exploiting the spatial clustering should be able to provide additional power and efficiency in detecting the outbreak.

There is much ongoing work in developing methods that are efficient at detecting outbreaks in a spatial context but these methods may still fail to deal with the latter fault mentioned above. When surveillance for bio-terrorism involves the monitoring of diseases or syndromes already present in the population then the detection of an attack may be delayed if it is introduced during a period of normal seasonal increased activity. For example, respiratory complaints are often much more frequent in the cooler months so detecting an intentional disease outbreak with respiratory symptomatology would need to differentiate between the usual and an unusual increase in cases. Therefore, it is often necessary to remove the influence of the expected behaviour of a disease to detect the signal of an introduced strain early.

Before presenting the method we are proposing in this chapter to deal with both of the above concerns, we begin by outlining some of the existing spatial disease detection methods. The current benchmark in spatio-temporal surveillance is the spatial SCAN statistic (Tango, 1995, Kulldorff, 1995, 1997, 2001, 2005). This method is a spatio-temporal moving average plan that systematically scans the target space applying a test to all windows of data up to a given fixed size in time and space. This presents an intuitive approach but has received some criticisms by Woodall *et al.* (2008) and Han *et al.* (2008), including: firstly that it is not as efficient as the cumulative SUM (CUSUM) (see Raubertas, 1989, and Rogerson and Yamada, 2004) for outbreak detection and secondly that its ability to detect outbreaks most effectively is dependent on the choice of shape and size of the scanning window. In addition, in some of the literature on the SCAN statistic, the focus is on whether diseases cluster rather than on early detection.

Some control chart methods have also been proposed such as the Multivariate Exponentially Weighted Moving Average (MEWMA) control chart method proposed by Joner *et al.* (2008). This approach could be extended to the lattice structure of counts discussed below but involving all cell counts in the lattice making it a high dimensional application of the MEWMA plan which is difficult to implement. Exponential weighted moving averages (EWMA) have also proved valuable in the early detection of persistent disease outbreaks (Steiner et al, 2010 and Sparks et al 2010a). However these methods are frequently unable to account for underlying changes that occur in the observation of disease instances through health services such as day-of-the-week or holiday effects. The removal of known trends, called nuisance variables, would reduce the noise in the departures of counts from expected, and as such provides the surveillance plans with a increased chance of early detection.

A bio-terrorist attack is likely to be initiated at several simultaneous disconnected locations causing clustered outbreaks of different size and shape. Having a technology that has the flexibility of finding outbreaks started at several disconnected locations is essential in this setting.

In this chapter, we explore the method EWMA Surveillance Trees that addresses the concerns outlined above and that has this flexibility. The approach taken here is to divide the geographical regions into a lattice structure so that the expected numbers of cases within the cells are as similar as possible. Expected counts are achieved by firstly building a model that describes the usual behaviour of disease counts (including any usual seasonal increases) and then using this model to produce a one day-ahead forecast for the expected counts (see Sparks, *et al.* 2010a). The method proposed then:

- Builds temporal memory of the disease process by smoothing the time series of cell counts using MEWMAs. This allows the method to build up memory of the process to detect slowly evolving changes.
- Uses exponentially weighted spatially smoothing of these temporal EWMA cell counts by smoothing across both the rows and columns of the lattice (very similar to MEWMA).
- Detects departures from expected value in the spatio-temporally smoothed lattice counts using a binary recursive partitioning approach that focuses in on specific areas of concern.
- Prunes these partitions in a way that leaves only the outbreaks, that is areas of significant departure from expected.

So this method should be able to detect outbreaks of varying size and shapes and incorporate the benefits of EWMA smoothing for early detection. Its performance will be measured against an implementation of the SCAN statistic.

The EWMA Surveillance Tree method proposed here also applies a smoothing in the spatial sense. If smoothing has the advantage of reducing spatial noise and more easily exposes spatial trends in disease outbreaks, then this could translate into earlier detection properties. This chapter will also evaluate when it is beneficial to spatially smooth counts for the early detection of diseases.

We will continue by giving a detailed overview of the spatial SCAN statistic. We will then propose the EWMA Surveillance Tree methodology in more detail and discuss the results of some simulation studies comparing this method to the SCAN statistic. Lastly we will briefly discuss the extension of these methods to a broader multivariate context which is the key in applications of these methods to syndromic surveillance for emerging diseases.

2. The SCAN statistic

Scan statistics are so described because they arise from the scanning of time and/or space looking for clusters of events. This section will present the details for an implementation of the spatial SCAN statistic that will be used as the benchmark in the simulation studies to follow. The SCAN statistic is similar to a spatio-temporal moving average plan that looks at the number of observations in cylinders of spatio-temporal space (e.g., see Figure 1), where the height of the cylinder is time. The SCAN plan used in this chapter is indistinguishable from the approaches used in Glaz *et al.* (2001) in the spatial dimension but uses a moving window for the temporal dimension. As such the results from Chen and Glaz can be used to get efficient starting estimates for the threshold used in the surveillance plan. For other literature on the SCAN plan see Tango (1995), Kulldorff and Nagarwalla (1995), Kulldorff (1997), and Kulldorff, M. (2001), Kulldorff *et al.* (2005), Woodall et al (2008) and Han *et al.* (2008).

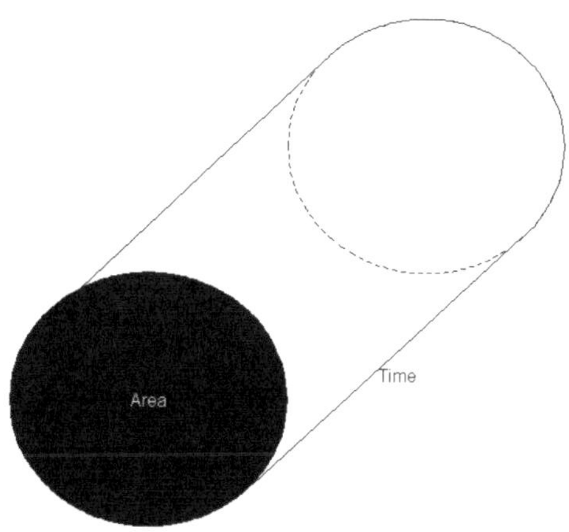

Fig. 1. Example of the scanned region - circular area is scanned and the depth is the number of days that counts are aggregated over.

The SCAN plan in this chapter is applied to a fixed lattice structure over the target area of the data for reasons which will become obvious later. Although this lattice structure may not be regular as in Figure 2 below, it is convenient at this stage to make it regular. In other words, in this lattice, individual cells are not taken to have a fixed volume; they are constructed so that the marginal total across each row/column spatial dimension has approximately the same expected number of counts. In addition the horizontal and vertical dividers of cells may be curved giving the design greater flexibility.

The lattice structure reduces the amount of multiple testing by forcing the scanned area to always include complete spatial ("square") cells. However, if a bio-terrorism event spans parts of some cells then some information about its signal is lost. The time window is arbitrarily taken as 10 days in this chapter, but could be taken as 7 days or 14 days to do away with the need for accounting for the influence of day-of-the-week effects.

The SCAN plan counts the number of disease cases within the scanned space-time window and compares this count to its expected count, assuming a Poisson distribution. Often autocorrelation of counts is ignored in this process which does cause inefficiencies in the inference of detecting bio-terrorism events. In this chapter we will also ignore the autocorrelation in the temporal counts. Since the SCAN plan involves significant amounts of multiple testing, we need to establish the false alarm rates for the level of multiple testing.

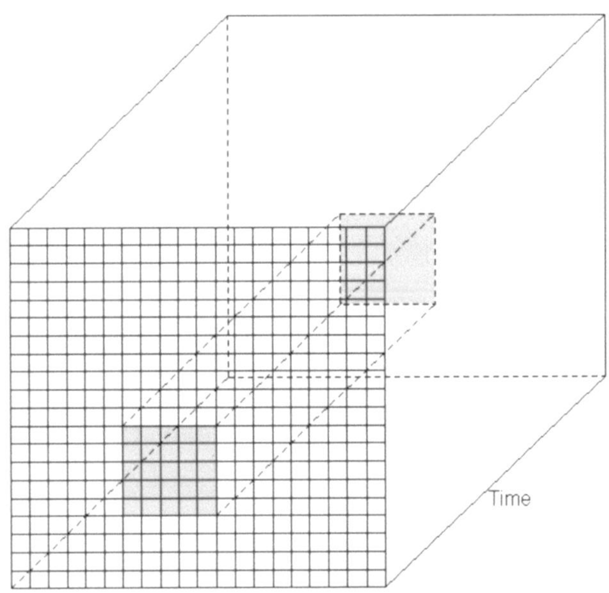

Fig. 2. The target region for assessing outbreaks is 20 by 20 cells by time and the scanned area is all 5 by 5 cells by time volumes - one example of which is illustrated in grey.

In this paper, we use a 40 by 40 cell target region. We examined two levels of spatial memory in the SCAN plans applied later in the chapter. The spatial cells scanned are either 5 by 5 or 10 by 10 both with a moving time window of 10 days. The 5 by 5 cell scan involves 36x36=1296 different (but overlapping) scanned regions, and the 10 by 10 cell scan involves 961 different (but overlapping) scanned regions. Clearly, the 10 by 10 cell scan involves fewer tests and so its level of significance for the fixed false alarm rate is larger than the 5 by 5 cell scan. This means that it should detect an outbreak close to 10 by 10 in dimensions earlier than the 5 by 5 cell scan. Therefore if the dimension of a future bio-terrorism outbreak is known in advance then it is best to use these dimensions precisely in designing the scanning window, unless the outbreak is sparse within the region. In this case a smaller window is needed (see Sparks, 2011c) to exploit this sparsity. Unfortunately, we seldom know the dimension of bio-terrorism outbreaks, and therefore we need methodology that is flexible enough for detecting unknown outbreaks quickly. The next section discusses such flexible technology that is not as dependent on the shape and size of the outbreak.

3. EWMA surveillance trees

The EWMA Surveillance Tree method proposed here for comparison against the SCAN plan uses an EWMA approach by smoothing counts first temporally to build in temporal memory of the process, and then spatially to average counts locally in space. Smoothing can also be viewed as an approach that reduces the noise in counts without reducing the signal too much. This makes the signal-to-noise ratio larger and therefore has early detection advantages. There are many examples of EWMA temporal smoothing of counts data aimed at early detection of diseases, for example see Sparks *et al.* (2010a) and Stiener *et al.* (2010) for Poisson counts, and Sparks *et al.* (2010b) and Sarka (2011) for negative binomial counts. There is no literature on spatial exponentially weighted moving average smoothing although there is some work by Rogerson et al (2006) using 2 dimensional kernel smoothers. The smoothed counts are then used in an outbreak detection procedure.

The EWMA smoothing process has computational advantages because only the last temporally smoothed cell counts are retained rather than the last 10 days as is necessary in the SCAN plan discussed in the previous section. Areas are searched for outbreaks by comparing their smoothed observed counts to their respective smoothed expected counts. An outbreak is signalled when the difference between observed and expected counts in a window exceeds a threshold. The value of the threshold is chosen to control the false alarm rate. Note that EWMA smoothed counts are no longer Poisson distributed, however EWMA smoothing (spatial and temporal) helps improve the approximation to a normal distribution of the smoothed counts.

The method consists of three major steps:

1. EWMA based smoothing of observed and expected counts, first temporally then spatially;
2. Growing a surveillance tree of departures from expected value in the spatio-temporally smoothed counts using a binary recursive partitioning approach
3. Pruning the surveillance tree to reveal outbreaks and control the false alarm rate.

Each of these steps is detailed in subsections 3.1, 3.2 and 3.3 respectively.

3.1 EWMA temporal and spatial smoothing

Define 40 by 40 matrices of counts and expected values for day t by $Y_t = \{y_{(\ell,k,t)}\}$ and $\Lambda_t = \{\lambda_{(\ell,k,t)}\}$ respectively. Temporal smoothing examines the exponentially weighted moving average (EWMA) to the counts according to

$$\bar{Y}_t = \alpha Y_t + (1-\alpha)\bar{Y}_{t-1}$$

($\bar{Y}_0 = \Lambda_1$) and similarly smooths the matrix of expected values of these counts using

$$\bar{\Lambda}_t = \alpha\Lambda_t + (1-\alpha)\bar{\Lambda}_{t-1}$$

where $\bar{\Lambda}_0 = \Lambda_1$, and $0<\alpha<1$ is a constant that determines how much memory to retain in the averages. Larger values of α retain less temporal memory.

Once the counts have been smoothed temporally, we then smooth over space to average counts locally. So the temporal smoothed counts and temporal smoothed expected values of $\bar{Y}_t$ and $\bar{\Lambda}_t$ respectively are now spatially smoothed using smoothing matrix defined by $\{A_{ij}\} = \{(1-\lambda)^{|i-j|} / \sum_{j=1}^{40}(1-\lambda)^{|i-j|}\}$. The spatial smoothing of counts is defined by

$$\tilde{Y}_t = A\bar{Y}_t A^t$$

and the spatial smoothing of their expected values is defined by

$$\tilde{\Lambda}_t = A\bar{\Lambda}_t A^t \, .$$

This EWMA spatial smoothing has the advantage over other smoothers of computational simplicity and is efficient in terms of early outbreak detection. Alternative spatial smoothing involving two dimensional kernel smoothers (Riedel, 1993, Rogerson *et al.* 2006) or splines (Currie *et al.* 2003, Lee and Durban, 2009) are more complex computationally. The EWMA smoother is similar to a kernel smoother using a double exponential distribution. The main reason for this choice is computational speed. We ignore the boundary problems with this EWMA smoothing approach. It is clear that the spatial smoothing employed here smooths boundary cell counts less. In addition, the recursive partitioning approach does not adjust for the differential smoothing. Therefore the surveillance trees detect outbreaks that hug a boundary very quickly. For this reason no clusters are considered that hug boundaries in the simulation section, because this would exaggerate the performance of surveillance trees.

3.2 Growing the surveillance trees

The recursive partitioning approach applied in this paper is very similar to that in Yu (2009) and identical to Sparks and Okugami (2010b). Surveillance trees generate offspring by recursively partitioning either longitudinal cells or latitudinal cells into rectangular regions. We start by finding the best partition of longitudinal cells in terms of having the highest signal to noise ratio, and then the best partition of latitudinal cells. Thereafter, select the partition with the highest signal-to-noise ratio between the best longitudinal cell partition and the best latitudinal cell partition.

The choice of the signal-to-noise ratio as the measure of departure from expected value was decided based on the fact that the square root of the smooth counts has roughly a constant variance and its mean is equal to the square root of the smoothed mean.

The mathematical summary of this process for the first generation of offspring is as follows: denote $\tilde{Y}_{i.} = \sum_{j\in P}\tilde{Y}_{ij}$ and $\tilde{Y}_{.j} = \sum_{i\in P}\tilde{Y}_{ij}$ where P defines the parent space, e.g., at the root node the parent space is $P = \{k : k = 1,2,...,40\}$ for both i and j ($\tilde{\Lambda}_{i.}$ and $\tilde{\Lambda}_{.j}$ are similarly defined)

1. **Latitudinal (row oriented) partitions:** Calculate $r_k = \sqrt{\sum_{i=1}^{k} \tilde{Y}_{i.}} - \sqrt{\sum_{i=1}^{k} \tilde{\Lambda}_{i.}}$ and $r_{\sim k} = \sqrt{\sum_{i=k+1}^{40} \tilde{Y}_{i.}} - \sqrt{\sum_{i=k+1}^{40} \tilde{\Lambda}_{i.}}$ for $k = 1,2,...,39$.
2. **Longitudinal (column oriented) partitions:** Calculate $c_\ell = \sqrt{\sum_{j=1}^{\ell} \tilde{Y}_{.j}} - \sqrt{\sum_{j=1}^{\ell} \tilde{\Lambda}_{.j}}$ or $c_{\sim\ell} = \sqrt{\sum_{j=\ell+1}^{40} \tilde{Y}_{.j}} - \sqrt{\sum_{j=\ell+1}^{40} \tilde{\Lambda}_{.j}}$ for $\ell = 1,2,...,39$.
3. **Select the best partition:** Partition on
   a. Row 1 to k and k+1 to 40 if $\max(r_k, r_{\sim k}) > \max(c_\ell, c_{\sim\ell})$ for all ℓ and $\max(r_k, r_{\sim k}) \geq \max(r_i, r_{\sim i})$ for all $i \neq k$.
   b. Column 1 to ℓ and ℓ+1 to 40 if $\max(c_\ell, c_{\sim\ell}) > \max(r_k, r_{\sim k})$ for all k and $\max(c_\ell, c_{\sim\ell}) \geq \max(c_j, c_{\sim j})$ for all $j \neq \ell$.
4. Define $z_1 = \max(c_\ell, c_{\sim\ell}, r_k, r_{\sim k})$ as partition score for the right-hand partition and let the other offspring have signal-to-noise ratio $z_{\sim 1}$. If $z_1 = c_{\sim\ell}$ then $z_{\sim 1} = c_\ell$; if $z_1 = c_\ell$ then $z_{\sim 1} = c_{\sim\ell}$; $z_1 = r_k$ then $z_{\sim 1} = r_k$; and if $z_1 = r_k$ then $z_{\sim 1} = r_k$.

Now we repeat the process for the next generation of offspring by considering each offspring of the partition above as a parent space made up of p rows and q columns defined by rows $i_1, i_1+1, ..., i_p$ and columns $j_1, j_1+1, ..., j_q$. Then a further two offspring are generated by the following steps:

1. **Latitudinal partitions:** Calculate $r_k = \sqrt{\sum_{i=i_1}^{k} \tilde{Y}_{i.}} - \sqrt{\sum_{i=i_1}^{k} \tilde{\Lambda}_{i.}}$ and $r_{\sim k} = \sqrt{\sum_{i=k+1}^{i_p} \tilde{Y}_{i.}} - \sqrt{\sum_{i=k+1}^{i_p} \tilde{\Lambda}_{i.}}$ for $k = i_1, i_1+1, ..., i_p - 1$.
2. **Longitudinal partitions:** Calculate $c_\ell = \sqrt{\sum_{j=j_1}^{\ell} \tilde{Y}_{.j}} - \sqrt{\sum_{j=j_1}^{\ell} \tilde{\Lambda}_{.j}}$ or $c_\ell = \sqrt{\sum_{j=\ell+1}^{j_q} \tilde{Y}_{.j}} - \sqrt{\sum_{j=\ell+1}^{j_q} \tilde{\Lambda}_{.j}}$ for $\ell = j_1, j_1+1, ..., j_q - 1$.
3. **Select the best partition**: Partition on:
   a. Row i_1 to k and k+1 to i_p if $\max(r_k, r_{\sim k}) > \max(c_\ell, c_{\sim\ell})$ for all ℓ and $\max(r_\ell, r_{\sim k}) \geq \max(r_i, r_{\sim i})$ for all $i \neq k \in (i_1, i_1+1, ..., i_p)$.
   b. Column j_1 to ℓ and ℓ+1 to j_q if $\max(c_\ell, c_{\sim\ell}) > \max(r_k, r_{\sim k})$ for all k and $\max(c_\ell, c_{\sim\ell}) \geq \max(c_j, c_{\sim j})$ for all $j \neq \ell \in (j_1, j_1+1, ..., j_q)$.
4. Define $z_g = \max(c_\ell, c_{\sim\ell}, r_k, r_{\sim k})$ as partition score for the right-hand partition and let the other offspring have signal-to-noise ratio $z_{\sim g}$.

The process is repeated for each new generation and only stops when the smooth counts are either

- Too small to alarm an unusually high count (this is discussed in more detail later).
- All cells in the parent space are less than expected.

- The best longitudinal partition and best latitudinal partition are both the parent space.

Latitude

2	4	3	2	1	2	3	4	4	3	1	2	3	2	1	2	2	1	2	2
2	5	3	2	1	2	4	7	6	3	1	2	3	3	2	4	4	3	2	4
3	4	3	4	2	3	3	4	4	4	3	1	2	1	2	4	5	4	3	3
2	3	6	7	5	4	4	3	2	2	1	2	2	3	4	2	1	1	2	2
1	2	3	3	4	6	4	2	3	1	1	2	2	4	5	3	1	1	3	3
2	4	2	0	2	4	4	3	4	2	1	1	3	5	4	4	3	2	3	3
1	3	2	1	3	4	3	2	2	3	2	1	3	3	3	3	3	3	3	3
2	3	3	1	2	2	2	3	2	3	3	2	1	2	1	2	3	3	4	3
2	3	1	1	2	2	3	2	2	1	3	1	0	1	2	3	7	4	3	3
0	2	2	2	3	3	4	2	1	1	2	1	0	1	2	3	3	2	2	4
2	1	1	3	5	3	2	2	1	1	1	2	3	2	2	2	3	2	1	1
5	2	1	2	3	1	2	1	1	1	1	1	2	4	4	5	3	1	1	2
4	4	2	2	2	2	3	2	2	1	1	1	1	2	2	2	1	0	2	4
3	3	5	3	3	3	3	1	2	2	1	2	3	2	1	1	2	2	5	4
4	3	4	4	5	3	1	1	3	3	2	5	5	4	2	4	6	2	2	2
3	2	2	3	3	1	1	2	2	2	4	4	3	3	3	6	7	2	2	2
4	3	2	2	3	1	1	2	3	2	3	3	1	3	2	4	5	2	2	5
3	2	1	2	4	3	1	4	3	1	2	3	2	3	3	2	2	2	3	4
1	1	2	5	4	1	1	2	3	1	1	3	2	1	2	3	2	4	4	3
0	0	2	2	2	2	1	1	3	3	2	1	2	2	1	2	2	2	2	3

Longitude

Fig. 3. An example of in-control counts when cell means are correlated.

Latitude

0	0	2	1	2	1	2	3	5	4	3	2	2	3	2	2	1	0	0	1
1	2	2	1	2	1	2	3	4	5	8	8	7	8	6	4	4	5	2	1
3	1	0	0	1	2	3	3	3	7	6	8	9	13	7	4	4	2	7	2
2	1	1	2	2	3	2	4	4	7	7	4	7	6	4	10	4	2	4	3
1	2	3	6	2	2	2	4	3	6	7	5	4	5	3	7	7	8	3	2
1	2	3	6	3	1	3	4	3	2	3	2	1	3	4	2	4	2	2	3
2	3	3	5	3	2	5	5	3	2	4	3	1	1	4	3	3	2	2	4
2	5	3	3	4	3	3	4	2	4	4	4	2	1	2	2	2	2	1	2
2	4	2	3	3	2	1	2	2	1	1	3	4	2	1	1	1	2	3	5
2	3	1	4	5	2	2	4	3	1	0	2	3	2	1	1	3	3	4	5
1	1	1	2	2	1	2	4	4	4	1	1	1	2	1	2	3	2	3	3
1	1	3	3	1	1	3	4	5	4	2	2	2	2	2	1	4	4	2	1
2	2	2	3	1	0	2	3	5	3	4	5	2	1	2	1	2	3	3	1
2	4	3	2	0	0	2	3	3	3	3	4	3	1	2	1	2	2	2	3
2	4	3	2	0	1	3	3	3	5	4	3	4	2	2	2	3	1	3	5
2	3	1	1	1	2	3	2	1	3	3	1	2	2	2	2	3	1	2	3
2	3	2	0	1	2	1	2	1	1	2	1	0	0	0	2	2	1	3	3
1	1	1	1	2	2	1	3	3	2	1	1	1	0	0	2	2	2	3	3
2	1	2	4	2	1	2	4	6	5	1	0	0	1	0	1	1	3	2	1
3	2	4	3	1	0	1	4	4	3	0	0	0	0	1	0	1	4	2	1

Longitude

Fig. 4. An example of a hypothetical bio-terrorism event.

An example, of the recursive partitioning when there is no smoothing of counts is now used to demonstrate the growing process for a 20×20 grid. Assume that the in-control Poisson counts for each cell in the grid (except boundary cells) have a mean of 2,5. An example of in-control counts is presented in Figure 3. Latitude (La) cells are numbered from the bottom of row as 1 to the top row as 20. Longitude (Lo) cells are numbered 1 (left) to 20 (right). Correlated cell counts are noted from Figure 3 by higher than expected cell counts (greater than 2,5) clumping together even when in-control, e.g., latitude number rows 18, 19 and 20 (La>17) and longitude columns 7, 8, 9 and 10 (6<Lo<11). This makes it more difficult to identify bio-terrorism events.

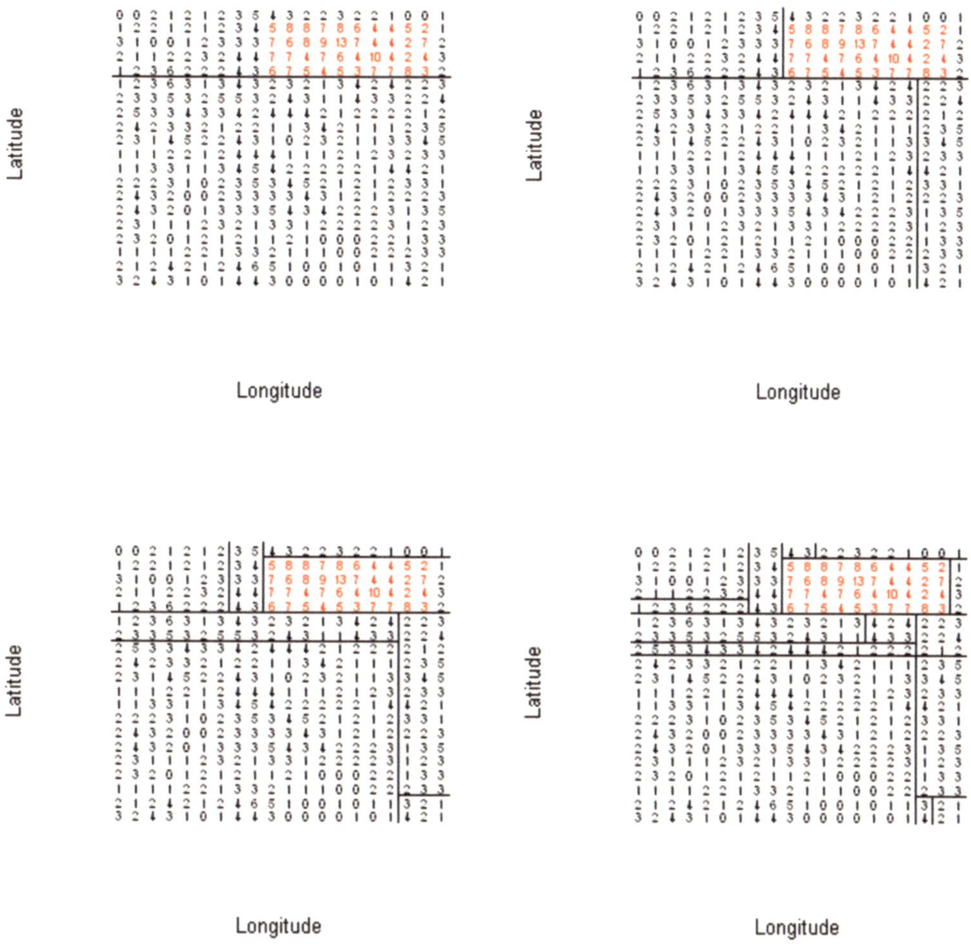

Fig. 5. Presenting offspring for 5 generations using recursive partitioning

We use transitional Poisson regression models to forecast the expected counts one day ahead. We assume that these forecasts, when no bio-terrorism event is present, produce unbiased estimates of the cell means. Therefore, in our application, the in-control count departures from the forecasts are assumed uncorrelated because the dependence is removed by the model forecasts, and the forecast errors are assumed spatially uncorrelated when in-control. The assumption here is that all the spatial correlation is in the mean of the Poisson counts, and the day ahead forecast is an unbiased estimate of this mean. As such, the differences between functions of counts and forecasts will be assumed to be uncorrelated.

Even if this is not true; provided the bootstrap population used to estimate the threshold is accurate, the simulation process will produce an unbiased estimate of the threshold (see Sparks et al. 2010b).

Figure 4 presents another representation of counts illustrated in Figure 3, except in Figure 4 a bio-terrorism event is simulated by adding additional (out-of-control) counts at Latitudes 16, 17, 18 and 19 $(15 < La < 20)$ and longitude 10, 11,..., 19 $(10 < Lo < 20)$. The additional counts were assumed to have a mean of 2 per cell. Red is used to highlight the simulated bioterrorism outbreak region in Figure 4. It is clear that the counts in red are higher than the counts for any other part of the 20×20 target region. We now demonstrate the recursive partitioning process in trying to find this outbreak.

The recursive partitioning starts by searching for the best partition of longitude and latitude in terms of maximizing the departure of the region's total counts from their expected value, i.e., maximising r_k and c_ℓ values, respectively. These are defined by rules La>15 and Lo>9, respectively. Generally the region with the greatest fraction of red will be the one with the highest departure from expected and this is true in this case. The best first partition of La>15 is represented by the black line in the top left-hand table in Figure 5. This first generation of offspring become parents for the next generation of offspring. Each region now grows two offspring by finding the partition that is best for each parent. For the parent region with La>15, it is clear that the best partition is Lo>9 (see the black line in top right-hand table of Figure 5 that separates the red counts from the black counts as best as possible). For the region with La<16, the best partition is less obvious - it turns out to be Lo>17. The bottom left-hand table in Figure 5 gives the next generation of offspring, and the bottom right-hand table in Figure 5 gives the generation that completely specifies the simulated outbreak. The z-score for the red region is $z_g = 10{,}6$ which is higher than any other partitioned region in the table of Figure 5. An exhaustive search of all regions of all different shapes and sizes in

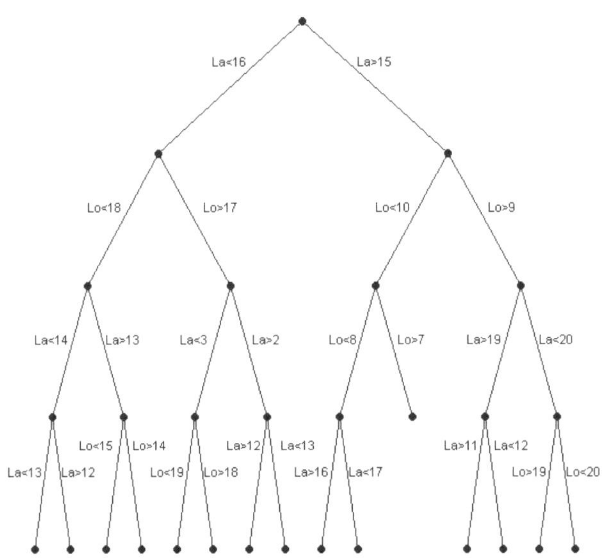

Fig. 6. Surveillance tree representation of the recursive partitions in Figure 5.

Figure 5 revealed that this gave the highest z-score of target region. Recursive partitioning is like stepwise variable selection when building parsimonious regression models - it does not always produce the same result as an exhaustive search. In this example, we have demonstrated that recursive partitioning found the largest outbreak area using significantly smaller number of computations than for example the SCAN statistic with multiple size windows. This balance between computational and detection efficiency is the most attractive feature of the recursive partitioning approach besides its ability to adapt with size and shape of the outbreak.

Figure 6 is a tree based representation of the recursive partitions made in Figure 5. Note that the terminal node defined by rules La>15, Lo<10 and Lo>7 does not have any offspring. The z_g for this node is $(\sqrt{36}-\sqrt{25})=1$ where $36=3+5+3+4+3+3+4+4+4+3$ and $25=2,5\times10$. No partition of this space produces a higher z-score than the parent node's z-score of 1. The closest to this is $(\sqrt{5+4+3+4+3}-\sqrt{5\times2,5}=0,825$. Ideally we would like to stop recursive partitioning at this node. In practice, the decision to stop unnecessarily growing of the tree is difficult. Generally we would keep partitioning until some stopping rule applies.

Once partitioning has stopped, then recursive pruning of the terminal nodes commences. The pruning process is outlined in the next section.

3.3 Pruning the surveillance tree to deliver a particular false alarm rate

The aim of pruning is to recursively trim away all terminal nodes with smoothed counts that do not differ significantly from their expected values. If all nodes in the tree are pruned away to leave no tree, then no outbreak is signalled. However, if terminal nodes remain after pruning, then an alarm is given. The geographical location of the outbreak is diagnosed by the set of partitioning rules for the remaining terminal nodes. This could involve several non-overlapping locations.

Pruning only starts after growing the tree has stopped. The pruning process is very simple. We prune terminal nodes recursively starting with the last generation offspring in the tree, and then repeat the process recursively with each remaining generation. Only branches with significantly higher than expected counts survive pruning. We prune the least significant offspring if $z_{\sim g}<h_z$ and prune and the generation if $z_g<h_z$ where h_z is a positive constant designed to deliver a specified false alarm. Pruning is used to control the false alarm rate measured by either specifying an in-control Average Run Length (ARL) or an in-control Recurrence Interval (RI). The Recurrence Interval (RI) is used to indicate the steady state false alarm rate. ARL and RI are defined more clearly in the simulation section (see Section 4). Pruning starts with the highest values of g (generations) and stops when either all generations are pruned or when at least one generation (terminal node) survives the pruning process.

The pruning process leaves only generations with smoothed counts significantly higher than expected, e.g., if we started pruning from generation 4 in Figure 5 then only two offspring containing the outbreak regions plus their parents, grandparents, etc would survive the pruning process. If pruning was applied to a tree for the data in Figure 3 with no outbreaks, then each generation in turn would be pruned away until no offspring remain. Even the target region (the original parent) would be pruned indicating no significant outbreak.

3.4 Using the example to demonstrate the stopping rules for the tree growing process

It is useful to stop partitioning when it is known that the threshold will not be exceeded with further partitions. Assume that the threshold is $h_z = 4{,}45$ then the node defined by rules La>15, Lo<10 and Lo>7 should be terminal because $(\sqrt{36} - \sqrt{2.5}) = 4{,}4$. No partition of this parent space is going to be greater than the threshold of 4,45. Two other nodes would terminate in generation three Figure 5 using $h_z = 4{,}45$. These would be:

a. Lo>9 and La>19 where

$$(\sqrt{4+3+2+2+3+2+2+1+0+0+1} - \sqrt{2{,}5}) = 2{,}9 < 4{,}45 .$$

b. La<3 and Lo>17 where

$$(\sqrt{3+2+1+4+2+1} - \sqrt{2{,}5}) = 2{,}0 < 4{,}45 .$$

Such a stopping rule stops the unnecessary growing of the surveillance tree, because all offspring will be pruned later. Generally this rule can be defined as stopping when the square root of the total of cell counts for a region is smaller than the threshold plus square root of the smallest cell mean in the region. If the threshold is quite low, then having a threshold on the lower limit for the smoothed count is sensible. Assume that our threshold turns out to be $h_z = 1{,}15$ then the above stopping rule does not help much in reducing the partitioning complexity. In the above example, it is sometimes helpful to specify when you would fail to respond, e.g., no response is made for any outbreak with counts less than 5 above expected per day. We would then stop if smoothed counts were below 7,5.

3.5 Lattice with cell means that are spatially non-homogeneous

Until now, we have assumed that all cells follow the same model. What if the same time trends persist across cells, e.g., the seasonal trend remains the same for each cell but the mean counts change from cell to cell? How does this influence the threshold for when the model is not homogeneous across all cells? Here we examined the in-control ARL and RI properties as we move the cell mean rate from an average of 0,7 to the current value used of 1,2 by examining its in-control ARL and RI using the same threshold of $h_z = 1{,}15$. The results are recorded in the Table 1 for counts generated using the R function in Appendix A with overall mean mu=0,1, day-of-the-week influences given by bweekday=(-0,025, -0,025, -0,025, -0,025, -0,025,0,05,0,075), seasonal influences given by bcos=0,1, bsin=-0,1, transitional influences of blags=(0,1,0,06,0,02,0,01), and k=-4.

This plan is also reasonably robust to changes in spatial non-homogeneity in means whereas other plans are not. From Table 1 it is clear that the in-control RI values are reasonably stable across a range of mean values. If these mean changes are not systematic as in table above, but random in space then these changes are expected to be ironed out by the spatial smoothing. Adaptive plans can be derived using the results in Table 1 based on Sparks (2000) and Sparks et al (2010a).

Average counts	0,7	0,8	0,9	1,0	1,1	1,27
h_z	1,15 1,2 1,25	1,15 1,2 1,25	1,15 1,2 1,25	1,15 1,2 1,25	1,15 1,2 1,25	1,15 1,2 1,25
In-control ARL	55,4 72,4 81,1	62,5 84,4 91,8	73,7 100,2 111,4	78,7 106,4 119,2	83,1 109,7 126,2	88,7 117,9 149,3
In-control RI	50,3 61,0 75,0	51,6 63,9 83,6	52,3 68,7 86,5	56,1 72,4 88,9	60,1 68,7 86,5	69,3 82,5 97,4

Table 1. In-control ARLs and RIs for specified thresholds of 1,15, 1,2 and 1,25

4. Simulation study

This section provides the results of simulation studies comparing the performance of the SCAN statistic with that of the EWMA Surveillance Trees for two outbreak shapes and locations using Average Time to Signal and Average Run Length as the measures of performance. When the size and shape of the scanning window matches that of the outbreak in the SCAN plan, then it remains optimal. However, the flexible partitions of EWMA Surveillance Trees result in robust performance across a range of outbreak dimensions, without being optimal for any specific outbreak size or shape.

We simulate uncorrelated Poisson counts on a 40x40 spatial grid using the R function in Appendix A as described in Section 3.4, with the exception that the mean value is bounded at a minimum of one (i.e., k=0) which makes the counts more homogeneous. Denote these counts by $\overline{c}_{i,j}$ for row i and column j. These counts are then aggregated locally as follows for non-boundary cells:

$$c_{i,j} = \text{floor}(\overline{c}_{i,j}+0,3\times(\overline{c}_{i-1,j}+\overline{c}_{i,j-1}+\overline{c}_{i+1,j}+\overline{c}_{i,j+1})+0,1\times(\overline{c}_{i-1,j-1}+\overline{c}_{i-1,j+1}+\overline{c}_{i+1,j-1}+\overline{c}_{i+1,j+1}))$$

where floor means round down to the nearest whole number. Boundary cells have smaller means and their counts are defined as in Table 2.

This generates more realistic spatially correlated in-control counts for infectious or contagious diseases. Note that these counts are not expected to be Poisson distributed, but tend to be under-dispersed counts relative to the Poisson distribution. We assume no knowledge of this under-dispersion in trying to forecast counts. We model the trends in the counts using transitional Poisson regression model and assume that if the counts are in-control then the one day ahead forecast errors are uncorrelated. In situations where spatial correlation persists in the forecast errors for in-control situations, an alternative approach is models which account for this spatial correlation, such as seeming unrelated Poisson regression models (King, 1989, and Grijalva, T., Bohara, *et al.* 2003), and multivariate Poisson regression model (Karlis and Meligkotsidou, 2005, and Bermudez and Karlis, 2011). However, here we model each of the 1600 cells separately using Poisson regression models very similar to that used in Sparks *et al.* (2010a) and Sparks *et al.* (2011a) that use explanatory variables: logarithm of lag counts plus 1, day-of-the-week, public holidays and harmonics. These models are used to produce one-day ahead forecasts which estimate the "Poisson" means for the next day.

$i=1,\ 1<j<40$	$c_{1,j}=\text{floor}(\bar{c}_{1,j}+0{,}3\times(\bar{c}_{1,j+1}+\bar{c}_{1,j-1}+\bar{c}_{2,j})+0{,}1\times(\bar{c}_{2,j-1}+\bar{c}_{2,j+1}))$
$i=40\ ,\ 1<j<40$	$c_{40,j}=\text{floor}(\bar{c}_{1,j}+0{,}3\times(\bar{c}_{40,j+1}+\bar{c}_{40,j-1}+\bar{c}_{39,j})+0{,}1\times(\bar{c}_{39,j-1}+\bar{c}_{39,j+1}))$
$1<i<40,\ j=1$	$c_{i,1}=\text{floor}(\bar{c}_{i,1}+0{,}3\times(\bar{c}_{i+1,1}+\bar{c}_{i-1,1}+\bar{c}_{i,2})+0{,}1\times(\bar{c}_{i-1,2}+\bar{c}_{i+1,2}))$
$1<j<40\ ,j=40$	$c_{i,40}=\text{floor}(\bar{c}_{i,1}+0{,}3\times(\bar{c}_{i+1,40}+\bar{c}_{i-1,40}+\bar{c}_{i,39})+0{,}1\times(\bar{c}_{i-1,39}+\bar{c}_{i+1,39}))$
$i=1,\ j=1$	$c_{1,1}=\text{floor}(\bar{c}_{1,1}+0{,}3\times(\bar{c}_{2,1}+\bar{c}_{1,2})+0{,}1\times\bar{c}_{2,2})$
$i=40,\ j=40$	$c_{40,40}=\text{floor}(\bar{c}_{40,40}+0{,}3\times(\bar{c}_{39,40}+\bar{c}_{40,39})+0{,}1\times\bar{c}_{39,39})$

Table 2. The process used to simulate cells counts that are spatially correlated.

The recursive partitioning process is then applied to the temporal or spatio-temporal smoothed counts. The z_g statistic is used to assess the departure of smoothed counts from smoothed day ahead forecasted counts. When in-control, z_g has mean zero and approximately a constant variance. The convenience of the statistic is discussed in Sparks *et al.* (2010b) and has been demonstrated to compare very well with the SCAN statistic.

The simulation process generated in-control counts. Simulated bio-terrorism outbreaks are generated by adding to these in-control counts additional Poisson counts for a fixed rectangular region. The outbreak region is then hidden and we examined how early the plans alarm this outbreak. Rectangular outbreak regions were generated involving either 10x4 cells or 20x2 cells. Zero-state in-control ARLs and the Recurrent Interval (RI) were estimated as follows:

- Start the Run Length (RL) at 1. Generate in-control cell counts for the first day, and perform the surveillance tree process. If no tree results after pruning then go to the next step.
- Increase the RL by 1. Generate in-control cell counts for the next day, perform the surveillance tree process, and if no tree results after pruning, then go to the next step.
- Repeat the previous step until some branches of the surveillance tree survive the pruning process. Record the RL (denote this RL_1) and go to the next step.
- Generating in-control cell counts for the several consecutive days until there are at least 7 consecutive days with no tree surviving, then set RI=7.
- Increase the RI by 1. Generate in-control cell counts for the next day, perform the surveillance process, and if no tree results after pruning, then go to the next step.
- Repeat the previous step until some branches of the surveillance tree survive the pruning process. Record the RI (denote this RI_1) and go to the next step.
- Repeat all steps above 1600 times to give $(RL_i, RI_i), i=1,2,...,1600$. Average these to give the in-control ARL and an estimate of the expected RI.

The 1600 simulations were selected balancing both computational effort and estimation accuracy. Traditionally, the standard deviation for RL with an in-control ARL=100 is about 100. The standard deviation from the in-control ARL is expected to be roughly $100/\sqrt{1600}=2{,}5$.

The out-of-control ARL are calculated in the same way as the in-control ARL, except with each run additional counts with the same mean are added to the outbreak region. The results are reported in Table 1. The recurrence interval for out-of-control situations was not very interesting because generally when a plan signalled it did not stop signalling. The out-of-control ARLs are therefore the zero state out-of-control ARLs. Reporting the in-control RI values provides readers insight into the steady state in-control performance.

Outbreak	Recursive partitioning with temporal smoothing ($\alpha=0{,}1$) $h_z=1{,}255$		Recursive partitioning with temporal smoothing ($\alpha=0{,}1$) $h_z=1{,}404$		Recursive partitioning with spatio-temporal smoothing ($\lambda=0{,}7,\ \alpha=0{,}1$) $h_z=1{,}15$	
Rows Columns	10:19 16:19	10:11 1:20	10:19 16:19	10:11 1:20	10:19 16:19	10:11 1:20
ARL/RI δ	108,9 / 37,5	108,9 / 37,5	201,5/70,6	201,5/70,6	108,3 / 69,6	108,3 / 69,6
1	**11,88**	**11,95**	13,25	12,00	15,42	16,26
2	6,78	**4,86**	7,96	4,91	**5,61**	6,39
3	4,51	**3,55**	5,12	4,11	**3,94**	3,95
4	3,72	**2,76**	3,80	3,20	**2,94**	2,93
5	3,02	**2,35**	3,24	2,55	**2,65**	2,44
6	2,51	2,12	2,72	2,19	**2,10**	**2,11**
7	2,44	**1,70**	2,50	1,77	**1,97**	1,79
8	2,40	1,55	2,41	1,60	**1,70**	**1,53**
9	2,34	**1,45**	2,36	1,50	**1,56**	**1,45**
10	2,10	1,31	2,12	1,32	**1,20**	**1,30**
11	2,02	**1,12**	2,04	1,16	**1,15**	1,16
12	1,91	**1,05**	1,91	1,07	**1,04**	1,08

Table 3. ARL performance of the surveillance tree plans when the outbreak spans regions of 40 cells δ is the increase in mean for cells in the outbreak region.

Recursive partitioning does well when the outbreak is located on the boundary of the target region, partially because fewer partitions are necessary to find it. Another reason is that the boundary cells are where counts are smoothed less and the mean rates are lowest on the boundary, and therefore the signal is the highest. In other words, boundary outbreaks are easier to find using recursive partitioning because fewer generations are needed to find them and the signal-to-noise ratio on the boundary in this simulation process is higher.

The robust performance of plans, i.e., when nothing is known about the shape and size of the outbreak, is an important consideration because in bio-terrorism nothing is known about the size or shape of the outbreak. Therefore, Table 3 looks at a variation in rectangular shaped outbreaks. The recursive partitioning plan's flexibility in partitions strengthens its robust performance across a range of outbreak sizes (see Sparks *et al.* 2011c). In other words, if the outbreak dimensions are known, then the SCAN plan can always be trained to be more efficient than the recursive partitioning plan, and therefore it is preferred in these circumstances. But when nothing is known about its size and shape recursive partitioning is a more flexible and robust approach than the SCAN plan.

Table 3 demonstrates that spatial smoothing prior to applying recursive partitioning of temporally smoothed counts has early detection advantages for the same in-control RI values of approximately 70, e.g., for large shift in mean counts of 12 per cell the ARL is 1,04 as opposed to 1,91 (almost a day later). The spatial smoothing also closes the gap between the in-control ARL and in-control RI, and therefore it is likely to have equivalent steady state early detection advantages.

The future research challenges are to investigate what levels of spatial smoothing are best for early detection. In these studies we only tried $\lambda = 0,7$. In addition, there may be an interaction between the temporal smoothing and spatial smoothing. Therefore this needs to be investigated in future work.

The SCAN plan was applied using two separate scanning window sizes: 5 by 5 cells and 10 by 10 cells. As nothing is known about future outbreaks, therefore we consider square m by m scans – for at least the first outbreak considered in Table 4 the 5 by 5 cells scans is close to the m by m scanning plan with the smallest out-of-control ARLs. Unlike the recursive partitioning for the scan plans the expected values were taken as known, and therefore this gives an advantage to the SCAN plan in this comparison. Note that there was less of a difference between the in-control ARL and in-control RI for the scan plans than the surveillance tree plan. This mostly occurs because of the way we estimated the RI. In addition, by not allowing a signal in the first 7 values after a outbreak signal means that there are only a correlation of 0,3 between the signalled time point and the start of the RI for the scan plan, whereas in plans using the temporal EWMA smoothing with $\alpha = 0,1$ this is 0,48. Hence the way we estimated RI is going to be more influenced by the previous signal in the surveillance tree plan and therefore its RI is smaller. Clearly, the more the outbreak matches the scanning region the earlier the SCAN plan detects outbreaks, but it is clear that it lacks the flexibility in terms of detecting outbreaks of unknown shape and size. It is worth noting that when the SCAN plan does perform better than the surveillance trees (comparing Tables 3 and 4), the surveillance trees are not far behind in performance whereas the reverse is not true. Figure 7 provides a graphical comparison of the ARL properties. From Figure 7, the SCAN plan 5 by 5 by 10 days is best on average for detecting a 10 by 4 outbreak which is near the centre of the target region but significantly worse for the 2 by 20 outbreak. The 2 by 20 outbreak is quite feasible, e.g., this shaped outbreak would result if the outbreak was started in railway carriages travelling along a specific route.

5. Conclusions

The recursive partitioning approach can easily be extended to deal with more than two or three dimensions. It is ideal for finding disease outbreaks which cluster in multivariate space that could also include variables such as triage category (severity), age or gender, whereas the SCAN plans become computationally infeasible in higher dimensions. However further research is required to determine whether we can extend the benefit found from spatial smoothing to other dimensions that are not spatial, for example smoothing over age groups.

An advantage of the ability to extend to higher dimensions is that Surveillance Trees could be used to monitor several related diseases or symptoms jointly using disease category as a variable searched over in the recursive partitioning process. This would mean having one false alarm rate for all disease groups being monitored. Such planning may be beneficial in terms of managing the effort an epidemiological unit can devote to investigating false alarms. Similarly the method could also be used for syndromic surveillance - the surveillance of public health records such as Emergency Department visits. Detecting increases in ill-defined syndromes that may indicate the use of new and unknown biological agents.

Because of the efficiency of computation, another advantage of recursive partitioning is that it could be implemented using a hand-held mini-computer in the field to assess whether say counts have increased more than expected for any cluster of a target region. It does not need a sophisticated computer, as opposed to the SCAN plan.

Ultimately the EWMA Surveillance Tree methodology is a promising tool for detecting spatio-temporal outbreaks when the size and location of the outbreak is unknown. By incorporating the benefits of temporal and spatial smoothing with a tool for efficiently locating outbreaks, the method is well suited for the surveillance of bioterrorism events.

Outbreak	SCAN plan for 5 by 5 scans Threshold p-value=0,9999999999999991		SCAN plan for 10 by 10 scans Threshold p-value=0,99999999999994	
Rows Columns	10:19 16:19	10:11 1:20	10:19 16:19	10:11 1:20
ARL/RI δ	94,5 / 77,2	94,5 / 77,2	80,5/65,6	80,5/65,6
1	14,22	49,66	32,38	59,95
2	5,63	8,14	5,80	15,26
3	**3,85**	5,31	4,08	5,97
4	**2,99**	4,39	3,28	4,88
5	**1,79**	3,55	2,54	3,99
6	**1,60**	3,07	2,23	3,39
7	**1,54**	2,63	1,85	2,92
8	**1,30**	2,30	1,78	2,53
9	**1,22**	2,09	1,56	2,31
10	**1,15**	1,98	1,43	2,11
11	**1,05**	1,78	1,30	1,91
12	**1,01**	1,68	1,19	1,72

Table 4. ARL performance of the SCAN plan when the outbreak spans regions of 40 cells.

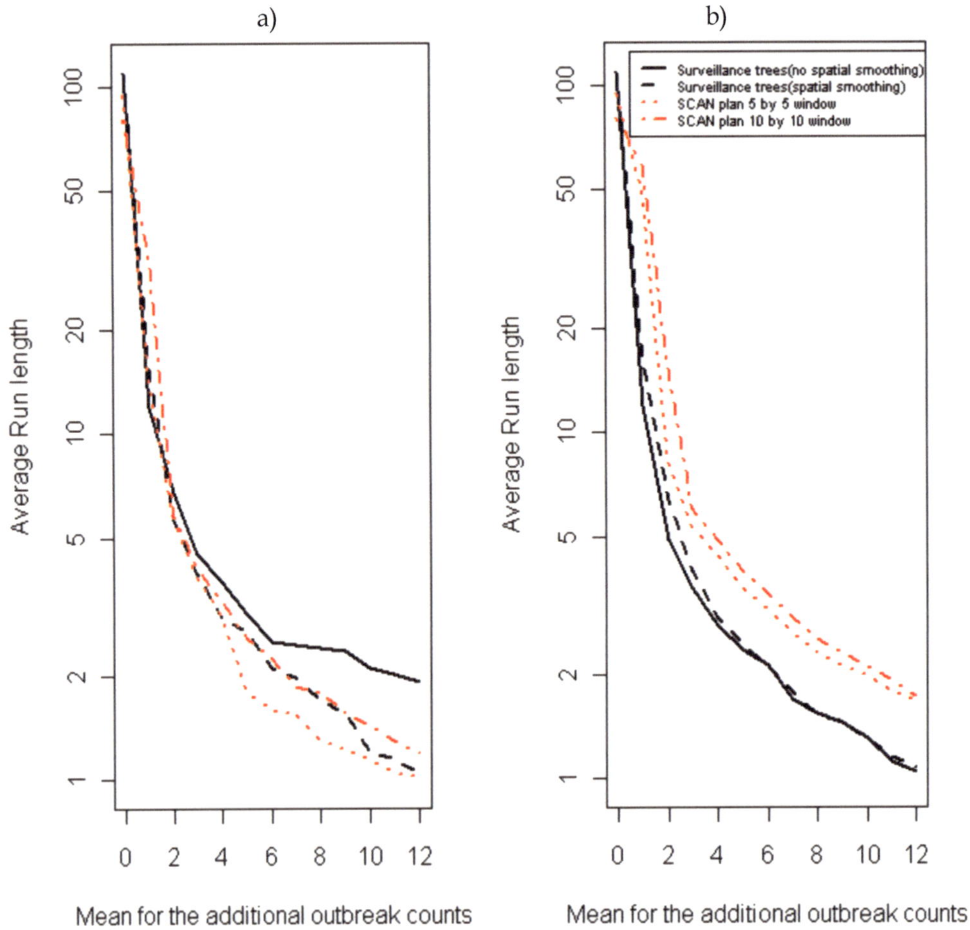

Fig. 7. In-control and out-of-control ARL for the SCAN plan and Surveillance Tree plan

6. Appendix

Inputs to the function are mu=overall mean; bweekday=day-of-the-week influence; bcos and bsin = influence of the season; blags = is the influence of previous counts; nob= number of counts generated; k is the threshold specifying the lowest expected count allowed (Poisson counts are truncated at times).

```
transitionalPoisson<-function(mu,bweekday,bcos,bsin,blags,nob,k){
nlag<-length(blags)
lcounts<-rep(0,nlag)
dw<-1
for(i in 1:nob){
temp<-
mu+bweekday[dw]+bcos*cos(2*pi*i/365.25)+bsin*sin(2*pi*i/365.25)+sum(blags*log(lcounts
+1))
```

```
temp[temp<k]<-k
if(i==1)ncount<-rpois(1,exp(temp)) else ncount<-c(ncount,rpois(1,exp(temp)))
lcounts[2:nlag]<-lcounts[1:(nlag-1)]
lcounts[1]<-ncount[i]
dw<-dw+1
if(dw>7)dw<-1}
ncount}
```

7. References

Bermudez, L. & Karlis, D. (2011). Bayesian multivariate Poisson models for insurance ratemaking. *Insurance: Mathematics and Economics*, 48:226-236.

Currie, I., Durban, M. & Eilers, P. (2003). Using p-splines to extrapolate two-dimensional poisson data. In Proceedings of the 18th International *Workshop on Statistical Modeling*, Verbeke, G. Molenberghs, A., & Fieuws, S. (Eds.). Katholieke Universiteit Leuven: 97–102.

Chen, J., & Glaz, J. (1996). Two-Dimensional Discrete SCAN Statistics, Statistics and Probability Letters, 3 1 : 59-68.

Glaz, J., Naus, J. & Wallenstein, S. (2001) *SCAN Statistics*. Springer, New York.

Grijalva, T., Bohara, A.K. & Berrens, R.P. (2003). A seemingly unrelated Poisson model for revealed and stated preference data, *Applied Economics Letters*, 10: 443-446.

Han, S. W., Mei, Y. & Tsui, K.-L. (2008). A comparison between SCAN and CUSUM methods for detecting increases in Poisson rates, *Technical Report*, School of ISyE, Georgia Institute of Technology.

Joner M. D., Woodall, W.H. Reynolds, M.R., Fricker, R.D. (2008). A One-sided MEWMA Chart for Health Surveillance. *Quality and Reliability Engineering International*. 24: 503-518.

Karlis, D. & Meligkotsidou, L. (2005). Multivariate Poisson regression with covariance structure. *Statistics and Computing*, 15: 255-265.

King, G. (1989), "A Seemingly Unrelated Poisson Regression Model," *Sociological Methods and Research*, 17: 235–255.

Kulldorff, M. & Nagarwalla N. (1995). Spatial disease clusters: Detection and Inference. *Statistics in Medicine*, 14:799-810.

Kulldorff, M. (1997). A spatial SCAN statistic, *Communications in Statistics: Theory and Methods*, 26:1481-1496.

Kulldorff, M. (2001). Prospective time periodic geographical disease surveillance using a SCAN statistic, *Journal of the Royal Statistical Society Series A-Statistics in Society* 164: 61-72.

Kulldorff, M., Heffernan R., Hartman J., Assunção RM., Mostashari F. (2005). A space-time permutation SCAN statistic for the early detection of disease outbreaks, *PLoS Medicine*, 2:216-224.

Lee, D-J. & Durban, M. (2009). Smooth-CAR mixed models for spatial count data. *Computational Statistics and Data Analysis*, 53: 2968-2979.

Raubertas, R.F. (1989). An analysis of disease surveillance data that uses the geographic locations of reporting units, *Statistics in Medicine*, 18: 2111-2122.

Riedel, K.S. (1993). Optimal data-based kernel estimation of evolutionary spectra. IEEE Transactions on signal processing, 41: 2439-2447.

Rogerson, P.A. & Yamada, I. (2004). Monitoring Change in Spatial Patterns of Disease: Comparing Univariate and Multivariate Cumulative Sum Approaches. *Statistics in Medicine*, 23 (14): 2195-2214.

Rogerson, P.A., Lee, G. & Yamada, I. (2006). Statistical methods for detection and monitoring of spatial clusters. Technical report. See www.acsu.buffalo.edu/~rogerson/technical%20report.doc

Sarka, III, J.L. (2011). Surveillance of negative binomial and Bernoulli processes. Ph.D. Thesis, Virginia Tech.

Sparks, R. (2000). CUSUM Charts for Signalling Varying Location Shifts. Journal of Quality Technology. 32(2):157-171.

Sparks, R., Carter,C., Graham, P.L., Muscatello, D., Churches, T., Kaldor, J., Turner, R., Zheng, W. & Ryan, L. (2010a). Understanding sources of variation in syndromic surveillance for early warning of natural or intentional disease outbreaks. IIE Transactions, 42(9): 613-631.

Sparks, R.S. & Okugami, C. (2010b). Surveillance trees: early detection of unusually high number of vehicle crashes, *InterStat*, January, see http://interstat.statjournals.net/YEAR/2010/abstracts/1001002.php

Sparks, R.S., Keighley, T. & Muscatello, D. (2011a). Exponentially weighted moving average plans for detecting unusual negative binomial counts. *IIE Transactions* 42:721-733.

Sparks, R.S., Keighley, T. & Muscatello, D. (2011b). Optimal exponentially weighted moving average(EWMA) plans for detecting seasonal epidemics when faced with non-homogeneous negative binomial counts. *Journal of Applied Statistics*. DOI: 10.1080/02664763.2010.545184.

Sparks, R.S. (2011c). Spatially clustered outbreak detection using EWMA SCAN statistics with multiple sized windows. *Communications in Statistics – Simulation and Computation*. To appear.

Steiner, S.H., Grant, K., Coory, M. & Kelly, H.A. (2011). Detecting the start of an influenza outbreak using exponentially weighted moving average charts. *BMC Medical Informatics and Decision Making*, 10:37.

Tango, T. (1995). A class of test for detecting general and focused clustering of rare diseases. *Statistics in Medicine*, 14: 2323-23334.

Woodall, W. H., Marshall, J. B. , Joner, M. D. Jr., Fraker, J. E. & Abdel-Salam, A. G. (2008). On the use and evaluation of prospective SCAN methods for health-related surveillance, *Journal of the Royal Statistical Society: Series A* 171: 223-237.

Yu, X., Tang, L.A. & Han, J. (2009). Filtering and Refinement: A two stage approach for efficient detection of anomalies. 9th IEEE International Conference on Data Mining.

9

Rickettsia and Rickettsial Diseases

Xue-jie Yu and David H. Walker
Department of Pathology, University of Texas Medical Branch, Galveston, Texas USA

1. Introduction

Rickettsia prowazekii and *R. rickettsii* are HHS and USDA select agents (http://biosafety.utk.edu/pdfs/salist.pdf), and *R. prowazekii* is a category B bioterrorism agent as determined by the Centers for Disease Control and Prevention (CDC) (http://www.bt.cdc.gov/agent/agentlist-category.asp). The criteria for CDC category B bioterrorism agents are that the organisms are moderately easy to disseminate, cause diseases with moderate morbidity and low mortality and require specific enhancements of diagnostic capacity and enhanced disease surveillance. However, the case fatality ratios of both *R. prowazekii* and *R. rickettsii* may exceed the CDC bioterrorism agent category B level. Epidemic typhus caused by *R. prowazekii* and Rocky Mountain spotted fever (RMSF) caused by *R. rickettsii* can reach up to 60% fatalities without antibiotic treatment and 4% even with antibiotic treatment (Raoult et al., 2004). *Rickettsia* had been explored for biowarfare use. The former Soviet Union developed *R. prowazekii* as a biologic weapon in the 1930s (Alibek K and Handelman S, 2009). During World War II, the Japanese performed human experiments with rickettsial agents for purposes of biologic weapon development during their occupation of China (Harris S, 1992).

Epidemic typhus, also known as louse-borne typhus, has been distributed worldwide, was one of the man's major scourges and frequently played a decisive role in wars in Europe from the 15th through 20th centuries, thus affecting the course of European history (Conlon JM, 2007). It killed millions of people through this period. Although worldwide epidemics of typhus may not occur again, the threat of louse-borne typhus is still real as small scale epidemics or large scale epidemics in settings of extreme poverty and natural and manmade disasters. Louse-borne typhus occurs in epidemics when social, economic, or political systems are disrupted exposing a large population such as refugees to louse infestation due to lack of hygiene. This situation has been observed in recent outbreaks of typhus in Burundi, Algeria, Peru, and Russia. In 1997, it was estimated that as many as 100,000 cases of typhus occurred in the refugee camps of Burundi during a civil war (Raoult et al., 2004).

RMSF originated as an emerging infectious disease on the western *frontier* in the Rocky Mountains. Now the disease is found all over the United States, and over half of the cases occur in the southeastern and south-central regions of the United States and in South America (Center for Disease Control and prevention[CDC], 2010).

2. Etiologic agents

Rickettsia are small (0.3 - 0.5 x 0.8 - 1.0 µm) gram-negative obligately intracellular bacterial parasites of eukaryotic cells. The genus is subdivided into the typhus group (TG) and spotted fever group (SFG) based on lipopolysaccharide (LPS) antigens. The TG rickettsiae include louse-borne *R. prowazekii* that causes epidemic typhus and flea-borne *R. typhi* that causes murine typhus. The SFG rickettsiae consist of more than 20 named species, which are transmitted by tick bite except for *R. akari* (mite-borne) and *R. felis* (flea-borne). Antibodies to LPS antigens cross-react among organisms within the same biogroup, but do not cross-react between the two groups (Vishwanath, 1991). There are two major outer membrane proteins in *Rickettsia* OmpA (Sca 0) and OmpB (Sca5). OmpB exists in all *Rickettsia* and OmpA exists only in SFG rickettsiae. Genomic sequencing identified additional 14 surface cell antigens (Scas) among *Rickettsia (Blanc et al., 2005)*. However, most *sca* genes are degenerated in *Rickettsia,* and only two Scas (Sca4 and Sca5 also called OmpB) present in all *Rickettsia*. Scas of gram-negative bacteria belong to the autotransporter protein family which are usually associated with virulence functions.

2.1 Pathogenesis and pathophysiology

In vitro experiments showed that *Rickettsia* attaches to the host cell through its surface proteins, OmpB, OmpA, Sca1, and Sca2, and host cell receptors (Martinez et al., 2005). After attachment, *Rickettsia* induces non-phagocytic endothelial cells to engulf it. Once it enters the host cell, *Rickettsia immediately* lyses the phagosomal membrane and escapes into the cytoplasm. *Rickettsia* multiplies by binary fission with a doubling time of 8 hours. Both TG and SFG rickettsiae multiply in the cytoplasm of host cells, but SFG rickettsiae can also invade and multiply in the nucleus of host cells. TG rickettsiae accumulate in cytoplasm until the host cell bursts, but SFG rickettsiae seldom accumulate in host cells. The difference in the quantity of organisms that accumulate in host cells between TG and SFG rickettsiae is believed to be caused by the facts that SFG rickettsiae move by actin-based mobility inside the cytoplasm and can spread to adjacent cells, but TG rickettsiae do not move and cannot spread. SFG rickettsiae hijack the cell's actin which they stimulate to polymerize at one bacterial pole to facilitate their own movement (Teysseire et al., 1992). Due to the actin-based movement, SFG rickettsiae spread from cell to cell eventuating in cell death and thus the formation of large plaques in cell culture. In contrast, typhus group rickettsiae accumulate in the host cell and form very small plaques when the heavily infected cells burst.

The target cell of *Rickettsia in vivo* is microvascular endothelium. The crucial pathophysiologic effect of rickettsial endothelial infection is increased microvascular permeability resulting from discontinuities in interendothelial adherens junctions. The pathogenic mechanisms of endothelial injury include endothelial cell production of toxic reactive oxygen species, damage to the cell membrane upon rickettsial exit, and cytotoxic T lymphocyte-induced apoptosis of infected endothelial cells. Rickettsial infections cause a procoagulant state, but only very rarely disseminated intravascular coagulation. Thrombi comprise non-occlusive hemostatic plugs that are appropriately located at foci of severe endothelial damage to mitigate hemorrhage (Walker DH, 2011).

2.2 Epidemiology and ecology

A part or the entire life cycle of rickettsiae is usually associated with one species of arthropod, including lice, fleas, ticks and mites. Arthropods are the vectors and, in most cases, the reservoir of rickettsiae. The distribution of tick-borne SFG rickettsioses are restricted to areas where their tick reservoirs are present, such as Rocky Mountain spotted fever in the Americas, Mediterranean spotted fever in Europe, Africa and Asia, and Japanese spotted fever in Japan and eastern Asia (Table 1). Human louse-, flea-, and mouse

Disease	Rickettsial agent	Vector	Geographic Distribution
SFG rickettsiae			
African tick- bite fever	*Rickettsia africae*	Ticks	Sub-Saharan Africa, Caribbean islands (Mediannikov et al., 2010)
Far eastern spotted fever	*Rickettsia heilongjiangensis*	Ticks	Far East of Asia (Mediannikov et al., 2004)
Flinders Island spotted fever	*Rickettsia honei*	Ticks	Australia and southeastern Asia (Graves S & Stenos J, 2003)
Mediterranean spotted fever	*Rickettsia conorii*	Ticks	Southern Europe, southern and western Asia, and Africa (Rovery et al., 2008)
North Asian tick typhus Lymphangitis-associated rickettsiosis	*Rickettisa sibirica* *Rickettsia sibirica mongolotimonae*	Ticks	Asia, Europe, and Africa (Fournier et al., 2005)
Japanese spotted fever	*Rickettsia japonica*	Ticks	Japan and eastern Asia (Chung et al., 2006)
Queensland tick typhus	*Rickettsia australis*	Ticks	Australia (Sexton et al., 1991)
Rocky Mountain spotted fever	*Rickettsia rickettsii*	Ticks	North, Central and South America (Galvao MA et al., 2003)
Tick-borne lymphadenopathy	*Rickettsia slovaca*	Ticks	Europe (Selmi et al., 2008)
Unnamed	*Rickettsia parkeri*	Ticks	North and South America (Nava et al., 2008)
Unnamed	*Rickettsia massiliae*	Ticks	Europe and North and South America (Labruna MB, 2009)
Unnamed	*Rickettsia aeschlimannii*	Ticks	Europe and Africa (Raoult et al., 2002)
Unnamed	*Rickettsia monacensis*	Ticks	Europe (Jado et al., 2007)
Unnamed	*Rickettsia helvetica*	Ticks	Europe and Asia (Fournier et al., 2004)
Rickettsialpox	*R. akari*	Mite	Worldwide
Cat flea rickettsiosis	*R. felis*	Flea	Worldwide
TG rickettsiae			
Epidemic typhus	*R. prowazekii*	Louse	Worldwide
Murine typhus	*R. typhi*	Flea	Worldwide

Table 1. Distribution of rickettsioses

mite-borne *Rickettsia* such as *R. prowazekii, R. typhi, R. felis,* and *R. akari* are distributed worldwide with their hosts and vectors.

Non-virulent or low virulence SFG rickettsiae may be maintained in nature largely via transovarian transmission in the arthropod hosts. However, highly virulent SFG rickettsiae such as *R. rickettsii* and *R. conorii* are pathogenic for the *Dermacentor* and *Rhipicephalus* ticks, respectively (Niebylski et al., 1999; Santos et al., 2002). Virulent rickettsiae such as *R. rickettsii* need an animal host to amplify the organisms for establishing new lines of transovarian rickettsial maintenance (e.g., *D. variabilis* ticks acquire *R. rickettsii* while feeding on rickettsemic cotton rats) (Niebylski et al., 1999). Each species of pathogenic SFG rickettsiae may have one or multiple tick vector species. The vectors of Rocky Mountain spotted fever are *D. variabilis* (American dog tick) in the eastern two-thirds of the US and regions of the Pacific coast states, *D. andersoni* (wood tick) in the Rocky Mountain states, *Rhipicephalus sanguineus* (brown dog tick) in the southwestern US, northern Mexico, and South America and *Amblyomma cajennense* and *A. aureolatum* in South America. The seasonal and geographic distribution of each rickettsiosis reflects the months of activity of the vector and its contact with humans. Over 90% of cases with Rocky Mountain spotted fever occur during April through September. Approximately 250-2000 cases of Rocky Mountain spotted fever have been reported annually in the United States (CDC, 2010).

Epidemic typhus is transmitted primarily by the human body louse, *Pediculus humanus corporis*. However, the louse is only a vector and not a reservoir because infected lice die 5-7 days after they become infected with *R. prowazekii. Rickettsia prowazekii* multiplies in louse gut epithelium, which detaches, ruptures and releases rickettsiae into the feces. The louse feces containing rickettsiae are scratched into the skin, rubbed into mucous membranes such as the conjunctiva, or inhaled. Humans can develop latent infection after acute louse-borne typhus and serve as reservoirs of *R. prowazekii. R. prowazekii* can be reactivated causing recrudescent typhus fever (Brill-Zinsser disease) when latently infected persons' immunity wanes. *Rickettsia prowazekii* is also maintained in a zoonotic cycle involving flying squirrels (*Glaucomys volans*) and their specific flea and louse in the United States. Sporadic epidemic typhus occurring in the United States is transmitted by fleas of flying squirrels (Duma et al., 1981). Murine typhus is transmitted by fleas including rat fleas and cat fleas.

3. Virulence determinants of *Rickettsia*

Rickettsia has no exotoxin, and rickettsial LPS is not toxic and apparently is not associated with the pathogenesis of *Rickettsia* infections. Since *Rickettsia* are obligately intracellular bacteria, their survival mechanisms involve proteins related to the attachment, to entry into and exit from host cells, and enzymes for protein and DNA modification and obtaining nutrition from the host.

Adhesins: The first step for obligately intracellular *Rickettsia* to establish infection is to adhere to and invade the host endothelium. These processes require the interaction of rickettsial surface proteins with mammalian host cell receptors. Three outer membrane proteins of *Rickettsia* OmpA, OmpB, and Sca2 have been identified as adhesins of *Rickettsia*(Li & Walker, 1998; Martinez et al., 2005; Cardwell & Martinez, 2009). OmpB has been demonstrated to interact with its mammalian receptor, Ku70. However, in Ku70$^{-/-}$ mouse embryonic fibroblasts *R. conorii* invasion is reduced only 50 to 60%, suggesting that *Rickettsia* may use multiple adhesins and receptors.

Membranolytic enzymes: Internalized rickettsiae are initially bound within a phagosome (Teysseire et al., 1995). *Rickettsia* quickly (<10 min) lyse the phagosomal membrane to escape from phagosomal vacuoles before phagolysosomal fusion occurs, which would result in the death of the *Rickettsia* through the activity of the lysosomal enzymes (Teysseire et al., 1995;Hackstadt, 1996;Feng & Walker, 2000;Walker et al., 2001a). *Rickettsia* are also required to exit the host cell by lysis of the host cell membrane. The mechanism of lysis of the phagosomal membrane and the host cell membrane has been hypothesized to be mediated by a phospholipase enzyme (Radulovic et al., 1999;Renesto et al., 2003). The genomic sequences of *Rickettsia* have revealed four proteins with potential membranolytic activities: patatin B1 precursor (*pat-1* gene), hemolysin A (*tlyA*), hemolysin C (*tlyC*), and phospholipase D (*pld*) (Andersson et al., 1998;Ogata et al., 2001;McLeod et al., 2004). TlyC has been demonstrated to have hemolytic activity, (Radulovic et al., 1999) and can mediate escape by *S. enterica* serovar Typhimurium from phagosomes (Whitworth et al., 2005). Patatin B of *R. typhi* (RT0522) has been implicated as a phospholipase A2. However, knockout of *R. prowazekii pld* gene does not prevent *R. prowazekii* escape from the phagosome or exit from host cells. Patatin B is truncated by an ISRpe 1 transposon in *R. peacockii*, which apparently does not affect the release of *R. peacockii* from phagosomes (Felsheim RF). These observations suggest that the multiple membranolytic enzymes of *Rickettsia* may be functionally redundant.

Actin-based mobility: Like other intracytosolic bacteria such as *Listeria monocytogenes* and *Shigella flexneri*, SFG rickettsiae exploit the host cell actin cytoskeleton to promote intracellular mobility and cell-to-cell spread by assembling distinctive 'comet tails' that consist of long, unbranched actin filaments(Tilney and Portnoy, 1989;Bernardini et al., 1989;Teysseire et al., 1992;Heinzen et al., 1993). The molecular mechanisms of actin polymerization by *L. monocytogenes* and *S. flexneri* primarily involve activation of the Arp2/3 complex, an actin nucleator that can initiate the polymerization of new actin filaments and organize filaments into Y-branched arrays (Mullins et al., 1998;Welch et al., 1998;Blanchoin et al., 2000). In host cells, the Arp2/3 complex is activated by nucleation-promoting factors including members of the Wiskott–Aldrich syndrome protein (WASP) family of proteins(Higgs & Pollard, 2001;Welch & Mullins, 2002). The mechanisms of activation of the Arp2/3 complex by intracellular pathogens are that they express surface proteins that recruit host WASP family proteins (e.g., *S. flexneri* IcsA), or they express functional mimics of WASPs (e.g., *L. monocytogenes* ActA) (Goldberg, 2001). It was proposed that actin in *Rickettsia* comet tails is nucleated by the host Arp2/3 complex, and the bacterial protein RickA has been shown to assemble branched actin networks *in vitro*(Jeng et al., 2004;Gouin et al., 2004) . Coincidently, RickA is inactivated by an ISRpe1 transposon in *R. peacockii*, which does not have actin-based mobility(Simser et al., 2005). However, a new discovery suggests that besides RickA Sca2 is also involved in the actin-based mobility of *Rickettsia*. Knocking out the *sca2* gene completely aborts actin-based mobility of *R. rickettsii*. Sca2 mimics eukaryotic formins to determine the unique organization of actin filaments in *Rickettsia* tails and to drive bacterial mobility, independently of host nucleators. Actin-based mobility is important for the virulence of some rickettsiae such as *R. rickettsii*, but it is not important for the virulence of TG rickettsiae because TG rickettsiae do not have actin-based mobility or have only erratic mobility. Even SFG rickettsiae with actin-based mobility are not all virulent such as *R. bellii*, a tick symbiont, which has actin-based mobility but has not yet been shown to cause disease in humans or animals.

Methyltransferase: The patterns of methylation of lysine in the surface antigens of avirulent Madrid E (E) strain, virulent revertant Evir strain, and wild type Breinl strain of *R. prowazekii* are different. The major surface antigen of the virulent Breinl and Evir strains contains more N^{ϵ}-Me3-lysine and less N^{ϵ}-Me-lysine than the avirulent E strain (Rodionov et al., 1991;Turco & Winkler, 1994). Outer membrane protein B (OmpB) is heavily methylated in the virulent strains, while OmpB from the attenuated strain is hypomethylated(Ching et al., 1992). The methyltransferase gene (Rp028/Rp027) is inactivated by a frameshift mutation in E strain, but the mutation reverts to wild type in the virulent revertant Evir strain. A single nucleotide mutation in the methyltransferase gene is the only mutation in E strain compared to Evir strain (Yu, unpublished data). Taken together our results and the previous discovery that E strain is deficient in methylation of OmpB suggests strongly that the reversible mutation in the methyltransferase gene determines the virulence state of E strain, i.e., the organisms become avirulent when the gene is inactivated in E strain, and the organisms become virulent when the gene function is restored in Evir strain.

3.1 Clinical spectrum/treatment

Spotted fever: Rocky Mountain spotted fever caused by *R. rickettsii* is a very severe disease, and fatal cases occur in association with delayed or ineffective antibiotic treatment in as many as 4% of cases. RMSF occurs 1 -2 weeks after feeding by an infected tick. The disease is characterized by acute onset of fever that may be accompanied by headache, malaise, myalgia, nausea/vomiting, or neurologic signs. A macular or maculopapular rash appears 3-5 days following onset in most (~90%) patients, and the rash has a centripetal pattern of spread, meaning that it begins on the extremities and spreads towards the trunk. In severe disease, petechiae appear in the center of the maculopapules. However, 10% to 15% of persons with RMSF never develop a rash, a condition referred to as "Rocky Mountain *spotless* fever"(Sexton & Corey, 1992). The target of *Rickettsia* is endothelium of blood vessels. Inflammation and damage of endothelia of capillary blood vessels by *Rickettsia* results in increased vacular permeability, which causes rash, hypovolemic hypotension, pulmonary and cerebral edema and organ failure.

Other spotted fevers may have similar clinical symptoms as RMSF, but are less severe. Rash is less frequent in less severe rickettsioses such as African tick bite fever and *R. parkeri* infection. Focal skin necrosis with a dark scab (an eschar) at the site of tick feeding is a common feature of boutonneuse fever, African tick bite fever, North Asian tick typhus, Queensland tick typhus, Japanese spotted fever, Flinders Island spotted fever, rickettsialpox, tick-borne lymphadenopathy, and the recently described infections in the US caused by *R. parkeri* and a novel strain 364 D, but is rare in Rocky Mountain spotted fever.

Typhus: Epidemic typhus and murine typhus are caused by *R. prowazekii* and *R. typhi*, respectively. Historically murine typhus and epidemic typhus were difficult to differentiate due to similar clinical symptoms, but epidemic typhus is more severe than murine typhus. Murine typhus occurs predominantly in summer and fall, and epidemic typhus usually occurs in winter. Symptoms of typhus may include high fever (105 - 106 degrees Fahrenheit), which may last up to 2 weeks, severe headache, severe muscle pain (myalgia), dry cough, delirium, stupor, and a dull red rash that begins on the trunk and spreads peripherally.

Tetracyclines are first-line treatment, and doxycycline may be used to avoid tooth staining in children. Tetracyclines are rickettsiostatic, not rickettsicidal. Chloramphenicol is a second line, less effective treatment that can be used in the rare instance of contraindication to use of doxycycline. Ciprofloxacin, other fluoroquinolones, azithromycin, and clarinthromycin are effective against certain rickettsiae but are not recommended for the severe rickettsioses. Because diagnostic tests can take time and may be insensitive, antibiotics are usually begun presumptively to prevent significant deterioration, complications, death, sequelae, and prolonged recovery.

3.2 Immune mechanisms of *Rickettsia*

Most of our understanding of the immune response against *Rickettsia* is derived from *in vitro* studies as well as the murine models of rickettsioses. Proinflammatory cytokines such as IFN-γ and TNF-α are essential for primary defense against rickettsial infection. These cytokines act in concert to activate endothelial cells, the major target cells of rickettsial infections, as well as other minor target cells to kill intracellular organisms via nitric oxide synthesis-dependent and indoleamine 2,3-dioxygenase-dependent mechanisms. The sources of these protective cytokines are hypothesized to be the T lymphocytes and macrophages that infiltrate the perivascular space surrounding the vessels with infected endothelium.

Cell mediated immunity plays a critical role in host defenses against rickettsial infections(Walker et al., 2001b). There are two important effector components of the acquired immune response against *Rickettsia*, namely IFN- γ production by $CD4^+$ and $CD8^+$ type-1 cells, which activates intracellular bactericidal mechanisms of endothelial cells and macrophages, and the generation of *Rickettsia*-specific cytotoxic $CD8^+$ T cells that induce apoptosis in infected target cells via pathways involving perforin and/or granzymes. $CD8^+$ T cells are more important in clearance of rickettsial infection than $CD4^+$ T cells(Walker et al., 2001b). Although adoptive transfer of either CD4 or CD8 immune T lymphocytes controls the infection and leads to survival, only depletion of CD8 T lymphocytes alters the outcome of infection, and depletion of CD4 cells has no observed effect on the course or outcome of infection(Walker et al., 2001c).

The humoral response may play an important role in protection against infection, and antibodies against surface protein antigens are very likely critical effectors of vaccine-associated protective immunity. In animal experiments, antibodies to Rickettsia or rickettsial outer membrane proteins can neutralize rickettsia (Anacker et al., 1987;Li et al., 1988). However, natural infection does not result in the production of protective antibodies prior to clearance of rickettsiae. Thus, humoral immunity may be more important in preventing reinfection and in vaccine-induced immunity than in clearance of primary infection.

4. Experimental vaccines and other potential vaccine prospects

Currently no commercial vaccine is available for any rickettsial disease. Infection with *R. rickettsii* and *R. conorii* is believed to confer long lasting immunity against re-infection. Thus, it is feasible to develop a vaccine against rickettsial diseases. In theory, a subunit vaccine targeting a conserved rickettsial protein such as OmpB may be developed to prevent all rickettsial diseases. An attenuated organism that can multiply, but does not cause disease in the host, has been proved to be effective in protection against rickettsial infections in humans and laboratory animals. Attenuated *Rickettsia* has been selected by passage in chicken egg yolk sacs in the past and was recently achieved by gene knockout technology.

Inactivated vaccine. The history of development of vaccines against rickettsial diseases contains numerous failures and limited success in preventing or ameliorating disease. Killed rickettsial vaccine was prepared from infected ticks in 1924, in yolk sac of embryonated chicken eggs in 1938 (Cox HR, 1939), and from cell culture in the 1970s (Gonder et al., 1979;Kenyon et al., 1979). The original tick-derived rickettsial vaccine produced severe local inoculation site reactions(Spencer RR and Parker RR, 1925). Evaluation of its protective effect in field use was impressive by the standards of the day. The fatality rate from Rocky Mountain spotted fever among vaccine recipients was reduced dramatically although illness and even death occurred in some vaccinated persons. The killed yolk sac-derived rickettsial vaccine was never field tested. When tested by challenge of human volunteers, neither the yolk sac vaccine nor the tick vaccine prevented the illness, which, of course, was treated to prevent severe illness or death. The yolk sac vaccine was withdrawn from the market in 1978. A subsequent challenge trial of a cell culture killed-*R. rickettsii* vaccine yielded protection of 25% of the volunteers who received it(Gonder et al., 1979).

Subunit vaccine for Rickettsia. Two surface protein antigens of *R. rickettsii*, OmpA and OmpB, have been identified as major protective antigens and are candidates for use as subunit vaccines. The first evidence that OmpA and OmpB contain protective epitopes came from the studies of monoclonal antibodies to heat sensitive epitopes of OmpA and OmpB, which neutralized *R. rickettsii* toxicity in mice and infection in guinea pigs (Anacker et al., 1987;Li et al., 1988). The *E. coli*-expressed OmpA N-terminal fragment partially protects guinea pigs against a lethal challenge dose of *R. rickettsii* (McDonald et al., 1988). A fragment from the N-terminus of *R. conorii* OmpA protects guinea pigs against experimental infection with *R. conorii* and partially protects guinea pigs from challenge with the heterologous *R. rickettsii* (Vishwanath et al., 1990). Fragments of the *ompA* and *ompB* genes have been tested as DNA vaccines. In a regimen of DNA immunization followed by boosters of the corresponding peptide, mice immunized with *R. rickettsii ompA* or *ompB* fragments are partially protected against a lethal challenge with heterologous *R. conorii*(Diaz-Montero et al., 2001). It is not known whether the incomplete protection of OmpA and OmpB against the heterologous *Rickettsia* species challenge in these experiments is caused by the antigenic differences between the rickettsial species, the immunization regimen, or the antigen composition.

Live vaccine. The attenuated Madrid E (E) strain of *R. prowazekii* was used in humans as an experimental vaccine from the 1950s to 1970s. E strain is a spontaneous laboratory variant of *R. prowazekii* that was isolated from a typhus patient in Madrid in 1941 and passed in rapid succession in embryonated chicken eggs 255 times. This strain has limited virulence for guinea pigs and low virulence for humans. E strain is protective and provides long term immunity against louse-borne typhus. Ninety-four percent (170/181) of immunized persons were protected from natural infection by epidemic typhus compared to the unvaccinated controls in a 14-month period after vaccination. Ninety-six percent (27/28) of volunteers who were vaccinated with E strain and subsequently challenged with Breinl strain at intervals from 2 months to 36 months remained healthy following challenge, and 83% (5/6) of the volunteers who were challenged at 48 to 66 months were protected(FOX et al., 1961). However, the E strain vaccine caused a late reaction in up to 14% of vaccinated persons 9-14 days after inoculation. The late reaction varied from simple malaise and mild headache to modified typhus characterized by fever, headache, malaise and occasionally a rash in a small proportion of subjects. The reason for the late reaction was not known at the time. In 1970s a virulent revertant Evir strain was isolated from guinea pigs by passage of E strain in guinea pigs or mice.

Attenuation of Rickettsia by gene knockout. Because of the difficulty of transforming *Rickettsia,* scientists were unable to knock out rickettsial genes to determine their function and to create an attenuated rickettsial vaccine until recently. The phopholipase D (*pld*) gene was the first rickettsial gene that was genetically knocked out. The *pld*-inactivated Evir strain is avirulent for guinea pigs at doses for which the Evir strain is virulent and stimulates protective immunity to virulent *R. prowazekii* (Driskell et al., 2009). Genetic inactivation of *sca-2* in *R. rickettsii* results in loss of actin-based mobility in cell culture (Kleba et al., 2010). Sca-2 deficient *R. rickettsii* lacks the ability to cause disease in guinea pigs, but stimulates protection against challenge with virulent *R. rickettsii* (Kleba et al., 2010). Thus, Sca-2 and phospholipase D-deficient strains should be further evaluated as vaccines for Rocky Mountain spotted fever and epidemic typhus. Genetically attenuated *Rickettsia* are the strongest future prospect for developing an effective rickettsial vaccine.

Differentiation of strains of *R. prowazekii* and *R. rickettsii*. *R. prowazekii* has been isolated from humans, flying squirrels, and ticks for more than half century. Due to different sources and different passages, *R. prowazekii* strain can be grouped in to three virulence groups: high virulence group represented by Breinl strain, medium virulence group represented by flying squirrel isolates and low virulence or non-virulence group represented by Madrid E strain and its revertant strains. All strains of *R. prowazekii* can be differentiated by sequencing several loci of the genome of *R. prowazekii* (Zhu et al., 2008). *R. rickettsii* strains were not genetically typed except for virulent R strain and nonvirulent Iowa strains, whose whole genomes were completely sequenced (Ellison et al., 2008).

5. Conclusion

There has been progress in molecular biology, cellular biology and immunology and pathogenesis of *Rickettsia*. However, diagnosis of rickettsial diseases is still difficult and is usually retrospective. Rapid diagnostic methods are required for diagnosis of rickettsial diseases and in response to bioterrorism.

6. References

Alibek K; & Handelman S. (2009). Biohazard: the chilling true story of the largest covert biological weapons program in the world told from the inside by the man who ran it. Hutchinson, London

Anacker; R. L., McDonald, G. A., List, R. H. & Mann. R. E. (1987). Neutralizing activity of monoclonal antibodies to heat-sensitive and heat-resistant epitopes of Rickettsia rickettsii surface proteins: Infect.Immun., v. 55, no. 3, pp. 825-827.

Andersson; S. G., Zomorodipour, A., Andersson, J. O., Sicheritz-Ponten, T., Alsmark, U. C., Podowski, R. M., Naslund, A. K., Eriksson, A. S. , Winkler, H. H. & Kurland, C. G. (1998) The genome sequence of Rickettsia prowazekii and the origin of mitochondria: Nature, v. 396, no. 6707, pp. 133-140

Bernardini; M. L., Mounier, J., d'Hauteville, H., Coquis-Rondon, M. & Sansonetti, P. J. (1989). Identification of icsA, a plasmid locus of Shigella flexneri that governs bacterial intra- and intercellular spread through interaction with F-actin: Proc.Natl.Acad Sci U.S.A, v. 86, no. 10, pp. 3867-3871

Blanc, G.; Ngwamidiba, M., Ogata, H., Fournier, P. E., Claverie, J. M. & Raoult, D. (2005). Molecular evolution of rickettsia surface antigens: evidence of positive selection: Mol.Biol.Evol., v. 22, no. 10, pp. 2073-2083

Blanchoin, L.; Amann, K. J., Higgs, H. N., Marchand, J. B., Kaiser, D. A. & Pollard, T. D. (2000). Direct observation of dendritic actin filament networks nucleated by Arp2/3 complex and WASP/Scar proteins: Nature, v. 404, no. 6781, pp. 1007-1011

Cardwell, M. M.; & Martinez, J. J. (2009). The Sca2 autotransporter protein from Rickettsia conorii is sufficient to mediate adherence to and invasion of cultured mammalian cells: Infect.Immun., v. 77, no. 12, pp. 5272-5280

Center for Disease Control and prevention, 2010, Rocky Mountain Spotted Fever, Website, <http://www.cdc.gov/rmsf/stats/>

Ching, W. M.; Carl, M. & Dasch, G. A. (1992). Mapping of monoclonal antibody binding sites on CNBr fragments of the S-layer protein antigens of Rickettsia typhi and Rickettsia prowazekii, Mol.Immunol., v. 29, no. 1, pp. 95-105

Chung, M. H.; Lee, S. H., Kim, M. J. , Lee, J. H., Kim, E. S., Kim, M. K., Park, M. Y.& Kang, J. S. (2006). Japanese spotted fever, South Korea, Emerg.Infect.Dis., v. 12, no. 7, pp. 1122-1124

Conlon JM. (2007). The historical impact of epidemic typhus, Website, <http://phthiraptera.info/sites/phthiraptera.info/files/61235.pdf>

Cox HR. (1939). Rocky Mountain spotted fever: protective value for guinea pigs of vaccine prepared from rickettsia cultivated in embryonic chick tissues: Public Health Rep, v. 54, pp. 1070-1077

Diaz-Montero, C. M., H. M. Feng, P. A. Crocquet-Valdes, & D. H. Walker. (2001). Identification of protective components of two major outer membrane proteins of spotted fever group Rickettsiae: Am.J Trop.Med.Hyg., v. 65, no. 4, pp. 371-378

Driskell, L. O.; Yu, X. J., Zhang, L., Liu, Y., Popov, V. L., Walker, D. H., Tucker, A. M. & Wood, D. O. (2009). Directed mutagenesis of the Rickettsia prowazekii pld gene encoding phospholipase D: Infect.Immun., v. 77, no. 8, pp. 3244-3248

Duma, R. J.; Sonenshine, D. E., Bozeman, F. M., Veazey Jr., J. M., Elisberg, B. L., Chadwick, D. P., Stocks, N. I., McGill, T. M., Miller Jr., G. B. & MacCormack, J. N. (1981) Epidemic typhus in the United States associated with flying squirrels: JAMA, v. 245, no. 22, pp. 2318-2323

Ellison, D. W.; Clark, T. R., Sturdevant, D. E. , Virtaneva, K., Porcella, S. F. & T. Hackstadt. (2008). Genomic comparison of virulent Rickettsia rickettsii Sheila Smith and avirulent Rickettsia rickettsii Iowa: Infect.Immun., v. 76, no. 2, pp. 542-550

Feng, H. M. & Walker, D. H. (2000). Mechanisms of intracellular killing of Rickettsia conorii in infected human endothelial cells, hepatocytes, and macrophages, Infect.Immun., v. 68, no. 12, pp. 6729-6736

Fournier, P. E.; Allombert, C., Supputamongkol, Y. , Caruso, G., Brouqui, P. & D. Raoult. (2004). Aneruptive fever associated with antibodies to Rickettsia helvetica in Europe and Thailand, J Clin.Microbiol., v. 42, no. 2, pp. 816-818

Fournier, P. E.; F. Gouriet, P. Brouqui, F. Lucht, & D. Raoult. (2005). Lymphangitis-associated rickettsiosis, a new rickettsiosis caused by Rickettsia sibirica mongolotimonae: seven new cases and review of the literature, Clin.Infect.Dis., v. 40, no. 10, pp. 1435-1444.

Fox, J. P.; Montoya J. A., Jordan M. E., Cornejo U., Llosa G. J., Arce E. S. T. R., Gelfand H. M., & Herrera L. (1961). Immunization of man against epidemic typhus by infection with avirulent "Rickettsia prowazekii" (strain E): Rev.Sanid.Hig.Publica (Madr.), v. 35, pp. 481-512

Galvao M.A.; Mafra C.L., Moron C., Anaya E., & Walker D.H. (2003). Rickettsiosis of the genus Rickettsia in South America. Ann N Y Acad Sci, v. 990, pp. 57-61

Goldberg, M. B. (2001). Actin-based motility of intracellular microbial pathogens, Microbiol.Mol.Biol.Rev., v. 65, no. 4, pp. 595-626

Gonder, J. C.; Kenyon R. H., & Pedersen Jr., C. E., (1979). Evaluation of a killed Rocky Mountain spotted fever vaccine in cynomolgus monkeys, J Clin.Microbiol., v. 10, no. 5, p. 719-723

Graves S. & Stenos J. (2003). Rickettsia honei: a spotted fever Rickettsia on three continents, Ann N Y Acad Sci, v. 990, pp. 62-66

Gouin, E., Egile, C., Dehoux, P., Villiers, V., Adams, J., Gertler, F., Li, R., & Cossart, P. (2004). The RickA protein of Rickettsia conorii activates the Arp2/3 complex: Nature, v. 427, no. 6973, p. 457-461

Hackstadt, T. (1996). The biology of rickettsiae, Infect.Agents Dis., v. 5, no. 3, pp. 127-143.

Harris S. (1992). Japanese biological warfare research on humans: a case study of microbiology and ethics, Ann NY Acad Sci, v. 666, pp. 21-52

Heinzen, R. A.; Hayes, S. F., Peacock, M. G.& Hackstadt, T. (1993). Directional actin polymerization associated with spotted fever group Rickettsia infection of Vero cells, Infect.Immun., v. 61, no. 5, pp. 1926-1935

Higgs, H. N. & Pollard, T. D. (2001), Regulation of actin filament network formation through ARP2/3 complex: activation by a diverse array of proteins: Annu.Rev.Biochem., v. 70, pp. 649-676

Jado, I.; Oteo, J. A., Aldamiz, M., Gil, H., Escudero, Ibarra, R.V., Portu, J., Portillo, A., Lezaun, M. J., Garcia-Amil, C., Rodriguez-Moreno, I., & Anda, P. (2007). Rickettsia monacensis and human disease, Spain, Emerg.Infect.Dis., v. 13, no. 9, pp. 1405-1407

Jeng, R. L., Goley, E. D., D'Alessio, J. A., Chaga, O. Y., Svitkina, T. M., Borisy, G. G., Heinzen, R. A., & Welch, M. D. (2004) A Rickettsia WASP-like protein activates the Arp2/3 complex and mediates actin-based motility: Cell Microbiol., v. 6, no. 8, p. 761-769

Kenyon, R. H.; Kishimoto, R. A., & Hall, W. C. (1979). Exposure of guinea pigs to Rickettsia rickettsii by aerosol, nasal, conjunctival, gastric, and subcutaneous routes and protection afforded by an experimental vaccine: Infect.Immun., v. 25, no. 2, pp. 580-582

Kleba, B.; Clark, T. R., Lutter, E. I., Ellison, D. W., & Hackstadt , T. (2010). Disruption of the Rickettsia rickettsii Sca2 autotransporter inhibits actin-based motility: Infect.Immun., v. 78, no. 5, pp. 2240-2247

Labruna, M.B. (2009). Ecologu of Rickettsia in South America, Ann N Y Acad Sci, v. 1166, pp. 156-166

Li, H., Lenz, B. & Walker, D. H. (1988). Protective monoclonal antibodies recognize heat-labile epitopes on surface proteins of spotted fever group rickettsiae, Infect.Immun., v. 56, no. 10, pp. 2587-2593

Li, H. & Walker, D. H. (1998). rOmpA is a critical protein for the adhesion of Rickettsia rickettsii to host cells, Microb.Pathog., v. 24, no. 5, pp. 289-298

Martinez, J. J.; Seveau, S., Veiga, E., Matsuyama, S. & Cossart, P. (2005). Ku70, a component of DNA-dependent protein kinase, is a mammalian receptor for Rickettsia conorii, Cell, v. 123, no. 6, pp. 1013-1023

McDonald, G. A., Anacker, R. L., Mann, R. E. & Milch, L. J. (1988). Protection of guinea pigs from experimental Rocky Mountain spotted fever with a cloned antigen of Rickettsia rickettsii, J Infect.Dis., v. 158, no. 1, pp. 228-231

McLeod, M. P.; Qin, X., Karpathy, S. E., Gioia, J., Highlander, S. K., Fox, G. E., McNeill, T. Z., Jiang, H. , Muzny, D., Jacob, L. S., Hawes, A. C., Sodergren, E., Gill, R., Hume, J., Morgan, M. , Fan, G., Amin, A. G., Gibbs, R. A., Hong, C., Yu, X. J., Walker, D. H. &Weinstock, G. M. (2004). Complete genome sequence of Rickettsia typhi and comparison with sequences of other rickettsiae, J Bacteriol, v. 186, no. 17, pp. 5842-5855

Mediannikov, O.; Trape, J. F., Diatta, G., Parola, P. , Fournier, P. E. & Raoult, D. (2010) Rickettsia africae, Western Africa, Emerg.Infect.Dis., v. 16, no. 3, pp. 571-573

Mediannikov, O. Y.; Sidelnikov, Y., Ivanov, L., Mokretsova, E., Fournier, P. E., Tarasevich, I. & Raoult, D. (2004). Acute tick-borne rickettsiosis caused by Rickettsia heilongjiangensis in Russian Far East, Emerg.Infect.Dis., v. 10, no. 5, pp. 810-817

Mullins, R. D.; Heuser, J. A. & Pollard T. D. (1998). The interaction of Arp2/3 complex with actin: nucleation, high affinity pointed end capping, and formation of branching networks of filaments: Proc.Natl.Acad Sci U.S.A, v. 95, no. 11, pp. 6181-6186.

Nava, S.; Elshenawy, Y., Eremeeva, M. E., Sumner, J. W., Mastropaolo, M., & Paddock, C. D. (2008). Rickettsia parkeri in Argentina: Emerg.Infect.Dis., v. 14, no. 12, pp. 1894-1897.

Niebylski, M. L.; Peacock, M. G., & Schwan, T. G. (1999). Lethal effect of Rickettsia rickettsii on its tick vector (Dermacentor andersoni): Appl.Environ.Microbiol., v. 65, no. 2, pp. 773-778.

Ogata H.; Audic S., Renesto-Audiffren P., Fournier P.E., Barbe V., Samson D., Roux V., Cossart P., Weissenbach J., Claverie J.M. & Raoult D. (2001). Mechanisms of evolution in Rickettsia conorii and R. prowazekii: Science, v. 293, no. 5537, pp. 2093-2098.

Radulovic, S.; Troyer, J. M., Beier, M. S., Lau, A. O. & Azad, A. F. (1999). Identification and molecular analysis of the gene encoding Rickettsia typhi hemolysin: Infect.Immun., v. 67, no. 11, pp. 6104-6108.

Raoult, D.; Fournier, P. E., Abboud, P. & Caron, F. (2002). First documented human Rickettsia aeschlimannii infection: Emerg.Infect.Dis., v. 8, no. 7, pp. 748-749.

Raoult, D; Woodward T. & Dumler, J.S. (2004). The history of epidemic typhus: Infect.Dis.Clin.North Am., v. 18, no. 1, pp. 127-140.

Renesto, P.; Dehoux, P., Gouin, E., Touqui, L., Cossart, P. & Raoult, D. (2003) Identification and characterization of a phospholipase D-superfamily gene in rickettsiae: J Infect.Dis., v. 188, no. 9, pp. 1276-1283.

Rodionov, A. V.; Eremeeva, M. E. & Balayeva, N. M. (1991). Isolation and partial characterization of the M(r) 100 kD protein from Rickettsia prowazekii strains of different virulence: Acta Virol., v. 35, no. 6, pp. 557-565.

Rovery, C.; Brouqui, P.& Raoult, D. (2008). Questions on Mediterranean spotted fever a century after its discovery: Emerg.Infect.Dis., v. 14, no. 9, pp. 1360-1367.

Santos, A. S.; Bacellar, F., Santos-Silva, M., Formosinho, P., Gracio, A. J. & Franca, S. (2002). Ultrastructural study of the infection process of Rickettsia conorii in the salivary glands of the vector tick Rhipicephalus sanguineus: Vector.Borne.Zoonotic.Dis., v. 2, no. 3, pp. 165-177.

Selmi, M.; Bertolotti, L., Tomassone, L. & Mannelli, A. (2008). Rickettsia slovaca in Dermacentor marginatus and tick-borne lymphadenopathy, Tuscany, Italy: Emerg.Infect.Dis., v. 14, no. 5, pp. 817-820.

Sexton, D. J. & Corey, G. R. (1992). Rocky Mountain "spotless" and "almost spotless" fever: a wolf in sheep's clothing: Clin.Infect.Dis., v. 15, no. 3, pp. 439-448.

Sexton, D. J.; Dwyer, B. , Kemp, R. & Graves, S. (1991). Spotted fever group rickettsial infections in Australia: Rev.Infect.Dis., v. 13, no. 5, pp. 876-886.

Simser, J. A.; Rahman, M. S., Dreher-Lesnick, S. M. & Azad A. F. (2005). A novel and naturally occurring transposon, ISRpe1 in the Rickettsia peacockii genome disrupting the rickA gene involved in actin-based motility: Mol.Microbiol., v. 58, no. 1, pp. 71-79.

Spencer R.R.& Parker R.R. (1925). Rocky Mountain spotted fever: vacconation of monkeys and man.: Public Health Rep, no. 40, pp. 2159-2167.

Teysseire, N.; Boudier, J. A. & Raoult, D. (1995). Rickettsia conorii entry into Vero cells: Infect.Immun., v. 63, no. 1, pp. 366-374.

Teysseire, N.; Chiche-Portiche, C. &Raoult D. (1992). Intracellular movements of Rickettsia conorii and R. typhi based on actin polymerization: Res.Microbiol., v. 143, no. 9, pp. 821-829.

Tilney, L. G. & Portnoy, D. A. (1989). Actin filaments and the growth, movement, and spread of the intracellular bacterial parasite, Listeria monocytogenes: J Cell Biol., v. 109, no. 4 Pt 1, pp. 1597-1608.

Turco, J. & Winkler, H. H. (1994). Cytokine sensitivity and methylation of lysine in Rickettsia prowazekii EVir and interferon-resistant R. prowazekii strains: Infect.Immun., v. 62, no. 8, pp. 3172-3177.

Vishwanath, S. (1991). Antigenic relationships among the rickettsiae of the spotted fever and typhus groups: FEMS Microbiol.Lett., v. 65, no. 3, pp. 341-344.

Vishwanath, S.; McDonald, G. A. & Watkins, N. G. (1990). A recombinant Rickettsia conorii vaccine protects guinea pigs from experimental boutonneuse fever and Rocky Mountain spotted fever: Infect.Immun., v. 58, no. 3, pp. 646-653.

Walker D.H. (2011). PATHOGENESIS OF RICKETTSIAL DISEASES, webpage, <http://www.uscap.org/site~/99th/pdf/companion05h02.pdf>

Walker, D. H.; Feng, H. M. & Popov, V. L. (2001). Rickettsial phospholipase A2 as a pathogenic mechanism in a model of cell injury by typhus and spotted fever group rickettsiae: Am.J Trop.Med.Hyg., v. 65, no. 6, pp. 936-942.

Walker, D. H.; Olano, J. P. & Feng, H. M. (2001b). Critical role of cytotoxic T lymphocytes in immune clearance of rickettsial infection: Infect.Immun., v. 69, no. 3, pp. 1841-1846.

Walker, D. H., Olano, J. P. & Feng, H. M. (2001c). Critical role of cytotoxic T lymphocytes in immune clearance of rickettsial infection: Infect. Immun., v. 69, no. 3, pp. 1841-1846.

Welch, M. D. & Mullins, R. D. (2002). Cellular control of actin nucleation: Annu.Rev.Cell Dev.Biol., v. 18, p. 247-288.

Welch, M. D.; Rosenblatt, J., Skoble, J., Portnoy, D. A. & Mitchison, T. J. (1998). Interaction of human Arp2/3 complex and the Listeria monocytogenes ActA protein in actin filament nucleation: Science, v. 281, no. 5373, pp. 105-108.

Whitworth, T.; Popov, V. L., Yu, X. J., Walker, D. H. & D. H. Bouyer. D.H. (2005). Expression of the Rickettsia prowazekii pld or tlyC gene in Salmonella enterica serovar Typhimurium mediates phagosomal escape: Infect.Immun., v. 73, no. 10, pp. 6668-6673.

Zhu, Y.; Medina-Sanchez, A., Bouyer, D., Walker, D. H. & Yu, X. J. (2008). Genotyping Rickettsia prowazekii isolates: Emerg.Infect.Dis., v. 14, no. 8, pp. 1300-1302.